Biological Relevance
of Immune Suppression
As Induced by Genetic, Therapeutic
and Environmental Factors

Biological Markers of Neoplasia: Basic and Applied Aspects
(Elsevier, New York, 1978)
Edited by
Raymond W. Ruddon, M.D., Ph.D.

Biological Relevance of Immune Suppression As Induced by
Genetic, Therapeutic and Environmental Factors
Edited by
Jack H. Dean, Ph.D. and Martin Padarathsingh, Ph.D.

Design of Models for Testing Cancer Therapeutic Agents
Edited by
Isaiah J. Fidler, Ph.D. and Richard J. White, Ph.D.

Biological Relevance of Immune Suppression As Induced by Genetic, Therapeutic and Environmental Factors

Edited by

Jack H. Dean, *Ph.D.*
Head, Immunology Section, Environmental Biology Branch
National Institute of Environmental Health Sciences
Research Triangle Park, North Carolina

Martin Padarathsingh, *Ph.D.*
Director, Department of Immunology, Litton Bionetics, Inc.
Kensington, Maryland

Second in a Series of
Technology Assessment Workshops Sponsored by
Litton Bionetics, Inc.

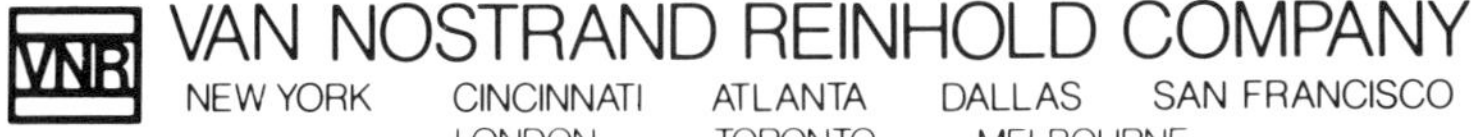

VAN NOSTRAND REINHOLD COMPANY
NEW YORK   CINCINNATI   ATLANTA   DALLAS   SAN FRANCISCO
LONDON   TORONTO   MELBOURNE

Van Nostrand Reinhold Company Regional Offices:
New York Cincinnati Atlanta Dallas San Francisco

Van Nostrand Reinhold Company International Offices:
London Toronto Melbourne

Library of Congress Catalog Card Number: 80–20553
ISBN: 0–442–24429–0

Manufactured in the United States of America

Published by Van Nostrand Reinhold Company
135 West 50th Street, New York, N.Y. 10020

Published simultaneously in Canada by Van Nostrand Reinhold Ltd.

15 14 13 12 11 10 9 8 7 6 5 4 3 2 1

Library of Congress Cataloging in Publication Data
Main entry under title:

Biological relevance of immune suppression as induced by
    genetic, therapeutic and environmental factors.

    Papers presented at a workshop held in Williams-
burg, Va., Nov. 13–14, 1979 and sponsored by Litton
Bionetics. Inc.
    Includes index.
    1. Immunosuppression—Congresses. 2. Immuno-
logical deficiency syndromes—Etiology—Congresses.
3. Immunosuppressive agents—Congresses. I. Dean,
Jack H. II. Padarathsingh, Martin. III. Litton
Bionetics, Inc. [DNLM: 1. Immunosuppression—Con-
gresses. QW920 B615 1979]
QR188.35.B67   616.07'9   80–20553
ISBN 0–442–24429–0

Foreword

"What art was to the ancient world, science is to the modern." These words by Benjamin Disraeli are of particular significance today as we witness an explosion of new scientific technologies—the results of which may eventually dwarf those of the past several centuries. Each new technological advance sets off its own chain reaction of opportunities and problems. The scope and speed of our current technological progress, particularly in the biomedical field, present an unprecedented challenge and opportunity to science, industry, government, and to all elements of our society. The U.S. Congress recognized this and has publicly expressed its concern for the scientific community's difficulty to rapidly translate new findings into practical applications for the good of society.

Litton Bionetics, as a major contributor to the development of basic research knowledge, has initiated a company-sponsored series of biomedical technology assessment workshops aimed at helping to meet this challenge. We believe that technology transfer, or translation of basic research findings into practical application, is necessary if the public is to benefit from basic research development and that organizations such as ours can uniquely contribute both to identifying high potential areas and to focusing the broad multidisciplinary talents needed to form a consensus on applicability.

This, our second workshop, is entitled Biological Relevance of Immune Suppression. Immunology was selected because, perhaps, no other contemporary field of research continues to provide more answers and insights which we believe could lead to improvements in our understanding of cancer and other diseases.

The first workshop in this series, held in the spring of 1978, addressed Biological Markers of Neoplasia: Basic and Applied Aspects. A subsequent conference is being planned for spring of 1980 concerned with the Design of Models for Testing Therapeutic Agents.

Sponsorship of this series is only one important tradition of our company's service to science, industry, government and society.

James C. Nance
President
Litton Bionetics, Inc.

April 14, 1980

Introduction

Robert E. Stevenson *

Litton Bionetics, Inc. Kensington, Md.

The biological relevance of immune suppression is the subject of this year's meeting and we are indebted to Drs. Jack Dean and Martin Padarathsingh for suggesting and organizing the topics and speakers.

A few weeks ago the nation observed the 100th anniversary of the birth of Will Rogers whose pertinent impertinences we still remember such as "Government is too important to be left up to the politicians." I wonder if today he would say technology transfer is too important to be left up to the scientists.

I don't think scientists deprecate technology transfer, but they are often caught in the situation depicted on the cartoon saying, "When you're up to your neck in alligators, you forget that your primary mission was to drain the swamp."

Nowhere has this been more evident than in the field of environmental toxicology and carcinogenesis with the public and political pressures demanding the identification of noxious agents and the control or elimination of them from the general and work environments.

To provide better tools to accomplish these aims has been the goal of a number of the people presenting papers at this meeting. You will hear their results and evaluate their accomplishments.

Others will show the significance of measuring and interpreting responses in the immune system and the results from strategically manipulating immune reactions for clinical objectives.

The broad range of topics and different perspectives represented on the program is the background of the meeting. The wide interests and responsibilities of the attendees should provide the basis for a lively dis-

* Dr. Stevenson is presently Director, American Type Culture Collection, Rockville, Maryland.

cussion and review of the current state of knowledge and applications of immunology to public health problems.

If this conference succeeds in its goals, those attending will go away with greater insight into the immune system's role in host defense, its characterization by various techniques, the significance of alteration in its states and the potential applications of this knowledge to problems of a highly practical nature. Failing that, a definition of work yet to be accomplished should justify your investment of time and energy during the next two days.

Acknowledgments

The editors wish to thank the chairmen who organized the individual sessions: Edmund Yunis (Harvard Medical School and Sidney Farber Cancer Institute), James L. McCoy (National Cancer Institute), and John Moore (National Institute of Environmental Health Sciences). Thanks go also to Frank Donnelly (Litton Bionetics, Inc.) for his attention to detail in coordinating the conference. We are grateful to Carolyn Fox, Kathy Murphy and Merlyne Ziaya (Litton Bionetics, Inc.) for their contributions to planning the conference and preparation of the proceedings. We express gratitude to Walter Brandenburg (Brandenburg and Hasty) who carefully reported the lively discussion sessions, to Jeanne Mowe (Frederick Cancer Research Center) who coordinated the proceedings and edited the discussion for this publication and to the staff of Document Preparation and Control (Litton Bionetics, Inc.) who assisted in preparation of the copy for publication. Finally, special thanks go to Robert Stevenson (Litton Bionetics, Inc.) who spearheaded the entire effort.

Jack H. Dean, Ph.D.
Martin Padarathsingh, Ph.D.
Co-editors

Contents

SECTION III—EXPERIMENTAL CHANGES IN IMMUNOLOGIC PARAMETERS FOLLOWING EXPOSURE TO ENVIRONMENTAL AGENTS

SECTION IV—HOST SUSCEPTIBILITY AND LUNG DEFENSE MECHANISMS

SECTION I
THE BIOLOGY OF IMMUNE SUPPRESSION AND IMMUNE REGULATION

1
Intrinsic and Extrinsic Regulation of Immune Responses

Richard J. Mahoney and Edmond J. Yunis

*Harvard Medical School, Sidney Farber Cancer Institute,
Boston, Massachusetts*

INTRODUCTION

Immune responsiveness requires the successful interactions of various types of lymphocytes and macrophages with antigen. Immunoregulation can also be mediated by the major cell types that promote immune responses, i.e., T cells, B cells and macrophages. These regulatory cells and their products are influenced intrinsically by a complex regulatory system of positive and negative factors that are under genetic control, especially by genes by the MHC. In addition, the regulatory components are capable of being manipulated extrinsically by therapeutic and environmental factors. The net effect of intrinsic and extrinsic immunoregulation is reflected by the state of health and ultimate life span of an individual. The purpose of this chapter is to review some of the natural and experimental factors that control and influence suppression and regulation of the immune system. Intrinsic factors include stimulatory signals from antigen-reactive T helper lymphocytes or macrophages, inhibitory signals from T suppressor cells, antibody itself, the aging process, and genetic influences. Extrinsic experimental factors used to manipulate immune regulation include thymectomy, pharmacologic agents, anti-lymphocyte serum, immunomodulatory agents, and diet.

RESULTS AND DISCUSSION

Intrinsic Immunoregulatory Factors

The immune system is designed to provide the host with resistance against a broad spectrum of infections. The operation and maintenance of the immune system requires the differentiation, interaction and regulation of multiple cell types. The activities of many genes and their products are required for the development and maintenance of a functional immune system. Biozzi and his associates (1979) have shown that at least 10 independent polymorphic loci can influence the immune response. However, one genetic system, the major histocompatibility complex, has a predominant influence on the immune response. Thus, the major histocompatibility complex (MHC) can control the ability to respond to selected antigens in an all-or-none fashion (Benacerraf and McDevitt, 1972).

The MHC, referred to as H-2 in mice, consists of a series of closely linked genes that primarily code for cell surface molecules. All higher species of vertebrates analyzed have a genetic system analogous to the MHC. McDevitt et al. (1972) were the first to note that genes within the MHC of mice could control the ability to respond to selected antigens. Subsequently, it was shown that these immune responses (Ir) genes could also influence a series of T cell functions to selected antigens. One fundamental characteristic of Ir genes is their exquisite antigen specificity. This led to an early hypothesis which suggested that the Ir gene product may actually represent the antigen-specific T cell receptor (Benacerraf and McDevitt, 1972). However, more recent evidence suggests that the Ir gene products represent specialized structures on the surface of macrophages or other antigen-presenting cells; these structures are termed the Ia molecules (Uhr et al., 1979). Some of the strongest evidence supporting this hypothesis involves the analysis of Ir genes in systems in which two distinct MHC-linked genes are required for immune responsiveness (Dorf and Benacerraf, 1975). Such gene complementation was explained at the molecular level by the finding that each of the complementing genes was coding for a separate chain of the Ia molecule (Uhr et al., 1979). Analogs of the murine Ia molecules have now been described in several species (Uhr et al., 1979; Ferrone et al., 1978). Presumably, specific T cell activation requires recognition of the neoantigenic determinants created by the interaction of Ia molecules with antigen (Benacerraf, 1978). This analysis of Ir genes has greatly facilitated our understanding of the molecular mechanism of helper T cell activation.

Genes of the major histocompatibility complex can also affect immune responsiveness by other mechanisms, expecially by regulation of immuno-suppression. It appears that the genetic control of immune responsive-ness and suppression are closely related, for in some Ir gene systems the inability to form an immune response is due to the predominance of antigen-specific T suppressor cells (Benacerraf and Germain, 1978). Furthermore, the generation of immune suppression to selected antigens is under genetic control by complementing MHC-linked genes (Bena-cerraf and Dorf, 1977). Antigen-specific T cell derived suppressor factors bear determinants coded for by the MHC (Tada et al., 1977) and H-2 compatibility is required for some of the interactions of these suppressor factors with cells of the immune system (Tada et al., 1977; Rich and Rich, 1976). At least some of the genes that regulate immune suppression appear to differ from the genes that regulate immune responsiveness, since they map to different positions within the MHC complex. Unfortunately, at this time comparatively little is known about the molecular mechanisms responsible for the induction of immune suppression. However, there is general agreement that suppressor cells play a key role in the regulation of the immune system. Suppressor T cells participate in different types of immunologic phenomena by limiting antibody responses and by interfering with cellular immunity.

Antibody itself also plays a regulatory role through its ability to in-hibit further production of antibody. While the mechanism of antibody-mediated suppression is not fully understood, it is important to note that the antibody molecule represents a copy of the antigenic recognition site on the antigen-reactive B cell and probably on antigen-specific T cells (Binz and Wigzell, 1977; Weinberger et al., 1979). An antibody can also act as an immunogen and thus may elicit an autologous anti-idiotypic re-sponse. Anti-idiotypic antibody or idiotype specific T cells directed against antigen-binding receptors on immunocompetent cells may play an im-portant regulatory role in limiting both humoral antibody formation and cellular immunity. Such idiotype anti-idiotype interactions are the basis for the network theory of immune regulation postulated by Jerne (1973).

The MHC also appears to be an important genetic system for regulating aging of the immune system and ultimate life span in mice. Because the immune system undergoes a series of marked changes with age, many of the MHC-associated functions that directly influence the immune system can be monitored in order to understand the exact relationship of these changes in immune function to survival. However, it is yet unknown whether the changes that occur in the immune system with age are re-sponsible for the decline in immune functional effectiveness seen in aging animals, or whether the primary aging process produces secondary changes in the immune system. Nevertheless, both humoral and cell-mediated immune responses decline with age in all animals. In mice, optimal humoral immunity is observed early in life. The activity then declines gradually, and in later life, the animals have only 5-10% of their peak activity (Makinodan, 1978). This decrease is found in both the primary and secondary responses to antigens that require thymic influences to elicit an immune response, as well as those that do not require thymic influences (Makinodan, 1978). In aging humans, the progressive decline of immune function and increased incidence of autoimmunity, malignancy, and infection suggest that the development of age-associated diseases may be controlled by immunologic factors.

Since H-2 linked immune response genes and H-2K/D molecules are expressed in dominant or codominant fashion, one likely mechanism for their role in survival would be to confer resistance to one or many environmental insults to which the laboratory mouse population is exposed. Because most individuals of an outbred mammalian population are heterozygous for many polymorphic alleles, including those of the MHC, we investigated whether a single copy of a particular I-region allele or H-2K/D gene product might confer a survival advantage under mouse colony conditions using F1 hybrid animals. The DBA/2J maternal strain and five congenic or recombinant congenic strains from the C57B1/10 genetic background were mated and their offspring were held for ultimate survival. Congenic strains provided an important approach for examining the influence of single copies of different H-2 haplotypes, H-2 subregion loci, and alleles of H-2 linked antigenic systems in animals that were otherwise genetically identical or nearly identical. Because the hybrids studied differed only by various portions of the paternally derived H-2 haplotype, it was possible to detect effects of H-2 subregions on survival. Survival data indicated that median survival times correlated with the H-2 haplotype of the paternal strain (Williams et al., in press). Thus, using the more biologically realistic F1 hybrid model, significant genetic determinants of survival appeared to be localized in the MHC. Smith and Walford (1977) also examined the aging MHC influence in congenic mice with three different genetic backgrounds: C57BL, C3H, and A strains. Their results showed that when the H-2 allele was the same, there were survival differences dependent on particularly H-2 haplotypes. Furthermore, immune response appeared to correlate with survival. For example, Meredith and Walford (1977) observed that among congenic strains of the C57BL/10 background, the longest-lived strain, B10.RIII, displayed the highest *in vitro* response to PHA throughout most of its life span. In contrast, the shortest-lived strain, B10.AKM, showed the lowest response. These findings support the hypothesis that the MHC, the principal gene complex that controls or regulates the immune system, also influences longevity.

Extrinsic Immunoregulatory Factors

There are several means by which one can modulate the immune response to specific antigens. Many of the procedures appear to preferentially eliminate or reduce helper-suppressor cell activity. One approach involves the induction of antigen-mediated immune suppression. Intravenous administration of syngeneic spleen cells, coupled with the palmitoyl derivative of protein antigens, results in a state of carrier-specific tolerance in mice (Sherr et al., 1979). Such antigen-induced immunosuppression is thought to be due to mechanisms involving the induction of both T cell tolerance and T cell suppression. The generation of T suppressor cells apparently has the effect of decreasing T cell help needed by the specific B cells.

Elimination of suppressor activity can also be demonstrated experimentally. Suppressor T cells (Murphy et al., 1976) and factors (Tada et al., 1976; Theze et al., 1977) produced by such cells contain antigenic products encoded by the I-J subregions of the H-2 complex in mice. Identification of these I-J products led to another approach by which immunoregulation was manipulated *in vivo*. Pierres and associates (1978) reasoned that administration of antiserum directed against I-J determinants on suppressor T cells should eliminate the activity of this T cell subset. They examined this hypothesis in tumor-bearing mice and found that, indeed, tumor growth did not progress in mice treated daily with small quantities of anti-I-J serum (Greene et al., 1977). Apparently, the immunologic balance in these mice shifted in favor of immunity following elimination of specific suppressor T cells by anti-I-J serum. Identification of I-J-like molecules on human suppressor T cells and the development of related antibody would allow for the possible elimination of suppressor cell activity associated with immunologic hyporesponsiveness in tumor-bearing patients.

Nonsensitized lymphoid cells referred to as natural killer cells are capable of lysing malignant cells (Haberman and Holden, 1978). Such natural killer cell activity works independently of antibody, complement and phagocytosis. NK cells, which lack characteristics of T cells, B cells and macrophages, are present in both normal and athymic mice. Athymic mice lack a T cell system but do not demonstrate a high incidence of spontaneous tumors (Moller and Moller, 1976). NK cells are capable of spontaneous cytotoxic activity directed against both normal cells and tumor targets *in vitro*. Thus, it is hypothesized that such cells play an important role in immunologic surveillance against neoplastic growth in athymic mice, as well as in mice with a normal T cell system. However, their control of spontaneous tumor development is open to question. Nevertheless, NK activity, like helper and suppressor T cell activity, is subject to manipulation. Antiserum that is specific for Ly5 antigens on NK cells allows for positive selection of such cells from nonimmune mice. These NK cells, upon adoptive transfer, can protect syngeneic mice against local growth of two different types of tumor cells (Kasai et al., 1979). NK cell activity can also be influenced by agents with opposing effects such as interferon and glucan. Interferon, which can affect many different aspects of the immune response (Epstein, 1977), augments NK activity (Santoli and Koprowski, 1979). Glucan, a B1,3-glucosidic poly-glucose, is a potent reticuloendothelial stimulant; however, this immuno-modulating agent apparently causes significant depression of NK cell activity in mice (Lotzova and Gutterman, 1979).

The thymus and the lymphoid cells derived from this organ have an important influence on immunoregulation as evidenced by the effect of adult thymectomy on the generation of suppressor T cells. When thymec-tomy is performed in adult life, humoral and cell-mediated immune re-sponses are increased (Simpson and Cantor, 1975), while T suppressor activity directed against malignant tissue *in vivo* is abrogated (Reinisch et al., 1977). Furthermore, spleen cells from mice that are thymectomized as adults exhibit an enhanced capacity to lyse syngeneic tumor cells *in vitro* (Reinisch and Andrew, 1978). These findings demonstrate that thymectomy serves as an important approach for analysis of function controlled by thymus-derived T cell subpopulations.

The nutritional state of an individual plays an important role in the function of the immune system. The influence of nutritional factors on malignancy, longevity, and immunity in experimental animals and man has been investigated extensively for years (Suskind, 1977). Most dietary manipulations shown to have an effect on immunity as it relates to dis-ease and aging involved either a caloric restriction (Walford et al., 1973–74; Fernandes et al., 1976), a deficiency in essential amino acids (Dubois et al., 1973; Hui et al., 1972), or a reduction of protein intake (Good et al., 1973). Polyunsaturated fatty acids (PUFA) also have been noted to have an apparent immunoregulatory effect (Mertin and Hunt, 1976). In contrast to caloric and protein restriction, the immunoregula-tion observed with PUFA dietary manipulation appeared to have a dual nature, i.e., immunoinhibition was observed with a deficiency of PUFA and immunopotentiation resulted with an excess of PUFA. Indeed, numerous studies have attempted to understand the immunoregulatory influence of nutrition on immune function and disease.

Restriction of food intake has been shown by Tannenbaum (1940) to reduce incidence of spontaneous mammary adenocarcinomas in C3H and DBA inbred strains of mice, as well as the incidence of spontaneous lung tumors in mice of various genetic backgrounds. Further, the incidence of chemically induced tumors also was reduced in mice on restricted diets (Tannenbaum, 1940; Tannenbaum, 1942). Substantial reduction of tumor risk was observed when the restricted diet was limited to only 7 weeks after weaning in rats (Ross and Bras, 1971), or when it was initiated as late as 9 months of age in mice (Tannenbaum, 1944). In a recent report, Tucker (1979) noted that restriction of food intake by only 20% increased longevity, reduced the incidence and delayed the onset of the most common tumor types in rats and mice (Tucker, 1979). Clearly, it would be of great value to understand the mechanisms underlying the relationship of reduced body weight and reduced cancer incidence.

Previous studies have examined the effect of diet on immune function and have noted profound influences. Chronic restriction of protein in the diet was shown by Jose et al. (1971) to result in depressed levels of antibody production. In contrast, cell-mediated immune responses were normal or increased as evidenced by the ability of animals to reject skin allografts, to produce cytotoxicity directed against syngeneic and allogeneic tumor cells and to resist virus infection (Jose, 1971; Jose, 1973; Cooper et al., 1974). However, both humoral and cellular immunity were depressed, following severe protein restriction (Jose, 1973). While immunodeficiency is generally a harmful physiologic condition in an organism, immunodepression induced by dietary restriction can have a beneficial effect on tumor incidence and autoimmune disease.

Autoimmune disease in NZB and (NZBxNZW)F1 mice is manifested by severe glomerulonephritis analogous to human system lupus erythematosus. Moderate calorie or protein restriction initiated at weaning or at 4–5 months of age in this autoimmune strain resulted in decreased levels of autoantibody formation, protection from the development of immune complex nephritis, and prolonged life span (Friend et al., 1978). A diet deficient in amino acids phenylalanine and tyrosine also has a beneficial effect on survival and nephropathy in NZBxNZWF1 mice (Dubois, 1973). Thus, the biological relevance of immunosuppression by dietary restriction is evidenced by its prophylactic and therapeutic effect on autoimmune disease in this model.

Fernandes et al. (1976) examined the influence of calorie restriction on the suppression of spontaneous mammary adenocarcinoma and alteration of immune function in C3H mice. They noted that calorie restriction prevented the development of mammary tumors and altered both cellular and humoral immunologic profiles. Antibody levels following *in vivo* immunization with sheep red blood cells were markedly depressed in the *in vitro* plaque-forming cell assay. Further, spleen cell stimulation by mitogens LPS, Con A and PHA was normal or increased as indicated by incorporation of tritiated thymidine into DNA of proliferating lymphocytes. In contrast, T cell suppressor activity was increased in the calorie restricted mice. Although dietary manipulation prevented tumor development and altered immune responses, there was no definitive evidence that dietary restriction prevented tumor development on an immunologic basis.

Indeed, immunologic control of susceptibility and resistance to tumor development is open to question. That is, while tumor antigens are capable of inducing specific immunity mediated by lymphoid cells, lymphoid cells also are capable of stimulating tumor growth. This concept of immunostimulation, first postulated by Prehn and Lappe (1971), holds that a low level of immune reactivity can stimulate tissue growth. T lymphocytes apparently are associated with tumor stimulation both *in vitro* and *in vivo* (Fidler et al., 1974; Small and Trainin, 1976; Small, 1977; Ruppert et al., 1979). The phenomenon of preventing tumor development through dietary restriction may possibly be due to the fact that the ability of lymphoid cells to stimulate a tumor growth is adversely affected by dietary manipulation. On the other hand, the cytotoxic capacity of the cytotoxic population may be augmented by dietary restriction. While the stimulatory and cytotoxic lymphoid populations appear to be different (Norbury, 1977), it is not yet known how dietary manipulation influences or regulates the function of each subset.

Dietary polyunsaturated fatty acids (PUFA) also have been shown to have a nonspecific immunoregulatory effect (Mertin, 1976). In contrast to caloric and protein restriction, however, immunoregulation observed with PUFA dietary manipulation can result in either immunoinhibition or immunopotentiation *in vivo*. That is, increase of dietary PUFA linoleic acid resulted in immunoinhibition as measured by increased survival of skin allografts and increased incidence of chemically induced tumors in mice; whereas, mice fed a PUFA-deficient diet exhibited an immunopotentiation as evidenced by accelerated skin allograft rejection and decreased incidence and rate of development of methylcholanthrene-induced tumors. Furthermore, spleen cells from mice treated with PUFA linoleic acid exhibited lower levels of cytotoxicity in the *in vitro* [51]Cr release assay. In a recent study (Hillyard and Abraham, 1979) rat and mouse mammary adenocarcinomas demonstrated increased growth when transplanted into recipients fed a diet high in polyunsaturated fat as opposed to a fat-free or saturated fat diet (Abraham and Rao, 1976). The presence of increasing concentrations of linoleic acid has been shown to result in a linear decrease in lymphocytotoxicity directed against a human breast carcinoma cell line (Samlaska, 1978). A common mechanism postulated in these PUFA diet studies is the possible decrease in lymphocytotoxicity directed against the growing tumor cells. Thus, PUFA dietary manipulation may directly affect the lipid components of cell membranes involved in the recognition and interactions of lymphocytes with tumor cells.

The dynamic state of cell surface membranes proposed in the fluid mosaic model (Singer and Nicolson, 1972) has generated interest in the relationship between membrane fluidity and function of membranes. Since most immunologic functions involve contact of lymphocyte membranes with membranes of other lymphoid or nonlymphoid cells, the fluid state of the lipid layer may play. a major role in cellular immunoregulatory mechanisms. Indeed, fatty acid levels of lymphoid cells have been found to be greater than levels in cells of other organs (Kigoshi and Ito, 1973). Because it is possible to substitute both saturated and unsaturated fatty acids into membrane phospholipids of lymphocytes and tumor cells in tissue culture (Mandel et al., 1978), the technique of altering membrane lipid composition of effector and target cells in cell-mediated immune reactions serves as a model for studying PUFA-mediated immunoregulation. Recent studies with both mouse and human leukemia have suggested that the development of the malignant state is accompanied by a significant alteration of the dynamics (Petitou et al., 1978) and composition of lipids, both in the cell plasma membrane and in serum lipoproteins. These lipid modifications resulted in a marked increase in the fluidity of both leukemic cells and leukemic serum. Moreover, since lipids can be translocated between cellular membranes and serum lipoproteins, it was suggested that changes in the dynamics and the composition of cellular membranes and serum complexes are interrelated parameters.

We have recently observed that a marked increase in serum fluidity is associated with the development of spontaneous mammary tumors in C3H mice (Lane et al., in press). The degree of lipid fluidity (LFU) was quantitatively monitored by fluorescence polarization analysis of the hydrocarbon fluorescent probe diphenylhexatriene when embedded in artificial and biological lipid complexes. An increase in serum LFU was

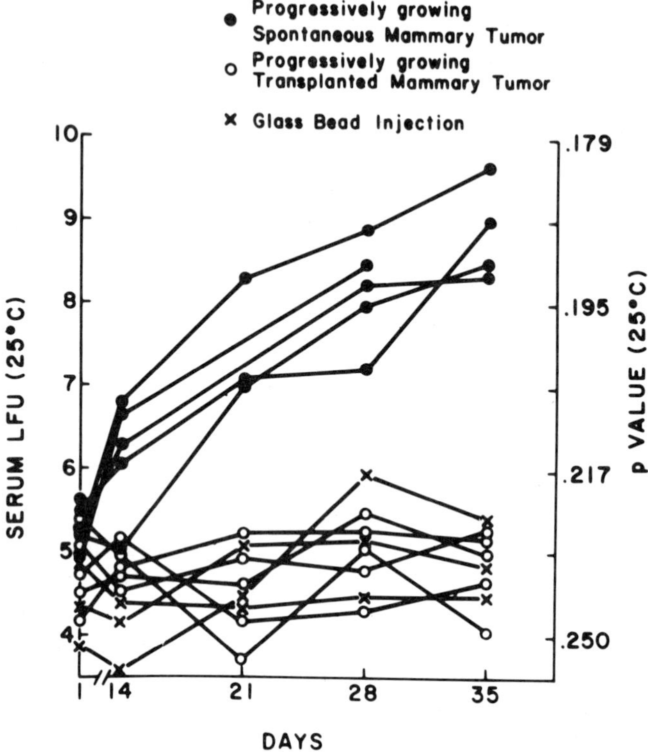

Figure 1. Individual serum samples from 3 groups of C3H female mice were assayed for serum lipid fluidity values. Sera were monitored on days 1, 14, 21, 28 and 35 following the observation of spontaneous mammary tumors in one group, transplantation of primary tumors in a second group, and subcutaneous injection of 10^3 antigenically inert glass beads in the third group of mice. Normal C3H female mice have a mean P value of $2.17\pm .009$ which corresponds to $5.97\pm .78$ mean LFU.

observed during the initiation of primary mammary adenocarcinomas in C3H mice. The serum LFU further increased as the tumor burden progressed in size. This increase was not observed in other groups of C3H mice that received transplants of syngeneic spontaneous mammary tumors or implants of antigenically inert glass beads (Figure 1). Since non-tumor bearing C3H mice had higher serum LFU values than non-tumor bearing C57BL/6, NZB and A/Jax strains, it is possible that alterations in the dynamics of serum lipids in the C3H model influenced the induction and/or growth of spontaneous mammary tumors.

CONCLUSION

Immune responsiveness requires the interactions of lymphoid cells and macrophages with antigen. The immune network, which is regulated by cells and mediators within the system, is primarily under genetic control by the major histocompatibility complex. The intrinsic regulatory control system can change with age causing alterations within the network. As a result, susceptibility to the development of autoimmune disease and cancer increases. There are several experimental approaches that can be used to manipulate immune regulation. These extrinsic factors include thymectomy, pharmacologic agents, anti-lymphocyte serum, immunomodulatory agents, and dietary manipulation. Many of these procedures will be discussed in this conference.

We have reviewed in some detail the use of diet as a means of manipulating immune regulation. Our discussion at the conference focused on the use of diet as a method to dissect immune regulation and to possibly prolong life span. Although dietary manipulation alters the immune status of experimental animals, it seems unlikely that life span will be prolonged far beyond the limits imposed by genetic influences. However, selective nutrition may allow for the full expression of the genetic potential for maximum life span by forestalling the appearance of diseases associated with aging. For instance, a high fat diet enhances the expression of autoimmunity in NZB mice (Fernandes et al., 1972). Chronic moderate protein restriction in these mice delays the onset of hemolytic anemia and prolongs the maintenance of thymic function. A more dramatic effect is observed using caloric restriction in (NZBxNZW)Fl mice. In this case increased life span is accompanied by sustained immunologic vigor, by inhibition of the development of cardiovascular and renal disease, by inhibition of anti-DNA production and by the inhibition of a spontaneous suppression cell population that occurs with age in (NZBxNZW)F1 mice (Fernandes et al., 1978). In addition, calorie restriction can also prolong life span in C3H mice that are susceptible to the development of spontaneous mammary tumors by preventing or reducing the incidence of tumors in these mice (Fernandes et al., 1976). Although it is possible to demonstrate significant changes in immunoregulation in mice given a low-calorie diet, it is difficult to determine whether diet affects the immune system directly or through nonimmunologic pathways. Dietary manipulation may indirectly affect the immune system through endocrine interactions. Thus, dietary influence on hormonal activity might affect both the target organ of mammary tumor development, and/or the immunologic response to neoantigens.

ACKNOWLEDGMENTS

This work was supported by grants from the National Institutes of Health, National Cancer Institute: IF32, CA06283, CA06516, CA 19589 and CA 20531. Richard J. Mahoney is a recipient of an NIH Fellowship (IF 32 CA 06283) from the NCI. We thank Dr. Martin E. Dorf for his contributions to and review of the manuscript.

REFERENCES

Abraham, S. and Rao, G. A.: Lipids and lipogenesis in a murine mammary neoplastic system. In, *Control Mechanisms in Cancer,* (W. E. Criss, T. Ono and J. R. Sabine, eds.), Raven Press, New York, pp. 363–378 (1976).

Benacerraf, B. and McDevitt, H. O.: Histocompatibility-linked immune response genes. Science, *175*:273–279 (1972).

Benacerraf, B. and Dorf, M. E.: Genetic control of specific immune responses of and immune suppressions by I-region genes. Cold Spring Harbor Symp. Quant. Biol., *41*:465–475 (1977).

Benacerraf, B.: A hypothesis to relate the specificity of T lymphocytes and the activity of I-region-specific Ir genes in macrophages and B lymphocytes. J. Immunol., 1809–1812 (1978).

Benacerraf, B. and Germain, R. N.: The immune response genes of the major histocompatibility complex. Immunol. Rev., *38*: 70–119 (1978).

Binz, H. and Wigzell, H.: Antigen-binding, idiotypic T lymphocyte receptors. Contemp. Top. Immunbiol., *7*:113–177 (1977).

Biozzi, G., Moutou, D., Heumann, A. M., Bouthillier, Y., Stiffel, C. and Mevel, J. C.: Genetic analysis of antibody responsiveness to sheep erythrocytes in crosses between lines of mice selected for high or low antibody synthesis. Immunology, *36*: 427–483 (1979).

Cooper, W. C., Good, R. A. and Mariani, T.: Effects of protein insufficiency on immune responsiveness. Amer. J. Clin. Nutr., *27*:647–664 (1974).

Dorf, M. E. and Benacerraf, B.: Complementation of H–2 linked IR genes in the mouse. Proc. Natl. Acad. Sci. USA, *72*:3671–3675 (1975).

Dubois, E. and Strain, L.: Effect of diet on survival and neuropathy of NZB/NZW hybrid mice. Biochem. Med., *7*:336–342 (1973).

Epstein, L. B.: The effects of interferons on the immune response *in vitro* and *in vivo*. In Interferons and Their Actions (W. Steward, II., ed.), CRC Press, Cleveland (1977).

Fernandes, G., Yunis, E. J., Smith, J. and Good, R. A.: Dietary influence on breeding behavior, hemolytic anemia, and longevity in NZB mice. Proc. Soc. Exp. Med., *139*:1189–1195 (1972).

Fernandés, G., Yunis, E. J. and Good, R. A.: Influence of diet on survival in mice. Proc. Natl. Acad. Sci. USA, *73*:1279–1283 (1976a).

Fernandes, G., Yunis, E. J. and Good, R. A.: Suppression of adenocarcinoma by the immunological consequences of calorie restriction. Nature (Lond), *263*:405–507 (1976b).

Fernandes, G., Friend, P., Yunis, E. J. and Good, R. A.: Influence of dietary restriction on immunologic function and renal disease in (NZBxNZW)F1 mice. Proc. Natl. Acad. Sci. USA, *75*:1500–1504 (1978).

Ferrone, S., Allison, J. P. and Pellegrino, M. A.: Human DR (Ia-like) antigens: Biological and molecular profile. Contemp. Topics in Molec. Immunol., 7:239–281 (1978).

Fidler, I. J., Brody, R. S. and Bech-Nielsen, S.: *In vitro* immune stimulation-inhibition to spontaneous canine tumors of various histologic types. J. Immunol., *112*: 1051–1060 (1974).

Friend, P. S., Fernandes, G., Good, R. A., Michael, A. F. and Yunis, E. J.: Dietary restrictions early and late. Effects on the nephropathy of the NZBxNZW mouse. Lab. Invest., *38*:629–632 (1978).

Good, R. A., Jose, D. C. and Cooper, W. C.: In, *Microenvironmental Aspects of Immunity* (B. D. Jankovic and K. Isakovic, eds.), Plenum, NY, pp. 321–326 (1973).

Greene, M. I., Dorf, M. E., Pierres, M. and Benacerraf, B.: Reduction of syngeneic tumor growth by an anti I–J alloantiserum. Proc. Natl. Acad. Sci. USA, *74*:5118–5121 (1977).

Haberman, R. B. and Holden, H. T.: Natural cell-mediated immunity. In, *Advanced Cancer Research.* (G. Klein and S. Weinhouse, eds.), Vol. 27, Academic Press (1978).

Hillyard, L. A. and Abraham, S.: Effect of dietary polyunsaturated fatty acids on growth of mammary adenocarcinomas in mice and rats. Cancer Res., *39*:4430–4437 (1979).

Hui, Y. H., DeOme, K. B. and Briggs, G. M.: Influence of dietary phenylalanine deficiency on the mammary tumor virus activity in C3H mice. Cancer Res., *32*: 2086–2088 (1972).

Jerne, N. K.: The immune system. Sci. Amer., *229*:52–60 (1973).

Jose, D. G. and Good, R. A.: Absence of enhancing antibody in cell-mediated immunity to tumor heterografts in protein deficient rats. Nature (Lond), *231*: 323–325 (1971).

Jose, D. G., Stutman, O. and Good, R. A.: Long term effects on immune function of early nutritional deprivation. Nature (Lond), *241*:57–58 (1973).

Kasai, M., Leclerc, J. C., McVay-Boudreau, L., Shen, F. W. and Cantor, H.: Direct evidence that NK cells in nonimmune spleen cell populations prevent tumor growth *in vivo*. J. Exp. Med., *149*:1260–1264 (1979).

Kigoshi, S. and Ito, R.: High levels of free fatty acids in lymphoid cells with special reference to their cytotoxicity. Experientia, *29*:1408–1410 (1973).

Lane, M. A., Mahoney, R. J., Watson, A. L. M., Yunis, E. J. and Inbard, M.: Increased fluidity of serum lipids and development of spontaneous mammary tumors in C3H mice. Cancer Immunol. Immunotherapy (in press).

Lotzova, E. and Gutterman, J. U.: Effect of glucan on natural killer (NK) cells: Further comparison between NK cells and bone marrow effector cell activities. J. Immunol., *123*:607–611 (1979).

Makinodan, T.: Mechanism, prevention, and restoration of immunologic aging. In, *Birth Defects* (D. Bergsma and D. E. Harrison, eds.), Original Article Series, Vol. XIV, pp. 197–212 (1978).

Mandel, G., Shimizu, S., Gill, R. and Clack, W.: Alteration of the fatty acid composition of membrane phospholipids in mouse lymphoid cells. J. Immunol., *120*: 1631–1636 (1978).

McDevitt, H. O., Deak, B. D., Shreffler, C., Klein, H., Stimpfling, J. H. and Snell, G. D.: Genetic control of the immune response. Mapping of the IR-1 locus. J. Exp. Med., *135*:1259–1278 (1972).

Meredith, P. J. and Walford, R. L.: Effect of age on response to T- and B- cell mitogens in mice congenic at the H-2 locus. Immunogenetics, 5:109–128 (1977).

Mertin, J.: Effect of polyunsaturated fatty acids on skin allografts survival and primary and secondary cytotoxic response in mice. Transpl. 21:1–4 (1976).

Mertin, J. and Hunt, R.: Influence of polyunsaturated fatty acids on survival of skin allografts and tumor incidence in mice. Proc. Natl. Acad. Sci. USA, 73:928–931 (1976).

Möller, G. and Möller, E.: The concept of immunological surveillance against neoplasia. Transpl. Rev., 28:3–16 (1976).

Murphy, D. B., Herzenberg, L. A., Okumura, K., Herzenberg, L. A. and McDevitt, H. O.: A new I subregion (I-J) marked by a locus (Ia-4) controlling surface determinants on suppressor T lymphocytes. J. Exp. Med., 144:699–712 (1976).

Norbury, K. C.: *In vitro* stimulation and inhibition of tumor cell growth mediated by different lymphoid cell populations. Cancer Res., 37:1408–1411 (1977).

Petitou, M., Tuy, F., Rosenfeld, C., Mishal, Z., Paintrand, M., Jasnin, C., Mathe, G. and Inbard, M.: Decreased microviscosity of membrane lipids in leukemic cells: Two possible mechanisms. Proc. Natl. Acad. Sci. USA, 75:2306–2310 (1978).

Phren, R. T. and Lappe, M. A.: An immunostimulation theory of tumor development. Transpl. Rev., 7:26–54 (1971).

Pierres, M., Germain, R. N., Dorf, M. E. and Benacerraf, B.: *In vivo* effects of anti-Ia alloantisera. I. Elimination of specific suppression by *in vivo* administration of antisera specific for I-J controlled determinants. J. Exp. Med., 147:656 (1978).

Reinisch, C. L., Gleiner, N. A. and Schlossman, S. F.: Supressor cell regulation of immune response to tumors: Abrogation by adult thymectomy. Proc. Natl. Acad. Sci. USA, 74:2989–2992 (1977).

Reinisch, C. L. and Andrew, S. L.: Regulation of cytotoxic T cell reactivity to syngeneic tumors by the thymus. J. Exp. Med., 148:619–623 (1978.

Rich, S. S. and Rich, R. R.: Regulatory mechanisms in cell-mediated immune responses. III. I-region control of supressor cell interaction with responder cells in mixed lymphocyte reactions. J. Exp. Med., 143:672–677 (1976).

Ross, M. H. and Bras, G.: Lasting influence of early caloric restriction on prevalence of neoplasms in the rat. J.N.C.I., 47:1095–1113 (1971).

Ruppert, B., Blazer, B., Medina, D. and Heppner, G.: IV. Comparison of functional activity of lymphoid cells separated from mammary tumors to that of spleen and lymph node cells of tumor-sensitized mice. J. Immunol., 122:2180–2183 (1979).

Samlaska, C.: Linoleic acid inhibition of lymphocytotoxicity. Fed. Proc., 37:1273 (1978).

Santoli, D. and Koprowski, H.: Mechanisms of activation of human natural killer cells. Immunological Reviews, 441:163 (1979).

Sherr, D. H., Heghinian, K. M., Benacerraf, B. and Dorf, M. E.: Immune suppression *in vivo* with antigen-modified syngeneic cells. III. Distinctions between T cell tolerance and T cell-mediated suppression. J. Immunol., 123:2682–2688 (1979).

Simpson, E. and Cantor, H.: Regulation of the immune response by T cell subclasses: The effect of adult thymectomy upon humoral and cellular responses. Europ. J. Immunol., 5:337 (1975).

Singer, S. J. and Nicolson, G. Z.: The fluid mosaic model of the structure of cell membranes. Science, 175:720–731 (1972).

Small, M. and Trainin, N.: Separation of populations of sensitized lymphoid cells into fractions inhibiting and fractions enhancing syngeneic tumor growth *in vivo.* J. Immunol. *117*:292–297 (1976).

Small, M.: Characteristics of the immature cells involved in T cell-mediated enhancement of syngeneic tumor growth. J. Immunol., 118:1517–1523 (1977).

Smith, G. S. and Walford, R. L.: Influence of the main histocompatibility complex in aging in mice. Nature (Lond), *270*:727–729 (1977).

Suskind, R. M. (ed.): *Malnutrition and the Immune Response.* New York, Raven Press (1977).

Tada, T., Taniguchi, M. and David, C. S.: Properties of the antigen-specific suppressive T-cell factor in the regulation of antibody response of the mouse. IV. Special subregion of the gene(s) that codes for the suppressive T-cell factor in the H-2 histocompatibility complex. J. Exp. Med., *144*:713–725 (1976).

Tada, T., Taniguchi, M. and David, C. S.: Suppressive and enhancing T cell factors as I-region gene products: Properties and the subregion assignment. Cold Spring Harbor Symp. Quant. Biol., *41*:119–127 (1977).

Tannenbaum, A.: Initiation and growth of tumors. I. Effects of underfeeding. Amer. J. Cancer, *38*:335–350 (1940).

Tannenbaum, A.: The genesis and growth of tumors. II. Effects of caloric restriction per se. Cancer Res., *2*:460–467 (1942).

Tannenbaum, A.: The dependence of the genesis of induced skin tumors on the caloric intake during different stages of carcinogenesis. Cancer Res., *5*:673–677 (1944).

Theze, J., Waltenbaugh, C., Dorf, M. E. and Benacerraf, B.: Immunosuppressive factor(s) specific for L-glutamic acid[50] (GT). II. Presence of I-J determinants on the GT suppressive factor. J. Exp. Med., *146*:287 (1977).

Tucker, M. J.: The effect of long-term food restriction on tumors in rodents. Int. J. Cancer, *23*:803–807 (1979).

Uhr, J. W., Capra, D., Vitetta, E. S. and Cook, R. G.: Organization of the immune response genes. Science, *206*:292–297 (1979).

Walford, R. L., Liu, R. K., Gerbase-Delima, M., Mathies, M. and Smith, G. S.: Long-term dietary restriction and immune function in mice: Response to sheep red blood cells and to mitogenic agents. Mech. Aging Dev., *2*:447–454 (1973–74).

Weinberger, J. Z., Germain, R. N., Ju, S. T., Greene, M. I., Benacerraf, B., and Dorf, M. E.: Hapten-specific T cell responses to 4-hydroxy-3-nitrophenyl acetyl (NP). II. Demonstration of idiotypic determinants on suppressor cells. J. Exp. Med., *150*:761 (1979).

Williams, R. M., Kraus, L., Lavin, P. T., Steele, L. L. and Yunis, E. J.: Genetics of survival in mice. (In press).

DISCUSSION

HELLMAN: Dr. Yunis, in your studies on nutritional deficiency have you looked at the immunological modifications, particularly in the NZB and the C3H mouse, brought about by the expression of retroviral glycoproteins?

YUNIS: No, we have not. One problem, which applies in general to nutritional experiments in relation to diseases and aging, is that each experiment is costly and takes a long time, as much as three years.

The present experiments were completed just about a year ago. Of course, our main purpose was only to dissect the different compartments of the immune response. The experiments were done delaying only the maturation of the lymphoid system to allow the investigator to compare strains in which involution of the thymus occurs earlier than it does in others. Perhaps someone in the audience could answer your question, because I am not aware that this has been done. Further, these studies were completed just about a year ago. I am not doing those experiments now, but I'm still trying to use nutrition, low calories, high fatty acids or circulation of fatty acids just to dissect the different compartments of the immune response.

HELLMAN: I am not familiar with the nutritional aspects. However, retroviruses do modify the lymphocyte surface by their glycoproteins, and we have performed evaluations during very early stages of viral infection. By linker experiments, we have demonstrated that the receptor sites for the H-2 histocompatibility antigen and viral glycoproteins are very close to each other. Thus, some of the antigenic modifications that you describe may very well be due to modification of the general protein turnover rate and the expression of some of these viral glycoproteins may not have anything directly to do with the genetics of the animal.

YUNIS: That is right. Let me see if I communicate correctly. What I was trying to do, first, was to introduce the main concepts for discussion this morning. I can see that lymphocyte modifications may be due to modifications of the general protein turnover rate and expression of some of the retroviruses, but, underlying that biological phenonmenon, there are also modifying genetic factors. Random individuals may be born with better genetic equipment to deal with that kind of situation; whereas others may have all kinds of problems such as defective immune response genes that could deal abnormally with the retroviruses. Although we have not studied these viruses, we have discussed immunoregulation changes in hopes that it is possible to manipulate the defect, not by genetic means, but at least by the kind of manipulation that will be discussed.

KERMAN: Since immune response is associated with HLA-D or DRw complex why do you think the data show that women over 70 without HLA-B8 antigen were lower responders? Was the association with the B8, and what do you think is happening in terms of that association?

YUNIS: These results have to be corroborated. I do not want people to think that our observations are definitive. This study was done on a selected group of women from a nursing home who had very distinct ethnic backgrounds (i.e., people in Minnesota in general have a German, northern European ethnic background). It does not imply that this response is going to be found in all the populations.

But talking about the B8, DRw 3, remember that we are measuring the immune responses in an aged population—perhaps beyond the possible measurement of genetic control of the immune responses. When one goes to the older population to find a few surviving women, one tries to rely more on a marker than on an immune function. As you know, in general, HLA-B8, DW3 persons have a propensity for hyperimmunity and/or autoimmunity as opposed to HLA-B7, DW2 persons. We found that lymphocytes from young or older women of HLA-B8 phenotype have lower responses to PHA which suggests that HLA-B8 women may have a propensity for autoimmunity and lesser T-cell vigor. It is of interest that HLA-B8 is the phenotype found to be associated with autoimmune and endocrine diseases. But these persons have not developed those diseases and lived to be 70 or older, thus this antigen may be under represented.

KERMAN: How do you envision the manipulation nutritionally of T-cell function?

YUNIS: Well, nutrition can modify genetic control of the immune system. Although dietary manipulation alters the immune status of experimental animals, it seems remote to anticipate prolongation of life far beyond limits imposed by genetic determinants. However, nutrition may offer possibilities to achieve expression of full genetic potential by forestalling appearance of diseases of aging. In man, genetically superior persons (from the longevity point of view) may live as long as 95 to 110 years in vigorous health. Arteriosclerosis, coronary vascular sclerosis, renal diseases, cancer, and autoimmunities including arthritis, vasculities, amyloidosis, and infections, shorten the potential life span. If these diseases of aging can be prevented or reversed, the possibility of achieving longer life with good health will be real. In animals, especially mice, there is a significant correlation between preservation of immune vigor and absence of autoantibodies in long-lived, pure genetic strains of mice. In humans, it is possible to find correlations between survival, preservation of immune vigor, and absence of autoantibodies in populations beyond the age of 70 years.

It is of interest that the thymus functions appear to be better indicators of a long life than some of the other immune functions, i.e., the thymus-clock concept. There are some suggestions that the main alteration related to the thymus clock is the deficiency of thymus-controlled immune regulation which is accompanied by autoimmunity and shorter survival. Dietary manipulations of adult or aged humans have not been attempted either to prevent or to reverse diseases. However, in the mouse, calorie restriction which decreases both cellular and humoral immune functions early in life, may lead to preservation of the immunological functions and immune vigor if applied later in life. In contrast, well-fed mice, that show vigorous immunological functions early in life, are characterized by early decline of immunological function and earlier death. It seems that the effect of diets in long-lived strains of mice is controlled through the thymus, but we do not know the biochemical or the physiological basis of what appears to be an effect on change in the maturation and senescence of the thymus and/or cells derived from it.

DEAN: Dr. Yunis, would you develop for us how you propose immunologically that a high-calorie diet might lead to reduced incidence of spontaneous mammary tumors?

YUNIS: First, as I stated, these experiments are not complete. One thing I can leave with you is the fact that we have corroborated the finding that calorie restriction has a significant effect in decreasing spontaneous tumor development. We added to the literature the fact that we measured suppressive function. Unfortunately, the measurements of suppressive function were done at the period of life of the animal when tumors had not yet appeared. So, we do not know what happens in terms of function of the lymphocytes later than three months of age; so far, no one has done this experiment. I believe that in this particular situation, formation of a spontaneous tumor, calorie restriction can change certain endocrine functions that alter the proportion of regulatory cells which will produce a positive network geared to kill tumors.

HADDEN: Dr. Yunis, I wanted to stress a point so that the audience does not go away with the impression that starving is good for the immune system. It should be pointed out that the degree of reduction of calories in the mouse experiments would be lethal for humans. Also in these experiments, one encounters immunodeviation, where there is a relative compromise of antibody-mediated function with an augmentation of cellular immunity; the latter seems to be the factor correlating with survival.

YUNIS: I go along with that. The main difference is that these mice receive fewer calories, but the diet is sufficient to allow the animal to survive—provided of course, that the animal receives normal amounts of minerals and vitamins. What John Hadden is saying is that it does not really mean that starvation is good, because these experiments show that one improves survival of the mice that are not on starvation diets. One way of looking at it is the only thing one observes, when animals are underfed with calories, is that they are smaller than the ones receiving the so-called normal amount of calories. In general, fat mice do not live any longer than skinny ones. However, the mice are not starved; they are just skinny.

The important point is that this diet, for unknown reasons, alters the maturation of the immune system because of its low caloric value. The optimal age at which the animal reaches highest immune vigor is delayed, therefore, hypothetically, there is also a decrease of other functions. In other words, the long-lived strain on a normal-calorie diet will attain maximum vigor by the age of 18 months, whereas, the mouse will not expire until 36 months of age. Thus, when one shifts production of optimal immunity to a later age, one also shifts the age at which thymus or T-cell functions will involute.

UTERMOHLEN: I wondered whether, in the process of shifting the immune function, one would also shift development of the mammary gland, and so forth—

YUNIS: Yes.

UTERMOHLEN: (continuing) —and change hormonal balance in a general way; and thus alter development of mammary tumors.

YUNIS: This is true. Apparently it is one explanation of why low-calorie diets in C3H-susceptible strains do not produce tumors—the endocrine system is altered to affect estrogen function in the mammary glands—perhaps changing the estrogen receptors or even the levels of estrogen.

The end result of these studies might not be necessarily immunological. It might be just an alteration of the target for tumor development. The changes of immune regulation by diets may be unrelated to tumor development. I repeat that the changes of immune regulation by diets perhaps more directly influence autoimmune diseases than tumor development. But, in general, dietary manipulation can be used to dissect the immune system. Low calories are relative immunostimulants for some functions, and relative immunosuppressants for other functions; also, unsaturated fatty acids or vitamin A can alter the immune responses. By using these diets, it is possible then to study experimentally several compartments of the immune system. As I have discussed, there are also genetic controls of immune response and immune suppression, but this genetic control can be altered; in other words, it can be modified by the use of diet.

2
The Immunopharmacology of Immunotherapy

John W. Hadden

*Laboratory of Immunopharmacology,
Memorial-Sloan Kettering Cancer Center, New York, New York*

INTRODUCTION

Although the initial rationale for the development of immunotherapy derived from the need to mobilize immune mechanisms in the treatment of cancer, it has become increasingly evident that immunotherapy has potential to benefit man in the treatment of a broad spectrum of disorders, including immunodeficiency, chronic infection and autoimmunity. In embarking on such "pro-host" forms of therapy, experimental therapists are leaving the traditional domains of pharmacology and entering the relatively undefined area of pharmacologic regulation of the immune system. In general, the application of immunotherapy has involved the administration of a bacterial product or a chemical to an animal or a patient with an existing tumor or infection and the determination of changes in longevity or survival. The empiricism of this approach rests upon the assumption that the therapy is active on the immune response, in a favorable manner, under the conditions employed, and that the effect of the agent on the immune system will result in destruction of the tumor or the offending organism. The accumulated results of this approach are conflicting and have yielded mixed interpretations. A single unanimous interpretation is that more information about the function of the immune system and how to regulate it is required in order to mobilize it effectively in any particular disease state. There is, thus, the need for an immunopharmacology—a basic, preclinical, and clinical science of therapeutic immune regulation.

The purpose of this paper will be to outline some of the basic areas of development of such a science and to summarize what is known about the cellular targets of immunotherapy and some of the intracellular mechanisms involved in the actions of various therapeutic agents. Of the diverse agents available, the crude bacterial preparations such as the mycobacteria (BCG), mixed bacterial vaccines, corynebacteria (C. parvum) and pseudomonas vaccine will not be discussed since their actions have been reviewed elsewhere; and since, as a result of their complex and antigenic nature, each preparation involves multiple mechanisms of action. From the ensuing discussion, it will become apparent that such bacterial preparations, when better defined as to their active constituents, will lend themselves to the analyses of the mechanisms of action described. The discussion will focus on: 1) The chemically defined bacterial products such as (a) endotoxin (LPS); (b) muramyl dipeptide (MDP), derived from BCG organisms and (c) polysaccharides of bacterial or fungal origin, like glucan, lentinan, and Krestin; 2) biological products of the imune system such as lymphokines, monokines, interferon, and the thymic hormones (thymosin, thymopoietin, facteur thymique serique, etc.); and 3) chemicals such as polynucleotides, levamisole, isoprinosine, tilerone, SM 1213, BM 12531, and lynestrenol. The reader is referred to more extensive reviews elsewhere (Chirigos, 1977a; Chirigos, 1977b; Chirigos, 1978; Dukor et al., 1975; Hadden et al., 1977; Hadden and Delmonte, 1978; Johnson et al., 1978) for information about the biochemistry and the *in vivo* effects of these agents on the immune system; the present discussion will restrict itself to cellular targets and biochemical mechanisms of action.

As a background for understanding the action of these immunologically active substances, it is important to emphasize that in employing any particular substance to modify immune response to a particular antigen, features of the agent itself, of the antigen, of the immune system, and the general status of the host, must all be taken into collective consideration in order to reliably predict the outcome (see Figure 1).

Characteristics of the Agent

Most substances which act on the immune system, particularly bacteria and their products and interferon and its inducers, have the capacity for both positive and negative actions; thus, "immunomodulator" is the best general term to employ for these immunotherapeutic agents. Some of the chemical agents, e.g., levamisole and isoprinosine, fulfill the criteria for the term "immunopotentiator" in that they have little action alone, but

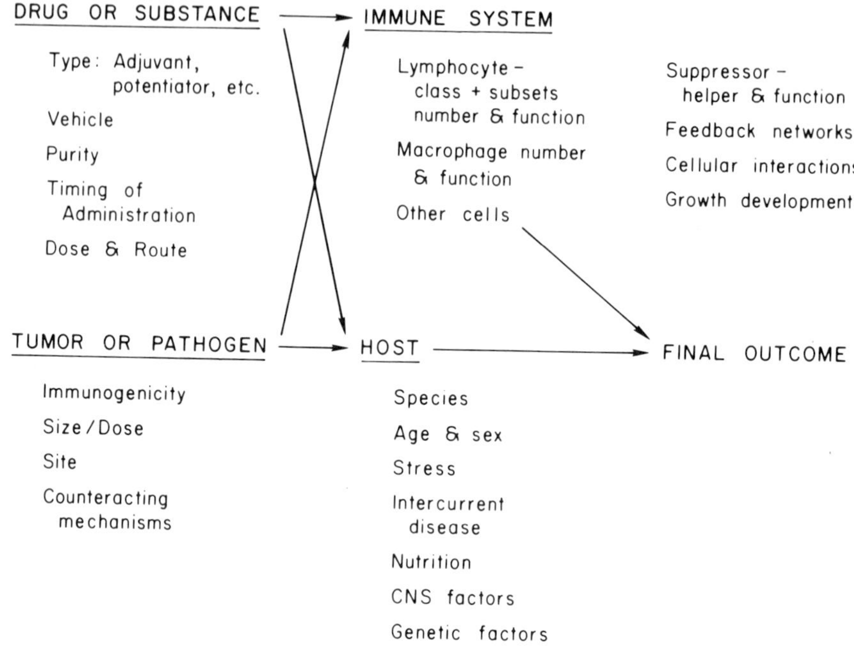

Figure 1.

in combination with antigenic stimulation, they augment the ongoing response. Still other agents, like polynucleotides, MDP, and alum, are "immunoadjuvants" in that their most effective use is in combination with a single administration with an antigen; many of these are immunosuppressive if given during the subsequent response to the antigen. The natural products of the immune system like the thymic hormones and the lymphokines constitute replacement therapy and might be classified as biological inducers of immune cell development or function. In general, agents which are A) proproliferative (i.e., they augment the proliferation of cells involved in the immune system) are immunopotentiating; B) antiproliferative or inductive of suppressor functions (i.e., they inhibit replication of immune cells) are immunomodulatory or immunosuppressive; C) activators (i.e., they directly induce proliferation of lymphocytes or activation of macrophages) are immunomodulators and/or immunoadjuvants. Agents such as the bacteria and their products are antigenic in addition to having one or more of the above characteristics. While simple, meaningful terminologies are in the process of evolving, these terms, currently in use, have functional significance in describing mode of action. One need only realize that the chronic administration of an immunoadjuvant without regard to the timing of antigen administration may lead to intolerable toxicity in order to understand that the mode of action is critical in deciding how and when to administer an agent.

Immunopotentiating agents are most effectively employed with and following antigen administration. Immunoadjuvants are best employed with antigen. Activators, particularly those acting on the macrophages, are effective before antigen administration and, in some cases, after. Inducers of cellular development, with some exceptions, can also be used both before or after antigen. In most circumstances of therapeutic application, the antigen is already in the host and the immune system is in reaction; antigen, however, can be reintroduced into the system in the form of a vaccine to allow more effective employment of immune adjuvants and activators.

Obviously issues of dose and the route and regimen of administration of an agent are critical in determining the response. Surprisingly little is known about these critical variables for any particular agent. In general, antigenic stimulation proceeds under principles of optimalization by which low antigenic as well as excessive antigenic stimulation leads to lack of response. Similarly, immunomodulators by nature of their dose, as well as timing of administration, can shift from a positive to a negative action. As a general rule, immunopotentiators lose their effect, and may induce toxicity, when higher doses are employed. In contrast with other forms of chemotherapy, if a little immunotherapy works, often more will not. Another characteristic of such agents acting on the immune system is that often doses or concentrations in the submicrogram or submicromolar range are effective (e.g., endotoxin, levamisole, thymopoietin) so that by prior therapeutic criteria, so-called "homeopathic doses" are active. Much more information is needed in this area of immunopharmacology before general principles of administration can be developed and applied with any confidence.

Characteristics of the Antigenic Challenge

The attempt to predictably modify response to an antigen involves knowledge of the degree of antigenicity, whether it will stimulate primarily a cellular or a humoral immune response, and the amount of antigen. Prior experience with the antigen may provide information about its antigenicity

FUNCTION
DEVELOPMENT
Levamisole
Isoprinosine
BMI2531
Interferon
Antigen
Mitogen
B. Pertussis
Proliferation
Cytotoxicity
Isoprinosine
BMI2531
MDP
Activation
Proliferation
Levamisole
Isoprinosine
Lymphokines
MMF
MAF
LPS
MDP
SMI213
Interferon
Antibody
Antigen
LPS
Antibody Secretion
T LYMPHOCYTE
MACROPHAGE
PLASMA CELL
THYMOCYTE
MONOCYTE
B LYMPHOCYTE
Monokines
Monokines
CSF
BONE MARROW
LYMPHOCYTE
PRECURSOR
MONOCYTE
PRECURSOR
Thymopoietin
Thymosin
FTS
Isoprinosine
Levamisole (in vivo)
Poly A:Poly U
LPS
LPS
Poly A:Poly U
Interferon
TNF

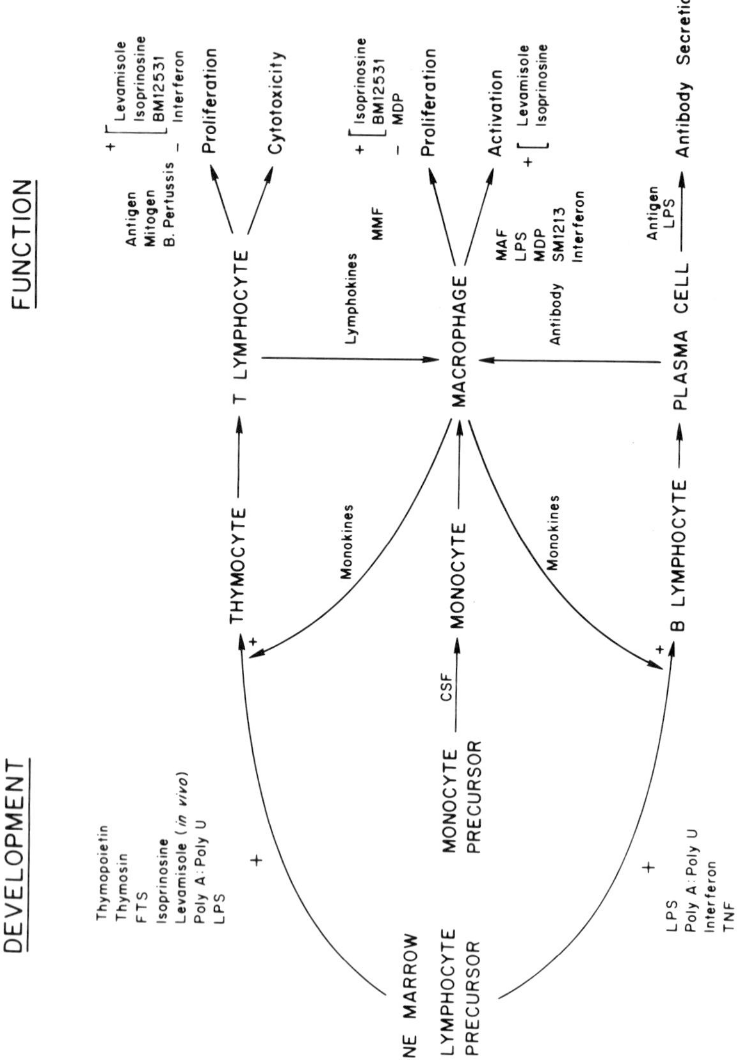

Figure 2.

and whether it elicits a cellular or a humoral immune response or both. In the case of pathogens, particularly those to which vaccines have been developed, much may be known; however, in the case of human tumors, little is known. In the case of therapeutic applications, the antigen, be it pathogen or tumor, has already been introduced into the system; therefore, its site and degree of dissemination may not be known and its amount may, therefore, not be calculable. Often, as a result of excessive amounts, immunosuppression and immunodeviation (imbalance in response, e.g., humoral»cellular or vice versa) may result. It may be that in certain circumstances, antigenic material must be reduced in amount in order to make immunotherapy effective. Thus in the case of cancer, bulk tumor must be removed by surgery, x irradiation, or chemotherapy, or in the case of pathogen, concomitant antimicrobial therapy may be essential. It is important to note that in the case of cancer therapy, each of the currently employed cytoreductive therapies are immunosuppressive and the concomitant administration of an immunosuppressive therapy with an immunopotentiating one will often lead to enhanced immunosuppression since immune cells like cancer cells are more susceptible to destruction when actively proliferating.

The presence of actively replicating antigen, either pathogen or tumor, in the host makes variables of unresponsiveness difficult to interpret. When a response to the antigen is defective, one must consider, in addition to factors to be discussed relative to the immune system, factors associated with the antigen which may be immunosuppressive. It is known that various tumors have the capacity to release low molecular weight substances such as peptides and prostaglandins which act to subvert the immune response. Many viruses, e.g., influenza, measles, varicella, mumps, Epstein-Barr virus, herpes virus, rubella, and polio, have been shown to be immunosuppressive by a variety of criteria and mechanisms including infection of lymphocytes and macrophages. Bacteria, particularly the facultative intracellular pathogens like those of tuberculosis, leprosy, listeriosis, brucellosis, and salmonellosis have the capacity to interfere with normal bactericidal mechanisms. In these cases, the immunotherapy may include efforts to inhibit the immunosuppressive mechanism, e.g., inhibitors of prostaglandin synthesis or agents which preferentially interfere with synthesis and secretion of suppressive substances. Nowhere is the need for more precise knowledge about the nature of antigenicity and of suppressive mechanisms better exemplified than in human cancer. Effective immunotherapy of any but minimal residual disease will require this knowledge to develop effective vaccines and antisuppressive therapy to be used in conjuction with immunotherapeutic agents.

Host Characteristics in Immunotherapy

It is natural to assume that non-immunologic aspects of host resistance will play a role in analyzing and predicting response to immunotherapy; however, only recently have we entertained the very great degree to which this is true. Remarkable differences among species, between sexes, and among age groups have been observed in response to antigens and in response to immunotherapy. While not yet catalogued nor understood as to their mechanism, these differences make immunotherapy a particularly unpredictable proposition. Clearly, man is not the facile substrate for immunotherapeutic manipulation that the mouse is, particularly in the case of cancer. Similarly, age and sex may prove to be critical determinants in the success of immunotherapy (Renoux, 1978). Understanding the reasons for this will be essential in overcoming the limitations they impose.

Host genetic factors are clearly critical. From work in mice, we know that high response, low response, or non-response to an antigen may be determined by specific immune response genes within the major histocompatibility complex. In addition, non-histocompatibility-linked genes are also critical in defining resistance to infection by viruses, intracellular bacteria, and to tumors (Hadden, 1979). This genetic predisposition defining response means that some strains of mice are very susceptible to certain diseases (e.g., DBA/2, Balb/c, C_3H) and others (e.g., C57B1/6 related strains) are highly resistant. Interestingly, those which are susceptible are most responsive to immunopotentiating therapy, while those which are resistant are also relatively unresponsive to such therapy (Cheers and McKenzie, 1978; Cotzias and Tang, 1977; Hadden, 1979; Lopez, 1975). These observations support the general impression that those patients with defective defense mechanisms are responsive to immunotherapy while those with normal defense mechanisms are not. This impression has led to the notion that some forms of immunotherapy should be considered "immunonormalizing". In any case, it is clear that clinical application of immunotherapy has yielded "responders" and "non-responders" within the same disease category, despite controlling for age, sex and disease stage, indicating that genetic and other host factors are important to consider.

Obviously, the general status of the host is critical. Nutrition is important. Protein-calorie malnutrition (Good et al., 1977) yields, when mild, immunodeviation and, when severe, immunosuppression. The immunodeviation is characterized by depressed humoral but augmented cellular immune response. Thus, in some circumstances, restriction of intake may itself be immunotherapeutic. Evidence indicates that excessive fat ingestion may be immunosuppressive. Specific vitamin and mineral deficiencies may be devastating for the immune system. Examples are vitamin C, biotin, and zinc.

Those who work with guinea pigs know that omission of "cabbage factors" in their diet will make impossible experiments of delayed hypersensitivity. No doubt, emphasis in this area will be important in the future.

Concomitant diseases and their therapies will obviously determine efficacy of immunotherapy. The obvious examples of cancer and infection have been discussed. However, organ dysfunctions, particularly of the renal, hepatic, cardiopulmonary and endocrine systems, are associated with impaired immune response and, logically, altered pharmacokinetics of the immunotherapeutic agent. Other drugs used to treat the organ dysfunction may also have actions to modify immune response of which we are not now aware. Psychic and central nervous system function, in a way suspected, but not well documented, may prove to be a critical determinant in immunotherapy. Certainly, stress has been shown to be a factor in immune function. In steroid-sensitive species like the mouse, this may mean that stress from blood drawing, poor sanitation or crowding may lead to lympholysis and profound immunosuppression and critically affect the outcome of immunotherapy experiments.

It must be emphasized that, in addition to having nutritional requirements equivalent if not more restrictive than the rest of the organism, the immune system is sensitive to a broad spectrum of hormones and neurotransmitter influences (Hadden, 1977); which allows for modifcation of the expression of immune response by any influence modifying body homeostasis.

Immune System

The immune system is a delicately balanced one involving responses of two major classes of lymphocytes (B & T), having at least 5 major B subsets subserving the function of antibody production and perhaps 4 major T subsets subserving the functions of allogeneic and antigen response, and helper and suppressor function. In addition, lymphocytes participate in the regulation of other cell types like macrophages, mast cells, platelets, and polymorphonuclear, basophilic and eosinophilic leukocytes. Involved in their interaction are multiple molecular communications resulting in the modulation of cellular function due to the liberation of a myriad of regulators including activated complement components, prostaglandins, lymphokines, and other allergic and inflammatory mediators. The specific response of the system is elicited by a foreign antigen. Central to an appropriate response is the digestion and processing of the antigen by phagocytic cells and its presentation to the respective class of lymphocytes. The lymphocyte response that results may involve predominantly one or the other class of lymphocytes or a combination of the two. In addition to a delicate balance of interactants, the integrity of the system is regulated by endocrine, neurological, and nutritional factors. Its development and replenishment involve growth- and differentiation-inducing factors and micro-chemical environments with regulatory influences yet to be clarified.

For the purposes of the present discussion, we will focus on the actions of immunotherapeutic agents on the ontogeny and function of lymphocytes and macrophages as revealed through *in vitro* studies. The emphasis on *in vitro* studies is justified for several reasons: A) Virtually all reviews of immunotherapeutic agents stress *in vivo* effects; B) Since regulation of the immune system involves such complicated networks of positive and negative feedback, *in vitro* studies are the only ones which allow a definitive statement that an agent acts directly on a particular cell at a particular stage of its development to modify a specific function; and C) knowledge of the foregoing is essential for interpreting the *in vivo* effects as to direct versus indirect actions, and ultimately for predicting outcome of modifications of therapeutic administration.

Effects of Agents on:

1) *Hematopoiesis.* Lymphocytes, macrophages and granulocytes develop from progenitor cells common to the hematopoietic lineage. The ontogeny of each line of cell has been demonstrated or is thought to be regulated by growth hormones often referred to as colony stimulating factors (CSF). To date no known immunotherapeutic agent has been demonstrated to act at this level. Candidate substances might be the lymphocytosis-producing factor derived from Bordetella pertussis (Morse, 1976), or monocytosis-producing factor derived from Listeria monocytogenes (Galsworthy et al., 1977). The mature macrophage is a major CSF producer and a number of agents to be discussed which activate the macrophage induce CSF production and would promote the development of macrophages and polymorphonuclear granulocytes from the precursors in the bone marrow. A CSF for lymphoid cells has been postulated but not yet isolated and characterized.

2) *Lymphocyte differentiation.* Lymphocytes destined for humoral or cellular immune response in mammals derive from a common precursor

under the influence of the microchemical environment of the thymus and of the bone marrow, respectively. Recent advances in the culturing of lymphocyte precursors and the serologic definition of cell surface markers which characterize the sequential maturation of the two lineages has made possible the *in vitro* assay of the induction of B & T lymphocyte differentiation. From the work of E. A. Boyse & colleagues (1978), we know that the T lymphocyte in the mouse progresses from no markers; to 0^+, TL^+, H_2^+ and Ly $^{1\ 2\ 3}$; to 0^+, TL^-, H_2^{++} and Ly^{1+} or $Ly^{2,3+}$ as intrathymic maturation occurs. Similarly, J. L. Touraine, R. A. Good, and I have shown in humans a similar evolution from no markers, to $HTLA^+$ E rosette$^+$, mitogen-responsive or alloantigen responsive (1977). Both mouse and human T lymphocyte development can be studied *in vitro* using precursor cells derived from spleen or bone marrow, respectively. The thymic hormones, thymosin (fraction V), thymopoietin, and facteur thymique serique have been demonstrated to induce these T cell surface markers within two hours of culture and with more prolonged culture the acquisition of allogeneic mitogen and proliferative responses can be demonstrated (Friedman, 1975). The action of the thymic hormones is quite specific on these cells and this effect accounts presumably for the *in vivo* effects of these hormones to replace thymic function in animals lacking a thymus (thymectomized or nude mice). Ultimately, the clinical application of these hormones now in development will be applicable to thymus immunodeficiency as occurs in cancer and aging.

In addition to these specific inducers, a number of nonspecific inducers have been uncovered including endotoxin, poly A: poly U, and isoprinosine (Scheid, 1978; unpublished observations of Hadden and Hämmerling). It is of note that sulfur-containing compounds including levamisole will *in vivo,* but not *in vitro,* induce a substance which will promote *in vitro* differentiation of T cells (Renoux and Renoux, 1977).

The development of the B cell lineage is characterized by the sequential acquisition of immunoglobulin, complement receptors, and plasma cell surface markers. The natural inducer of this development is bursapoietin in the chicken and a yet undiscovered hormone in mammals. Immunotherapeutic agents which have been demonstrated to induce B cell differentiation *in vitro* include endotoxin, a related endotoxin induced *in vivo,* called tumor necrosis factor, and interferon (Old, 1976; Scheid, 1978; unpublished observations of Hadden and Hämmerling).

The differentiation of both T and B cell to proliferative or secretory function can be further promoted by factors derived from the macrophage (monokines), lymphocyte activating factor (LAF) (Waksman and Wagshal, 1978) and B cell differentiation factor (BDF) (Calderon et al.,

1975), respectively, so that activators of the macrophage can promote lymphocyte differentiation indirectly.

3) *T Cell function.* Immunotherapeutic agents have been studied on a variety of T cell functions. The most common function is proliferation induced by mitogen such as phytohemagglutinin (PHA) and Concanavalin A (Con A) or by allogeneic cells. Only one agent studied is directly mitogenic for T cells and that is a yet uncharacterized substance from Bordetella pertussis (Morse, 1976). Many agents promote proliferation induced by mitogenic or allogeneic stimulation. These include: levamisole, thymopoietin, thymosin, isoprinosine, BM12531 (Azimexon), and lynestrenol (Cohen et al., 1975; Hadden et al., 1975; Hadden et al., 1976; Sunshine et al., 1978; Wybran and Govaerts, 1977; unpublished observations of Hadden), while others inhibit, including interferon Poly A: Poly U, tilerone (Chirigos, 1977a; Chirigos, 1977b; Chirigos, 1978). To a lesser extent lymphokine production by T cells has been studied and stimulants include levamisole, isoprinosine, and thymic hormones (Hadden et al., 1977).

Another assay of post-thymic lymphocyte function is the promotion of erythrocyte (E) rosette receptor display on circulating null cells (generally HTLA$^+$) or the increase in receptor avidity in the active rosette assay. Agents which augment E rosette binding include thymosin, levamisole, isoprinosine, and lynestrenol (Wybran et al., 1975; Wybran et al., 1977; Wybran and Govaerts, 1977). T cell helper function for antibody response is generally determined by the mouse spleen cell plaque assay in the mouse. In this assay, endotoxin, poly A: Poly U, thymosin, thymopoietin and levamisole will promote T helper function (Goidl et al., 1976; Hadden et al., 1977; Johnson et al., 1978; Renoux, 1978). T cell suppressor function is less well studied as a result of the lack of convenient assays. Levamisole, thymosin and thymopoietin are all thought to promote this function of T cells (Horowitz et al., 1977; Renoux, 1978; Sunshine et al., 1978). T cell killer function is promoted by levamisole (Renoux, 1978).

4) *B Cell functions.* B cell proliferation and antibody production are conveniently studied *in vitro* using endotoxin or pokeweed as mitogens and inducers of secretion. In addition to stimulation by endotoxin, only interferon inhibition (Epstein, 1977) and lack of effect of levamisole and isoprinosine have been reported (Renoux, 1978; Vecchi et al., 1978). The lack of information about these functions reflects the relatively greater emphasis on cellular immune response in the study of immunotherapeutic agents.

5) *Macrophage functions.* Macrophage migration and chemotaxis have

been shown to be modulated by T cell-produced lymphokines such as macrophage migration inhibitory factor (MIF) and macrophage chemotactic factor (MCF). Levamisole has been shown to modulate chemotaxis (Anderson et al., 1976).

Macrophage proliferation has been shown to be induced by a lymphokine macrophage mitogenic factor (MMF). Isoprinosine augments and muramyl dipeptide inhibits MMF-induced proliferation while levamisole & SM1213 have relatively little effect (Hadden, 1979; Hadden et al., 1979).

Macrophage activation to kill facultative intracellular pathogens or to kill tumor cells has been shown to be induced by one or more macrophage activating factors (MAF) of which MMF and interferon both appear to be examples. In addition to the natural inducers, endotoxin, poly A: poly U, a listeria factor, muramyl dipeptide, and SM1213, all act directly to induce activation (Alexander and Evans, 1971; Hadden and Englard, 1979; Hadden et al., 1979). While relatively inactive alone, both levamisole and isoprinosine promote lymphokine-induced activation. Another manifestation of activation, phagocytosis, is generally promoted by these agents.

In general agents which induce macrophage activation also induce secretion of enzymes and monokines by macrophages, thus effecting the secondary modulation of lymphocytes discussed. The natural inducers of macrophage activation (MAF, interferon, etc.) are in general less toxic than the bacteria-derived substances LPS, glucan, etc.), with the exception of muramyl dipeptide. However, MDP's potent antiproliferative action for macrophages suggests that it has a capacity to induce prostaglandin (PG) production since PG's are regulatory for macrophage proliferation (Hadden and Englard, 1979). The lymphokines in having considerable potency in the absence of great toxicity offer therapeutic potential particularly in cancer where macrophage dysfunction is emerging as a central defect in immune responses.

The foregoing represents a sweeping and admittedly incomplete summary of the studies of the *in vitro* actions of various immunotherapeutic agents. These studies allow clear-cut demonstration of the action of the agents on cellular targets and functions and they begin to allow comparisons of efficacy on a concentration basis. They have sorted the agents out into those principally active on lymphocytes and those active on macrophages, and into those which induce proliferation and activation; and those which promote the response to a mitogen or antigen. They have reflected and predicted both toxicity and inhibitory effects. They begin to predict which agents might be effectively employed in combination.

In general, each of the assays that has been described as being modified directly *in vitro* by a particular agent has reflected a similar change after *in vivo* treatment with the agent—that is, the tests have reliably predicted *in vivo* activity. This statement has been less true for certain classes of agents like the sulphur-containing compounds (Renoux and Renoux, 1977). These assays do not adequately reflect the cell-cell interactions and molecular communications which occur *in vivo;* however, when interpreted in conjunction with *in vivo* data, as space will not allow here, they begin to provide a complete and comprehensive view of primary and secondary events in host modulation by these agents.

Evident from a review of these studies is that better tests are needed for suppressor functions of both lymphocytes and macrophages and for the analysis of ontogeny and functions of subpopulations of lymphocytes and macrophages. It is apparent from the *in vivo* studies, particularly in man where, generally, the tests are restricted to cells and molecules obtainable from blood, that more sensitive tests for the action of immunotherapeutic agents are needed. Far more accurate substantiation of immunopotentiator action on the immune system of man is necessary before the first goal of immunotherapy can be achieved, i.e., reliable and predictable modification of immune response. With the primary goal adequately achieved, the secondary goal, the effective interaction of the host's immune system and his pathogen or cancer, can be realized.

Mechanisms of Action of Immunotherapeutic Agents

It is not within the scope of this limited review to analyze all that is known about the mechanisms of action of the immunotherapeutic agents under discussion; however, a discussion of some important generalizations which have emerged from recent studies seems warranted. The reader is referred to other reviews for more extensive treatment of this area (Hadden et al., 1977; Hadden and Delmonte, 1978). Perhaps the greatest insight into mechanisms of immunoregulation has been provided by the development of the biological roles of the cyclic nuleotides, cyclic 3'5' adenosine and guanosine monophosphates (cyclic AMP and cyclic GMP, respectively). These cyclic nucleotides appear to mediate diverse influences acting on cells of the immune system. The conventional understanding of the second messenger roles of the cyclic nucleotides derived from analyzing the primary hormone messengers on the functions of immune cells. It became clear early in these studies that the hematopoietic system had a rather unique regulation compared to other endocrine-responsive tissues. In most endocrine target organs, lack of proliferation is the mode and dominant functions like secretion are promoted by agents which increase cyclic AMP, and opposing or lesser functions are promoted by agents which increase cyclic GMP. In the hematopoietic system where proliferation is the mode, dominant functions like proliferation, secretion, and cytotoxicity are promoted by agents increasing cellular levels of cyclic GMP and these functions are inhibited or suppressed by agents which increase cyclic AMP. For this system, as in other systems, cyclic AMP plays an antiproliferative role associated with the induction or promotion of the differentiated state. These concepts provided important components for the development of the "yin-yang" hypothesis proposed by N. D. Goldberg, myself and coworkers (Goldberg et al., 1974). The development of these concepts in immunopharmacology is the topic of a textbook by the same name (Hadden et al., 1977) and the many studies referenced therein attest to the usefulness of these concepts in understanding the regulation of immune function not only by hormones but by biological factors and immunotherapeutic agents.

The recent developments of the understanding of actions of thymic hormones, lymphokines, monokines, and interferon demonstrate that the immune system is an endocrine microcosm in which a myriad of intercellular molecular communications are acting via mechanisms traditionally associated with the endocrine system. Each type of these molecular mediators has been demonstrated and strongly suspected to act via specific cell surface receptors on their target cells. Thymic hormones (thymosin and thymopoietin) have been linked to cyclic AMP in their capacity to induce prothymocyte differentiation (although the pharmacologic evidence is strong, actual increases in cyclic AMP levels have not been reported) (Scheid et al., 1978). Thymosin and thymopoietin have been linked to cyclic GMP in promoting proliferative and rosetting functions in mature T cells (Naylor et al., 1976; Sunshine et al., 1978). The lymphokines MCF, MMF, MAF have been linked to cyclic GMP in their effects on chemotaxis, proliferation and activation of macrophages (Hadden, 1979; Hadden and Englard, 1979; Hatch et al., 1977). The monokines CSF and LAF have been linked to cyclic GMP in effects to promote the proliferation of monocyte precursors and thymocytes (Kurland et al., 1977; Hadden, Coffey and Oppenheim, unpublished observations). Interferon as an antiproliferative agent and an inducer of B cell differentiation may be linked to cyclic AMP, although these actions do not appear to pertain to those involved in the antiviral action. In addition, the action of interferon to induce macrophage activation is antagonized by cyclic AMP (Schultz et al., 1978), in contrast to the antiproliferative and antiviral activities (Lopez, Hadden, unpublished observations), suggesting a cyclic GMP related mechanism. Thus, the biological factors acting to subserve intercellular communication in the immune system appear to act as hormones and to follow the "yin-yang" principles of conventional hormone action.

It is not surprising, then, that derivatives of bacteria and drugs were found to modulate lymphocyte and macrophage functions through these mechanisms. Endotoxin has been shown by us to increase cyclic AMP levels in lymphocyte precursors in association with induction of differentiation (Scheid, Hadden, Coffey, unpublished observations); it has also been shown to increase cyclic GMP levels in B lymphocytes for which it is mitogenic (Watson, 1975). MDP induces cyclic GMP increases in association with macrophage activation and cyclic AMP levels in relation to its action to inhibit macrophage proliferation presumably via prostaglandins (Hadden and Englard, 1979; Hadden et al., 1979). Complex polysaccharides like dextran sulphate induce cGMP increases in conjunction with B-cell activation (unpublished observation). One presumes that the other polysaccharides like lentinan, glucan and Krestin will share this cyclic GMP mechanism since they activate B cells, macrophages, or both.

Of the chemical agents, levamisole's proproliferative actions on lymphocytes have been paralleled to imidazole and the actions of both have been linked to decreases in cyclic AMP levels and increases in cyclic GMP levels (Hadden et al., 1975). Effects of levamisole on monocyte and neutrophil cyclic GMP levels correlate with effects on chemotaxis, phagocytosis, and bactericidal capacity (Anderson et al., 1976; Renoux, 1978). *In vivo* effects of levamisole, particularly on T cell differentiation, appear to result from yet unexplained actions of the sulphur aspect of this compound (Renoux and Renoux, 1977; Renoux, 1978). Other actions include effects on furmarate reductase and alkaline phosphatase (Renoux, 1978).

Isoprinosine, to date, has been shown not to modify nucleotide levels at least at early times of incubation. Based upon similarities to interferon action, later changes are suspected and experiments are in progress to determine if this is the case. Effects on RNA metabolism have been demonstrated (Gordon et al., 1974; Hadden unpublished).

Poly A: Poly U has been shown to increase cyclic AMP levels in association with its antiproliferative and differentiation-inducing effects in lymphocytes (Hadden and Delmonte, 1978). Other agents like tilerones, BM 12531, lynestrenol, etc., have not been examined in this context.

A rather consistent set of observations with hormones, biological factors, pharmacologic substances indicates that lymphocyte differentiation is induced by cyclic AMP. Both lymphocyte and macrophage proliferative functions are promoted by cyclic GMP and antagonized by cyclic AMP; and macrophage activation is also promoted by cGMP and antagonized by cAMP. The consistency of the cyclic nucleotide immunopharmacology indicates its usefulness in predicting effects of agents not yet studied, based on their biological effects, and in suggesting its potential usefulness in the design of new agents for immunotherapy.

CONCLUSIONS

In the future, the development of an effective immunopharmacology will service clinical immunotherapy by removing the current empiricism in which the latter is steeped. By dissection of critical features of the cell targets of action and intracellular mechanisms of action and relating these to primary effects to modify host immune responses, in a predictable, consistent manner, the primary goal will be achieved. Once achieved and appropriate nonimmunological aspects of host resistance and status are taken into account, the secondary goal of effective delivery of a restored or enhanced immune system to combat the invading tumor or pathogen can be made. Finally, by overcoming the resistance and suppressor mechanisms derived from the pathogen or tumor, immunotherapy will achieve an efficacy and safety which will ultimately justify a more general use. To date, cyclic nucleotide pharmacology and *in vitro* analysis of cellular targets and function have provided important first steps towards achieving these goals. Once achieved, the clinical potential for therapeutic benefit in cancer, immunodeficiency, aging, chronic infection and auto-immune disorders seems great.

REFERENCES

Alexander, P., and Evans, R.: Endotoxin and double stranded RNA render macrophages cytotoxic. Nature (New Biol.), *232*:76–78 (1971).

Anderson, R., Glover, A., Koornhof, H. J., and Rabson, A. R.:*In vitro* stimulation of neutrophil motility by levamisole. J. Immunol., *117*:428–432 (1976).

Boyse, E. A., and Old, L. J.: Immunogenetics of differentiation in the mouse. Harvey Lecture Series, *71*:23–35 (1978).

Calderon, M., Kiely, J. M., Lelko, J. L., and Unanue, E. R.: The modulation of lymphocyte functions by molecules secreted by macrophages. J. Exp. Med., *142*: 151–158 (1975).

Cheers. C., and McKenzie, I. F. C.: Resistance and susceptibility of mice to bacterial infection: genetics of listeriosis. Infection and Immun., *19*:755–770 (1978).

Chirigos, M.: *Modulation of Host Immune Resistance.* Washington, D.C.: U.S. Gov't Printing Office, 1977.

Chirigos, M.: *Control of Neoplasia by Modulation of the Immune System.* New York: Raven Press, 1977.

Chirigos, M.: *Immune modulation and control of neoplasia by adjuvant therapy.* New York: Raven Press, 1978.

Cohen, G. H., Hooper, J. A., and Goldstein, A. L.: Thymosin-induced differentiation of murine thymocytes in allogeneic mixed lymphocyte cultures. In: Thymus factors in immunity, Friedman, H., ed., New York: *New York Academy of Sciences,* 249:145–153 (1975).

Cotzias, G. C., and Tang, L. C.: An adenylate cyclase of brain reflects propensity for breast cancer in mice. Science, 197:1094–1096 (1977).

Dukor, P., Vasella, S., Schläfli, E., Perren, B., Gisler, R. H., Dietrich, F. M., and Bitter-Suermann, D.: Immunopotentiating agents: activity profiles and possible modes of action. In: *Host defense against cancer and its potentiation.* Mizuno, D., *et al.* eds., pp. 97–109. Baltimore: Univer. Park Press, 1975.

Epstein, L. B.. The effects of interferons in the immune response *in vitro* and *in vivo.* In: *Interferon and their actions,* Stewart, W. E., ed., pp. 91–132. New York: CRC Press 1977.

Friedman, H.. Thymus factors in immunity, 284, New York: *New York Academy of Sciences,* 1975.

Galsworthy, S. B., Gurofsky, S. M., and Murray, R. G. E.. Purification of a mono-cytosis-producing activity from Listeria monocytogenes. Infection and Immunity. 15:500–505 (1977).

Goidl, E. A., Innes, J. B., and Weksler, M. E.. Immunological studies of aging. II. Loss of IgG and high avidity plaque-forming cells and increased suppressor cell activity in aging mice. J. Exp. Med., 144:1037–1042 (1976).

Goldberg, N. D., Hadden, M. K., Dunham, E., Lopez, C., and Hadden, J. W.: The Yin Yang hypothesis of biological control: opposing influences of cyclic GMP and cyclic AMP in the regulation of cell proliferation and other biological processes. In: *Control of proliferation in animal cells,* I. Clarkson, B., Baserga, R., eds., pp. 600–626. New York: Cold Spring Harbor Press, 1974.

Good, R. A., Jose, D., Cooper, W. C., Fernandes, G., Kramer, T. R., and Yaines, E.: Influence of nutrition on antibody production and cellular immune responses in man, rats, mice and guinea pigs. In: *Malnutrition and the immune response.* Suskind, R. M., ed., pp. 169–183. New York: Raven Press, 1977.

Gordon, P., Ronsen, B., and Brown, E. R.: Antiherpesvirus action of isoprinosine. Antimicrob. Agents Chemother., 5:153–160 (1974).

Hadden, J. W., Coffey, R. G., Hadden, E. M., Lopez-Corrales, E., and Sunshine, G. H.: Effects of levamisole and imidazole on lymphocyte proliferation and cyclic nucleotide levels. Cellular Immunol., 20:98–103 (1975).

Hadden, J. W., Hadden, E. M., and Coffey, R. G.: Isoprinosine augmentation of phytohemagglutinin-induced lymphocyte proliferation. Infection and Immun., 13:382–391 (1976).

Hadden, J. W., Delmonte, L., and Oettgen, H.: Mechanisms of immunopotentiation. In: Immunopharmacology, Hadden, J. W., Spreafico, F., Coffey, R. G., eds., pp. 279–313. New York: Plenum Publish. Corp., 1977.

Hadden, J. W., Spreafico, F., and Coffey, R. G.: Immunopharmacology. New York: Plenum Publish. Corp. 1977.

Hadden, J. W., and Delmonte, L.: Cyclic nucleotides in immunopotentiator action.

In: *Handbook of cancer immunology* V. Water, H., ed., pp. 109–134. New York: Garland Publishing, Inc., 1978.

Hadden, J. W.: Immunopharmacology of mice and men. Internat. J. of Immunopharmacol., *1*:5–8 (1979).

Hadden, J. W.: The action of immunpotentiators *in vitro* on lymphocyte and macrophage activation. In: *Pharmacology of Immunoregulation,* Werner, G., and F. Floc'h, eds., pp. 369–384. London: Academic Press, 1979.

Hadden, J., and England, A.: Molecular aspects of macrophage activation and proliferation. In: *Pharmacology of Immunoregulation,* Werner, G., and F. Floc'h, eds., pp. 273–282 (1979).

Hadden, J. W., Englard, A., Sadlik, J. R., and Hadden, E. M.: The comparative effects of isoprinosine, levamisole, muramyl dipeptide, and SM1213 on lymphocyte and macrophage proliferation and activation *in vitro*. Internat. J. Immunopharmacol., *1*:17–23 (1979).

Hatch, G. E., Nichols, W. K., and Hill, H. R.: Cyclic nucleotide changes in human neutrophils, induced by chemoattractants and chemotactic modulation. J. Immunol., *119*:450–456 (1977).

Horowitz, S., Borchending, W., Moorthy, A. V., Chesney, R., Schulte-Wisserman, H., Hong, R., and Goldstein, A.: Induction of suppressor T cells in systemic lupus erythematosus by thymosin and cultured thymic epithelium. Science, *197*: 999–1001 (1977).

Johnson, A. G., Audibert, F., and Chedid, L.: Synthetic immunoregulating molecules: A potential bridge between cytostatic chemotherapy and immunotherapy of cancer. Cancer Immunol. Immunother., *3*:219–226 (1978).

Kurland, G., Hadden, J., and Moore, M. A. S.: Role of cyclic nucleotides in the proliferation of committed granulocyte-macrophage progenitor cells. Cancer Res., *37*:4535–4538 (1977).

Lopez, C.: Genetics of natural resistance to herpes virus infections in mice. Nature *258*:152–153 (1975).

Morse, S. I.: Biologically active components and properties of Bordetella pertussis. Adv. Applied Microbiol., *20*:9–27 (1976).

Naylor, P. H., Sheppard, H., Thurman, G. B., and Goldstein, A.: Increase of cyclic GMP induced in murine thymocytes by thymosin fraction 5. Biochem. Biophys. Res. Commun. 73:843–849 (1976).

Old, L. J.. Tumor necrosis factor. Clin. Bull., *6*:118–119 (1976).

Renoux, G. and Renoux, M.. Thymus-like activities of sulphur derivatives on T cell differentiation. J. Exp. Med., *145*:466–471 (1977).

Renoux, G.: Modulation of immunity by levamisole. Pharmac. Ther., *2*:397–423 (1978).

Sampson, D., and Lui, A.: The effect of levamisole on cell-mediated immunity and suppressor cell function. Cancer Res., *36*:952–955 (1976).

Scheid, M. P., Goldstein, G., and Boyse, E. A.: The generation and regulation of lymphocyte populations. Evidence from differentiative induction systems *in vitro.* J. Exp. Med., *147*:1727–1743 (1978).

Schultz, R. M., Pavlidis, N. A., Stylos, W. A., and Chirigos, M. A.: Regulation of macrophage tumoricidal function: a role for prostaglandins of the E series. Science, *202*:320–322 (1978).

Sunshine, G. H., Basch, R. S., Coffey, R., Cohen, G., Kenneth, W., Goldstein, G., and Hadden, J. W.: Thymopoietin enhances the allogeneic response and cyclic GMP levels of mouse peripheral derived lymphocytes. J. Immunol., *120*:1594–1599 (1978).

Touraine, J. L., Hadden, J. W., and Good, R. A.: Sequential stages of human T lymphocyte differentiation. Proc. Nat. Acad. Sci., *74*:3414–3418 (1977).

Vecchi, A., Sironi, M., and Spreafico, F.: A preliminary characterization in mice of the effect of inosiplex on the immune system. In: *Modulation of host immune resistance in the prevention or treatment of induced neoplasias.* Cancer Ther. Reports, *62*:1975–1980 (1978).

Waksman, B. H., and Wagshal, A. B: Lymphocytic functions acted on by immuno-regulatory cytokines; significance of the cell cycle. Cell Immunol., *35*:180–186 (1978).

Watson, J.: The influence of intracellular levels of cyclic nucleotides on cell pro-liferation and the induction of antibody synthesis. J. Exp. Med., *141*:97–111 (1975).

Wybran, J., Levin, A. S., Fudenberg, H. H., and Goldstein, A. L: Thymosin: Effects on normal human blood T cells. Ann. N.Y. Acad. Sci., *249*:300–307 (1975).

Wybran, J., Van Bogaert, E., and Govaerts, A.: Lynestrenol, an amplifier of stim-ulation. Biomedicine, *27*:16–19 (1977).

Wybran, J., and Govaerts, A.: Levamisole and human lymphocyte marker. Clin. Exp. Immunol., *27*:319–321 (1977).

Wybran, J., Govaerts, A., and Appelboom, T.: Inosoplex, a stimulating agent for normal human T cells and human leukocytes. J. Immunol., *121*:1184–1187 (1978).

ACKNOWLEDGMENTS

The National Cancer Institute and The American Cancer Society are acknow-ledged for their support of Dr. Hadden and his work. This manuscript is republished from Springer Seminars in Immunopathology *Immune Stimulation* (L. Chedid, Ed.) by permission of the publisher Springer Verlag.

3
The Heterogenous Interaction of Cytotoxic Immunodepressants with Immunocyte Subpopulations

Federico Spreafico

Department of Oncology and Immunology,
Instituto di Ricerche Farmacologiche 'Mario Negri'
Via Eritrea, 62, 20157 Milan, Italy

INTRODUCTION

The scope of this paper is to review some of our recent work on the characterization of the effects on the various cell types composing the immune system and their dependent effector mechanisms of cytotoxic antineoplastic agents. Although our original objectives in becoming engaged in this type of study were not directly related to immunotoxicology since our aims were directed at investigating the role of host resistance in the antineoplastic activity of chemotherapeutic agents and at studying approaches towards less empirical design of chemoimmunotherapy strategies, in the course of this research it became apparent that some of the results could also have an immunotoxicological relevance. In view of their well known immunodepressive capacity (Spreafico and Anaclerio, 1977), antitumorals can in fact be considered as useful model agents for the study of various immunotoxicological problems. An in-depth discussion of the lessons of immunotoxicological relevance, which the investigations conducted over the years have produced, is however beyond the limits of this chapter, in which only one specific theme will be essentially considered, namely that of the heterogeneity of cytotoxins on the various cellular components of the immune complex. This heterogeneity is therefore to be taken into account not only in the testing of xenobiotics for their possible immunotoxicological activity but also in the strategic planning of tests and conditions for the assessment of this activity.

RESULTS AND DISCUSSION

The Immunodepressive Effect of Adriamycin and Daunomycin

These two anthracycline drugs, widely used in cancer chemotherapy, can be regarded as very illustrative model chemicals for discussing heterogeneity of immunological effects among chemicals. As shown in fact in Figure 1, the chemical analogy between Adriamycin (AM) and its parent compound Daunomycin (DM) is very close, and the two analogs are believed to share a common biochemical mode of cytotoxic action on cells, exerted chiefly through direct binding to DNA. The two compounds have quantitatively and qualitatively superimposable general toxicity *in vivo*

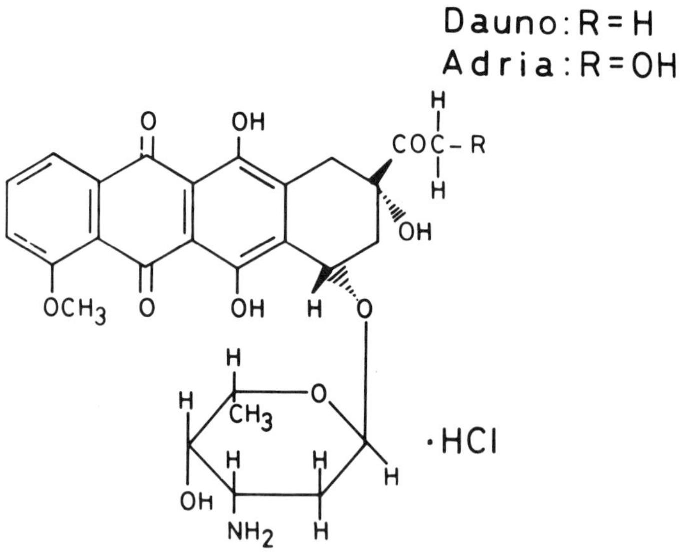

Figure 1. Comparison of structural relationships between Adriamycin and Daunomycin.

**Table 1.   In Vitro Cytotoxic Activity of
Adriamycin and Daunomycin
on Different Cells.**

		ED_{50} ($\mu g/ml$)	
CELL TYPE	TECHNIQUE	AM	DM
SL2 lymphoma	^{125}IUdR uptake	0.05	0.05
spleen lympho-cytes	^{125}IUdR uptake	0.17	0.15
murine macro-phages	^{86}Rb uptake	0.78	0.12

Exposure time: 24 hours.

(for instance, we demonstrated equivalent effects on bone marrow stem cells in rodents). On a series of *in vitro* tumor cells, they express comparable levels of cytoxic activity when relatively long exposure times stimulating their relatively long persistence *in vivo* are used (Table 1). On the other hand, AM is significantly more active *in vivo* than DM on a large series of experimental leukemia-lymphomas and solid neoplasms and this is generally believed to hold true also in man. Since this differential therapeutic effectiveness could not be satisfactorily explained by the known differences in metabolism and pharmacokinetics between the two agents, the hypothesis was advanced that the analogs may possess a different immunodepressive activity thus resulting in different capacities on the part of the host reactivity against the tumor to interact and synergize with the direct antineoplastic activity of the drugs. Evidence in support of this hypothesis was obtained by experiments showing that in tumor-bearing animals, which had previously been immunodepressed by various means, the therapeutic advantage of AM was lost, its antineoplastic effectiveness becoming comparable to that of DM. It was thus of interest to investigate in more detail the effects of these anthracyclines on different types of immune reactivities. Table 2 represents a schematic summary of results obtained in a series of earlier studies (Vecchi et al., 1976a; Mantovani et al., 1976a,b) and shows that the limited chemical variation existing between AM and DM imparts to these chemicals substantial qualitative and quantitative differences in immunodepressive activity. It can also be seen that with these analogs a measure of their effects on models of cell-mediated reactivities (e.g., resistance to i.p. tumor allografts) gives a better correlation with *in vivo* therapeutic efficacy than assays of effects on humoral antibody production. It is well known that cell-dependent

Table 2.   Effects of Adriamycin and Daunomycin on Various Parameters of Immune Responsiveness in Mice.

PARAMETER	AM	DM
Primary resp. T– depend. antigen	– – –	–
Primary resp. T– independ. antigen	– –	0
Allograft rejection	–	– – –
C M C	–	– – –
ADCC: cellular arm	– –	– – –
ADCC: humoral arm	±	– –
c'depend. cytolytic ab	– –	– –
spleen cellularity	–	– –
bone marrow cells	–	–
LD_{50} acute (mg/kg i.v.)	–	–

mechanisms are believed to be more important to tumor control. It could also be shown that the higher inhibition by DM of resistance to tumor allografts correlated with significantly lower levels of cell-mediated cyto-toxicity (CMC) against tumor cells measured in the peritoneal cavity of DM-treated mice than seen in AM-treated hosts. It is of note that whereas this *in vivo-in vitro* correlation was evident when CMC was assayed in the peritoneal cavity, i.e., at the site where direct tumor-host interaction was occurring in these experimental conditions, no such correlation was observable testing other lymphoid organs, e.g., the spleen. This is a further indication that the choice of the lymphoid organ or site to be examined can be of relevance in the reaching of truly representative con-clusions on the immunological effects of exogenous compounds.

In the attempt to further dissect the interaction of these drugs with host defence mechanisms, their effects on different immunocyte sub-populations were examined. Whereas no differences were detected between AM and DM on *in vitro* lymphocytes whether resting or stimulated by T or B-cell specific mitogens, a striking difference was seen on macro-phages in the sense that DM was significantly more inhibitory than AM on these cells *in vitro* (measured by both reduction of phagocytosis or number of surviving cells estimated by ^{86}Rb uptake (Table 1) as well as *in vivo*. Not only, in fact, are significantly lower numbers of macrophages recovered from DM than from AM-treated mice, but also the functional capacity of the recovered cells is lower after DM, as shown for instance

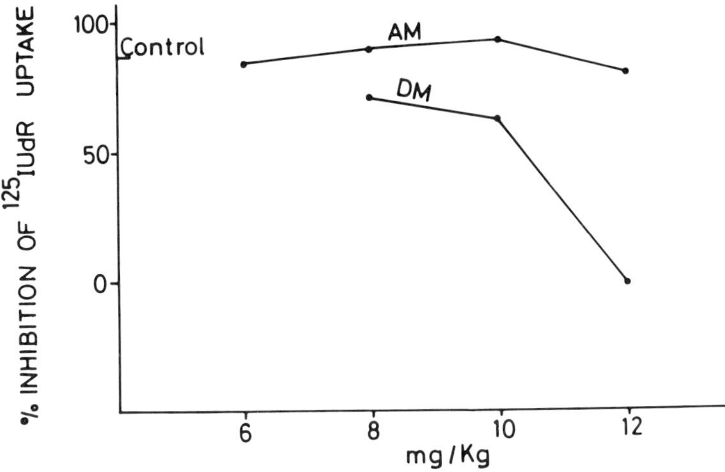

Figure 2. Comparison of nonspecific cytoxicity between AM- and DM treated mice.

in Figure 2 measuring the levels of nonspecific cytotoxicity versus cultured cancer cells elicited in macrophages by pretreatment with *C. parvum.*

The Heterogeneity of Cytotoxicity Drug Effects on Immunocyte Subpopulations

The findings described above were a stimulus to analyze the possibility that these anthracyclines, as well as additional cytotoxic agents, varied in their effects on other cellular components of the immune complex. A first immunocyte subpopulation investigated consisted of suppressor cells, i.e., elements increasingly regarded as pivotal in both the regulation of normal responses and the pathogenesis of various disease states ranging from cancer to autoimmunity.

The experimental system employed involved firstly inducing specific T suppressors by overloading mice with supraoptimal numbers of sheep erythrocytes, these animals acting as donors of splenocytes for secondary hosts subsequently challenged with optimal doses of the same antigen (Anaclerio et al., 1980). Inhibition of suppressor cell generation by drug treatment of donor mice can be revealed by the counting of higher numbers of specific antibody-producing cells in recipients transfused with splenocytes from treated donors in comparison to non-drug-treated sup-

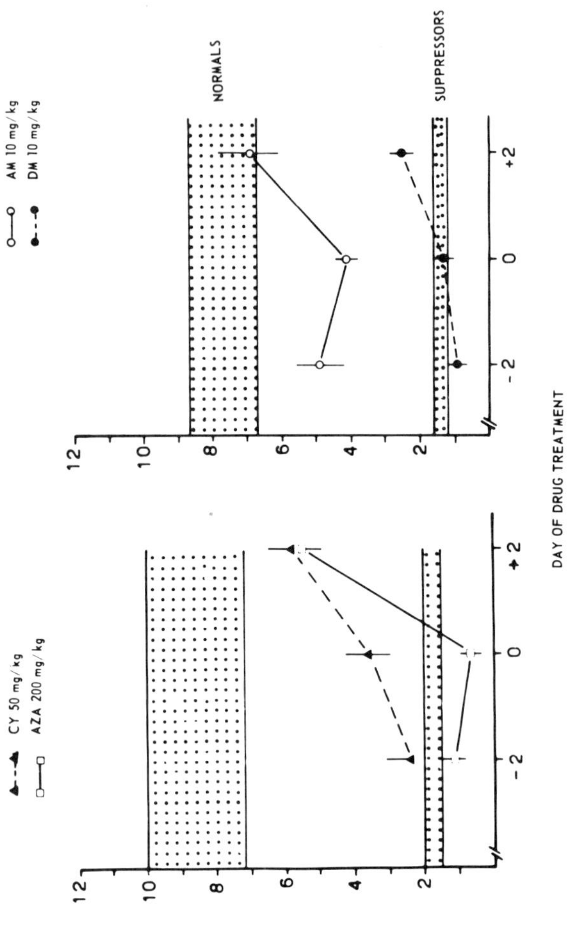

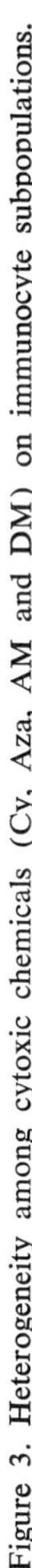

Figure 3. Heterogeneity among cytoxic chemicals (Cy, Aza, AM and DM) on immunocyte subpopulations.

pressor controls. In these conditions, it was found that DM had little inhibitory activity observable moreover only after repeated injections, whereas AM could produce significant, dose-dependent inhibition not only when administered after the induction of suppressor cells but also when injected before antigen overloading, suggesting an effect also on the precursors of T suppressor cells. Figure 3 shows further evidence of the heterogeneity among cytotoxic chemicals in their effects on immunocytes. It can be seen in fact that in the inhibition of T suppressor activity by Cyclophosphamide (Cy) and Azathioprine (Aza) not only quantitative but also qualitative differences exist since a significant inhibition is apparently seen with Aza only with injections after the suppressor-inducing stimulus, whereas with Cy this timing is less important. It is now well established that elements of the monocyte-macrophage lineage can exert a powerful nonspecific suppressive activity, which can be estimated for instance by measuring their capacity to reduce lymphocyte blastogenesis. When the effect of AM or DM on macrophage suppression was evaluated, it was seen that DM activity contrasted with that of AM, as could have been expected on the basis of the previously described differential sensitivity of these cells to the two analogs.

More recently, a significant degree of heterogeneity among cytotoxic agents was again observed testing their effects on natural cell-mediated killer (NK) activity (Mantovani et al., 1978). This activity should be of prime interest in the immunotoxicological evaluation of xenobiotics considering that this mechanism is currently believed to play a front-line role in immunosurveillance not only against neoplasms but also vis-a-vis infections (Herberman et al., 1980). Table 3 shows that AM injection

***Table 3.* Effect of Different Cytotoxic Agents on Spleen NK Activity.**

| | | % DECREASE IN SPECIFIC CYTOTOXICITY AT: A:T RATIO | | |
DRUG	DOSE (mg/kg)	10:1	20:1	50:1
AM	10	8	4	2
DM	10	20 *	22 *	15 *
AD 32	80	34 *	31 *	36 *
Aza	250	43 *	48 *	38 *
Cy	150	78 *	58 *	38 *
DITC	150	5	6	3

* = p < 0.01; tests were performed 2 days after drug injection i.p. or i.v.

Table 4.   Effect of Adriamycin on NK Activity in Different Organs.

AM (mg/kg i.v.)	SOURCE OF LYMPHOID CELLS	% SPECIFIC LYSIS					CELL NUMBER ($\times 10^4$)
		50:1	20:1	10:1	5:1	2:1	
—	Lymph nodes [a]	14	10	8	—	—	24 ± 1
10		14	7	5	—	—	10 ± 1 *
—	Spleen	44	24	17	—	—	89 ± 2
10		41	22	14	—	—	62 ± 3 *
—	PEC [b]	—	—	20	18	17	2.6 ± 0.2
10		—	—	20	14	12	2.4 ± 0.3

C57B1/6 mice were treated 2 days before assay performed using YAC-1 target cells.
* = $p < 0.05$.
[a] Pooled axillary and inguinal.
[b] Unstimulated peritoneal exudate cells.

does not significantly impair NK activity in the mouse spleen whereas the administration of similar and otherwise equitoxic doses of DM is followed by clear reductions in activity. Table 4 indicates that this lack of AM inhibition was also observed when NK cell activity was measured in mouse lymph nodes or peritoneal exudate cells at different times after a range of drug doses. It is to be noted that although NK cell activity per unit number of cells was not reduced by AM, lower total numbers of mononuclear cells were recovered from these organs, the greatest and lowest depletions being observed in this species in the lymph nodes and peritoneal cavity, respectively. This type of result again emphasizes the importance of the organ or site in which the effects of given substances are investigated. In this connection, it should be stressed that for all these investigations, AM and DM were always injected intravenously. This complexity may therefore be expected to be compounded when other routes of exposure are employed with obvious differences in organ distribution and persistence as well as in biotransformation of the foreign compound. The differential effect on lymphoid sites is probably related to pharmacokinetic mechanisms since significant differences in AM levels were seen among these organs (Figure 4). Of interest is the fact that the greater the macrophage content in these organs (40%, 8% and 2% for peritoneal exudate, spleen and lymph nodes, respectively), the lower the AM-associated cytopenia and the drug concentrations. Table 3 shows that differential sensitivity of NK-cell activity can also be found employing

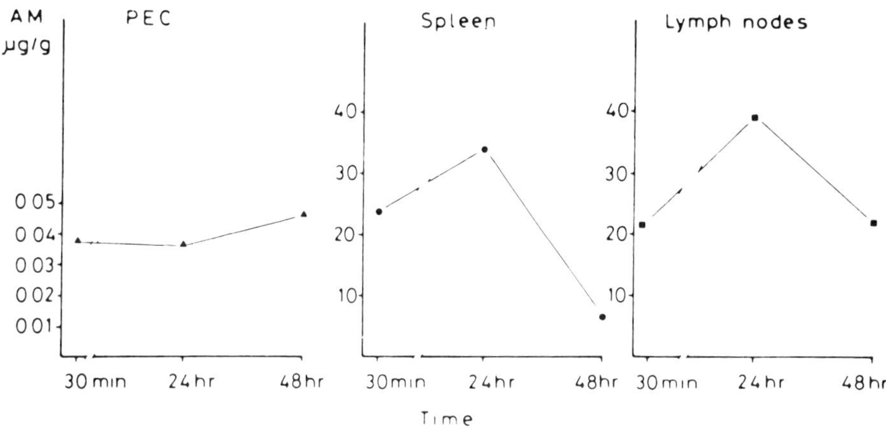

Figure 4. Distribution of AM levels in cells of the reticuloendothelial system.

other drugs. It is evident that Cy and Aza are marked inhibitors of this cell population whereas another cytotoxic drug of wide use in cytoreductive therapy and previously shown to have potent and long-lasting immunodepressive activity on this same species (Vecchi et al., 1976b), i.e., Dimethyltriazenoimidazole carboxamide (DTIC) produces no inhibition of NK activity per unit cell number.

In these studies another AM-related anthracycline was also investigated, i.e., N-trifluoroacetyl-Adriamycin-14-valerate (AD 32), a compound recently found to possess a better antineoplastic activity in animals than AM (Vecchi et al., 1978), which produced marked inhibition of NK activity, indeed greater than seen with DM even at high, already toxic doses. This type of observation is also an example that this kind of investigation can be of help in elucidating aspects of the mechanism of action of cytotoxic agents. In fact, the high activity of AD 32 on NK cells and on macrophages *in vitro* does not support the possibility that AD 32 may act *in vivo* essentially as a slow-release form of AM as could have been hypothesized from the drug's chemical characteristics. Indeed, recent studies of this group have confirmed that AM is not significantly found after the administration to rodents of AD 32, which has metabolic and pharmacokinetic characteristics quite distinct from those of AM (Salmona et al., 1980). A more in-depth discussion of the effects of AD 32 on immunity is presented elsewhere (Vecchi et al., 1980).

Very recently, evidence has been obtained that natural defense mechanisms against cancer may also be sustained by another cell type in addition to NK cells, i.e., unstimulated macrophages. The capacity of normal murine and human macrophages to exert a cytotoxic damage on transformed (but not on untransformed) cells has been described by this group and the similarities and differences of this activity with respect to NK-mediated resistance discussed (Mantovani et al., 1979a; Tagliabue et al., 1979). Table 5 shows the effects of various agents on this activity. The variability in the susceptibility of this mechanism to different cytotoxic agents is again clear and the heterogeneity of these compounds in affecting two natural defense mechanisms having a number of common aspects needs not to be especially emphasized.

The *in vivo* Relevance of Anthracycline Differential Interaction with Host Defense Mechanisms

In the preceding sections, evidence was provided that cytotoxic agents can markedly differ among themselves in affecting immunocyte subpopulations and dependent antitumor immune effector mechanisms. The question could thus be advanced of whether such differences have relevance in influencing the *in vivo* activity of these compounds, a question of not minor importance also in a purely immunotoxicological context.

An answer to this question can be obtained from results found in investigating again AM and DM. When the antineoplastic activity of AM

Table 5. **Effect of Selected Anticancer Agents on NK Cell and Macrophage-Mediated.**

DRUG	NK CELL [a] ACTIVITY	MACROPHAGE-CYTOTOXICITY	
		NATURAL [b]	BCG-ACTIVATED [c]
AM	=	=	=
DM	++	++	++
Aza	+++	+++	+++
Cy	+++	=	=
DTIC	+	++	++

+ and = indicate significant depression or no effect on a per cell basis.
[a] Measured in a short-term ^{51}Cr release assay using YAC-1 lymphoma target cells.
[b] Measured in a 48 hrs ^{3}H-thymidine release assay with mKSA-TU5 target cells.
[c] Measured in a 48 hrs ^{3}H-thymidine release assay with mF56 sarcoma target cells.

Table 6. **Antitumoral Effectiveness of Adriamycin and Daunomycin on Murine Tumors of Different Immunogenicity.**

DRUG	TUMOR [a]	IMMUNOGENICITY [b]	% ILS [c]	% CURES [c]
AM				
(10 mg/kg i.v.)	L 1210 Cr	10^2	42	0
	SL 2	10^3	85	10
	L 1210 Ha	10^5	150	45
DM				
(10 mg/kg i.v.)	L 1210 Cr	10^2	38	0
	SL 2	10^3	48	0
	L 1210 Ha	10^5	44	0

a 10^5 cells i.p. on day 0, drugs on day 1.
b Number of tumor cells rejected on challenge 10 days after i.p. immunization with 10^7 x-irradiated lymphoma cells.
c Mean of 5 experiments expressed as % increase in lifespan (ILS) and % cures (over 90 days survivors).

and DM was compared to leukemias of different immunogenicity (i.e., the moderately immunogenic SL 2 lymphoma, the highly immunogenic L1210 Ha and the non-immunogenic L1210 Cr subline), it was observed that in contrast to DM, the effectiveness of DM was clearly influenced by tumor immunogenicity (Table 6). It is to be noted that the syngeneic hosts for these leukemias do not show significant natural cytotoxicity against these tumor cells. The correlation between tumor immunogenicity and *in vivo* AM efficacy and its reduction in previously immunodepressed hosts leads to the conclusion that a response to tumor-associated antigens is contributory to the antineoplastic activity of AM and gives support to our starting hypothesis on the possible basis for AM superiority over DM. It was thus also of interest to examine the relative role of the various immunocyte subpopulations previously shown to be differentially affected by the two analogs. Such an effort is difficult and can at best only give relative indications considering the complex web of functional cell interactions physiologically existing in the immune system, as exemplified by the reciprocal influences operative between T lymphocytes and macrophages. A possible *in vivo* role of the differential sensitivity of NK cells to AM and DM could be suggested by preliminary findings showing that against a NK-sensitive tumor, AM has greater activity in mouse strains having "high" NK activity than in "low" NK strains. However, in view of the known regulatory influence exerted by macrophages on NK cells, the importance of this differential interaction of AM and DM on this natural cellular mechanism is uncertain. Although the sensitivity to AM and relative resistance to DM of suppressor T cells could in principle be a determinant of the higher efficacy *in vivo* of AM, no direct evidence is available on this point. On the other hand, more direct evidence has been obtained in favor of the importance of the differential sensitivity of macrophages to these drugs. In fact, in animals bearing the highly immunogenic L1210 Ha tumor and treated with silica particles, which are known to accumulate and kill macrophages, the effectiveness of optimal AM doses was significantly reduced. Conversely, no changes in AM activity were seen with the non-immunogenic Cr subline and, as expected, the efficacy of DM was equal in normal and silica-treated animals (Mantovani et al., 1979b). Further support for the reasoning that the differential toxicity of AM and DM for macrophages, elements currently believed to be pivotal in cancer control, was obtained investigating the association of these compounds with macrophage activators. On the basis of the previous data it could have been expected that the combination of AM with a macrophage stimulant such as *Corynebacterium parvum (C. parvum)* should have resulted in therapeutic synergism whereas no synergism should have followed the DM-*C. parvum* combination. As shown in Figure 5 by representative data, this prediction was supported by experimental evidence in a series of different murine tumor models (Tagliabue et al., 1977) since the DM-*C. parvum* combination had essentially no more effect than DM alone, whereas consistently high levels of synergism were seen with AM-*C. parvum*. The interval between the two drugs was however an important variable significantly affecting therapeutic activity. In the system presented in Figure 5, optimal degrees of synergism were in fact seen when AM preceded *C. parvum* by 5–6 days, whereas shorter or longer intervals produced significantly lower or no synergism. In investigating the possible reasons for the latter finding, a clear correlation between the presence of *in vivo* therapeutic synergism or its absence and the levels of macrophage-mediated nonspecific cytotoxicity versus neoplastic cells was observed. As shown, in fact, in Table 7, treatments with AM 1 or 2 days after, or up to 3 days before *C. parvum* (i.e., *in vivo* non synergistic schedules) were associated with very low levels of macrophage cytotoxicity, a dose-dependent inhibition observed using a range of attacker to target cell ratios. In contrast, *in vivo* synergistic schedules (e.g., AM preceding *C. parvum* by 5 days) were associated with cytotoxicity levels similar, and on certain days even higher, than seen after treatment with *C. parvum* alone whose capacity to stimulate nonspecific cytotoxicity in macrophages is well known. It would thus appear that maximal synergism was obtainable when AM was combined with *C. parvum* according to schedules not interfering with the induction or expression of the cytotoxic activity of macrophages. Further evidence of the importance of the right

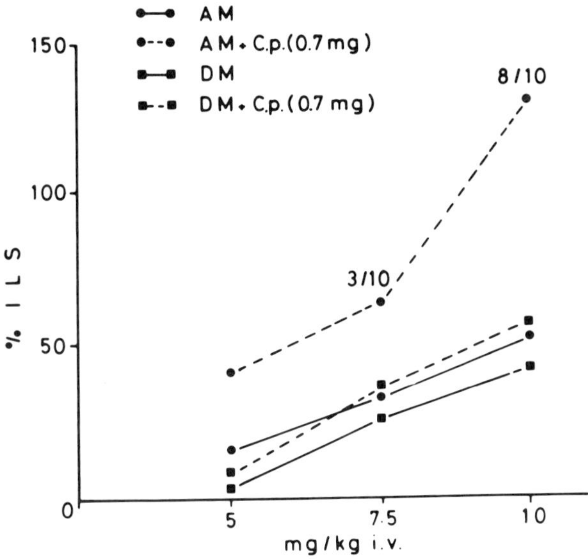

Figure 5. Therapeutic synergism of AM when combined with *C. parvum*.

matching of cytotoxic drugs and immuno-modifying agents in combined chemoimmunotherapy is presented elsewhere (Tagliabue et al., 1977; Spreafico, 1980), an importance which could have easily been expected given the heterogeneity in the mode of action on immunity known to exist for both categories of agents.

Table 7. Time Course of the Effect of Adriamycin on the Induction of Macrophage Cytotoxicity by *C. parvum.*

DAY OF AM RELATIVE TO *C. parvum*	% INHIBITION OF ^{125}IUdR UPTAKE ON DAY			
	6	7	12	18
—	55	77	91	68
−1	12 *	52 *	69 *	65
−5	65 *	83	88	72

Nonspecific cytotoxicity by macrophages was evaluated through ^{125}IUdR uptake by target SL2 tumor cells.
AM: 10 mg/kg i.v.; *C. parvum:* 0.7 mg i.v.

CONCLUSION

From the data presented, at least one general conclusion appears to emerge having direct relevance for a better approach to the study and evaluation of the effects of foreign compounds on immunity. Not only, in fact, does complexity of the immune system provide a multiplicity of levels and mechanisms through which interference can be exerted, but in addition, chemicals, even as structurally closely related as AM and DM, can significantly differ quantitatively and, more importantly, qualitatively in their interaction with the various components of the system. In the case of cytotoxic antineoplastic drugs discussed here as model immunotoxic compounds, these differential interactions can be of importance not only in helping to unravel their mode of action and in the rational development of novel analogs, but can also act as important determinants of the *in vivo* activity of these agents. Since it needs not to be especially emphasized here that the true scope of immunotoxicology is larger than just the study of immune "depression," in view of the fact that health risks can potentially be associated with significant deviations in either direction from a normal, balanced immune capacity, it is of relevance to note that a similar, if not greater heterogeneity can also be recognized among "immunostimulatory" compounds (Spreafico, 1980; Hadden, this volume). The existence of this heterogeneity can thus be expected to be found also among xenobiotics of immunotoxicological interest, a concept having a series of obvious practical implications in devising approaches and strategies in this research field of evident importance and clear potential.

ACKNOWLEDGMENT

The work described in this paper was supported by Contracts NCI–CM–53826 and NCI–CM–67064.

REFERENCES

Anaclerio, A., Conti, G., Gotti, Honorati, M. C., Ruggeri, A., Moras, M. L. and Spreafico, F.: Effect of cytotoxic agents on suppressor cells in mice. Eur. J. Cancer (in press) (1980).

Herberman, R. B., Holden, H. T., Bonnard, G. D., Kay, D., Tagliabue, A., Djeu, J. Y., Mantovani, A. and Riccardi, C.: Natural cell-mediated cytotoxicity against tumors: Nature of effector cells and factors affecting activity. In, *Annual Meeting and Symposium of the Immunology Area US-Japan Cooperative Cancer Res. Program,* (in press) (1980).

Mantovani, A., Tagliabue, A., Vecchi, A. and Spreafico, F.: Effects of adriamycin and daunomycin on spleen cell populations in normal and tumor allografted mice. Eur. J. Cancer, *12*:381–387 (1967a).

Mantovani, A., Vecchi, A., Tagliabue, A. and Spreafico, F.: The effects of adriamycin and daunomycin on antitumoral immune effector mechanisms in an allogeneic system. Eur. J. Cancer, *12*:371–379 (1976b).

Mantovani, A., Luini, W., Peri. G., Vecchi, A. and Spreafico, F.: Effect of chemotherapeutic agents on natural cell-mediated cytotoxicity in mice. J. Natl. Cancer
Inst., *61*:1255–1261 (1978).

Mantovani, A., Tagliabue, A., Dean, J. H. Jerrells, T. R. and Herberman, R. B.:
Cytolytic activity of human monocytes on transformed and untransformed human
fibroblasts. Int. J. Cancer, *23*:28–31 (1979a).

Mantovani, A., Candiani, P., Luini, W., Salmona, M., Spreafico, F. and Garattini,
S.: Effect of chemotherapeutic agents on host defense mechanisms: Its possible
relevance for the antitumoral activity of these drugs. In, Current Trends in Tumor
Immunology, Ferrone, S., Gorini, S., Herberman, R. B. and Reisfeld, R. A. (eds.),
New York: Garland STPM Press, pp. 139–159 (1979b).

Salmona, M., Donelli, M. G., D'Incalci, M. and Spreafico, F.: Pharmacokinetic-
activity correlations with N-trifluoroacetyl-adriamycin-14-valerate in tumor-bearing
mice. Cancer Pharmacol. Chemother. (in press) (1980).

Spreafico, F. and Anaclerio, A.: Immunosuppressive agents. In, *Immunopharmacology*, Hadden, J. W., Coffey, R. G. and Spreafico, F. (eds.), New York: Plenum
Press, pp. 245–278 (1977).

Spreafico, F.: Current problems with immunopotentiating agents. In, *The Immune
System: Function and Therapy of Dysfunction*, Doria, G. and Eshkol, A. (eds.),
New York: Academic Press (in press) (1980).

Tagliabue, A., Polentarutti, N., Vecchi, A., Mantovani, A. and Spreafico, F.: Combination chemo-immunotherapy with adriamycin in experimental tumor systems.
Eur. J. Cancer, *13*:657–665 (1977).

Tagliabue, A., Mantovani, A., Kilgallen, M., Herberman, R. B. and McCoy, J. L.:
Natural cytotoxicity of mouse monocytes and macrophages. J. Immunol., *122*:
2363–2370 (1979).

Vecchi, A., Fioretti, M. C., Mantovani, A., Barzi, A. and Spreafico, F.: The immunodepressive and hematotoxic activity of imidazole-r-carboxamide, 5-(3,3-dimethyl-
1-triazeno) in mice. Transplantation, *22*:619–624 (1976a).

Vecchi, A., Mantovani, A., Tagliabue, A. and Spreafico, F.: A characterization of
the immunosuppressive activity of adriamycin and daunomycin on humoral antibody production and tumor allograft rejection. Cancer Res., *36*:1222–1227
(1976b).

Vecchi, A., Cario, M., Mantovani, A., Sironi, M. and Spreafico, F.: Comparative
antineoplastic activity of adriamycin and n-trifluoroacetyladriamycin-14-valerate.
Cancer Treat. Rept., *62*:111–117 (1978).

Vecchi, A., Spreafico, F., Sironi, M., Cario, M. and Garattini, S.: The immunodepressive and hematotoxic activities of N-trifluoroacetyl-adriamycin-14-valerate.
Eur. J. Cancer (in press) (1980).

DISCUSSION

McCOY: I would like to pose a question to Dr. Hadden. He in-
ferred that interferon is a down regulator. Since there is wide interest in
interferon today, in the treatment of cancer patients, I think that it would

be wrong for the audience to go away with the impression that interferon is only a down regulator.

Quantitatively, as far as treatment regimens including dosages and so forth are concerned, one can see enhancing effects of interferon as well as depressive effects. Would Dr. Hadden like to expand on this issue?

HADDEN: I'm happy to. I didn't mean to cast aspersions on interferon, I was referring quite specifically to proliferation.

Let me summarize briefly some of interferon's activities. Interferon, as you know, is an antiviral substance which has been demonstrated to be antiproliferative in a number of cell systems; this includes the analysis of *in vitro* parameters of immune response. It is this antiproliferative activity that constitutes a major rationale for the use of interferon as an anticancer agent. Interferon or related substances have rather profound ability to activate cells, such as natural killer cells and macrophages. The full spectrum of these activities I think has not been brought out. We've observed that interferon will induce B-cell differentiation. (Hämmerling, Stewart and Hadden, unpublished observations).

Thus, interferon is a prime example of an immune modulator. It has the capacity to act in both directions. As I indicated in my talk, the clinical responses to interferon are akin to those observed with lymphokine preparations. If you remember that the interferon that we were using in the clinic is derived from leukocytes and is in a relatively impure state, it may be that some of the biological activities reported can be attributed to other biological substances in the interferon preparation and not to interferon itself.

The degree of biological response that we are obtaining *in vivo* would suggest that there is a great effect on the immune system. I say this because the degree of antiproliferative activity that interferon has at the levels that we are achieving in treated patients would be calculated to be relatively minor. For example, clinical levels of 100 units of interferon per ml (not considering issues of specific binding), is a low level for growth inhibition of many malignant cell lines *in vitro*. My own interpretation of the clinical data is that interferon activates the immune system. If so, this means that there are aspects of interferon action on the immune system which are greater than those which we would expect based upon *in vitro* parameter analyses. There are aspects either of interferon action or other biological substances present in interferon preparations that we don't yet understand.

YUNIS: You are talking about interferon decreasing proliferation in one sense, but I understand there is also an opposite effect on natural killers; right?

HADDEN: I don't have any information about proliferation of natural killer cells. As I said, interferon increases killing functions: both natural killer cell and macrophage—provided those experiments employed different cell populations. There are important aspects of the mechanism of interferon action that would relate to an antitumor potential.

McCOY: To follow up on your latter comments: We have to take into account that these are all *in vitro* experiments. We don't really know what the *in vivo* relevance of natural killer cells is. There are no published studies except some negative selection experiments performed by Harvey Kanter's group. These studies give some indication as to what the *in vivo* role of natural killer cells may be. I would like to question Dr. Spreafico, regarding his *in vitro* studies with natural killer cells. What does he think the biological relevance (since that term is in the workshop title) of natural killer cells really is.

SPREAFICO: I can answer you as regards the importance of a differential interaction with the NK cells of Adriamycin and Daunomycin. Everything considered, we think that the differential interaction of the two drugs with NK cells is of minor importance in the case of Adriamycin and Daunomycin differential antitumor activity. We think that the differential sensitivity of other cells, i.e., macrophages, is more important here.

GHAFFAR: Dr. Spreafico, did you notice any differences in binding or localization between Adriamycin and Daunomycin within macrophages or on macrophage surfaces. Are they both soluble?

SPREAFICO: Yes, they are both soluble. Some people suspect that *in vivo* daunomycin might have tendency to form micelles more easily than Adriamycin. However this is not yet substantiated. We ourselves have done studies on neither the uptake, nor, especially, the retention of the two drugs within macrophages. It is possible that Daunomycin may stay in the lysosomes longer. This is the best explanation so far. However, since it is based on indirect data, it might not be a true explanation. Essentially I would say that the basis for the differential sensitivity of macrophages to the drugs is still unknown.

GHAFFAR: And a second clarification on the same two drugs: What was the timing of the drug administration in relation to *C. parvum* treatment?

SPREAFICO: Which type? The last one?

GHAFFAR: Well, where you find the abrogation of cytotoxicity as well as the lack of synergism between the two.

SPREAFICO: The timing between the administration of Adriamycin and *C. parvum* is indeed critical for observing whether or not there is therapeutic synergism *in vivo*. When *C. parvum* is given following

Adriamycin to mice with leukemia-lymphomas and solid tumors, we have found the best interval between the drugs is 4 to 7 days. We have also observed the highest levels of macrophage cytotoxicity on culture cancer cells when *in vivo* synergistic intervals are used. Conversely, low levels of macrophagic cytotoxicity are seen when *in vivo* nonsynergistic intervals are employed.

GHAFFAR: So you use cyclic treatment for both models?

SPREAFICO: No, in these systems in mice we use one single injection of Adriamycin followed by one single injection of *C. parvum,* or preceded by one single injection of *C. parvum.*

GHAFFAR: You didn't find any differences between the two schedules?

SPREAFICO: Provided one maintains a certain interval between the two drugs, the same degree of synergism *in vivo* is noted. If one gives them close in time, therapeutic synergism is not seen. One sees only the effect of Adriamycin as given per se.

LUSTER: Dr. Spreafico, I think you may have alluded to the answer to this in the previous question somewhat, but I was curious as to whether you had any feelings about why you are seeing these differences, and what may be happening at the molecular level to account for these differences. Is it their activity, different receptors, different binding sites to DNAs?

SPREAFICO: I am afraid there is no answer yet to your question. With regard to the molecular mode of action of Adriamycin and Daunomycin, it is well known that these drugs bind to an intercalate in DNA. More recently, it has been shown that these molecules also exert damage on cell membranes, although the importance of the latter mechanism in tumor cell inhibitory activity is still unknown. It is also not known if these two analogs may differ, qualitatively and/or quantitatively, in exerting their effect on structures and systems other than DNA.

MUNSON: Dr. Hadden, I was interested in your comments, from a pharmacologist's point of view, on the evidence that there may be both alpha and beta adrenergic receptors, cholinergic receptors, and histamine receptors on lymphocytes, macrophages, and even bone marrow cells. There is a body of literature developing that some neurotransmittons may be able to modulate the immune system. Is it relevant here, and is there a future in investigations based on the hypothesis that the immune system may be modulated through these receptors?

HADDEN: That's a very good question. One of the first observations we made in science had to do with the demonstration that alpha and beta adrenergic receptor mechanisms regulated lymphocytes. At that time, Robert Good was slightly disbelieving because the effects we were observing were only 10 to 15 percent above background. He said, "Give me something that changes the log, and then I'll pay attention!" The evolution of events since that time has supported the existence of many hormonal agents which have modest effects on altering immune function. When you talk about physiologic modulation of the system, i.e., how you might manipulate it in a way that it's used to being manipulated and therefore not do harm as a part of that manipulation, it does indeed focus your thinking on these kinds of receptor mechanisms. Not very much has been done in an effort to make a therapeutic pharmacology of that. Some of the prostaglandins have been modified to make them therapeutically useful with longer half-life. Thus, the anti-proliferative effects of prostaglandin, presumably mediated by cyclic AMP, might be useful in a therapeutic sense. To this date, no one has modified catecholamines, histamine, or cholinergic substances with expressed attempt to make them more biologically active in the context of the immune system. It is notable that the H_1 histamine blocker, cimetidine, may have significant immunostimulating activity on cell-mediated immunity.

Also, levamisole has cholinergic kinds of activities as part of its action, perhaps related to the presence of imidazole in its structure. I think one of the current interpretations of the mechanism of action of levamisole on cyclic GMP levels indicates cholinergic receptors are involved. The thymic hormones are currently receiving considerable preclinical and clinical attention as immunotherapeutic agents. These are examples of natural hormonal regulators. I have no crystal ball, so I am giving you only random thoughts on your question. I agree that it's an important area for thought.

MUNSON: I don't think that the pharmacologist has generally become involved in this area. Pharmacologists look at the interactions of immune competent cells and soluble proteins and see similarities to other systems in the organism.

HADDEN: Yes, I would like to make one statement about your very welcome comment: The immune system is indeed structured like the central nervous system. It has reactivity. It has memory. It modulates other populations. It is fascinating to me that several immunologically active substances have central nervous system side effects. As you know theta antigen, as a surface marker, is common to the two systems. Cotzias, among others, has suggested that there is a strong association in the regulation of the two systems.

SIGEL: A question to Dr. Spreafico: Cyclophosphamide also fails to inhibit response to pneumococcal polysaccharide if given prior to stimulation by antigen, but does suppress it if given following antigen. What about your Adriamycin which depress the B-cell response?

SPREAFICO: It is Daunomycin which failed to depress the response. Adriamycin did depress it. I might also mention, however, that those effects are seen both pre- and post-treatment in respect to antigen.

SIGEL: Dr. Hadden, among your activators of cyclases and cyclic AMP, you mentioned that LPS does increase AMP cyclase. I wonder how do you reconcile this increase in cyclic AMP with potentiation of various immune responses?

HADDEN: Yours is not a simple question. Endotoxin has an interesting ambivalence to it. At the level of both pre-T and pre-B cell it's an inducer of differentiation within the context of producing surface marker display. This is the work of my colleagues Hämmerling, Scheid, and Boyce at the Sloan-Kettering Institute. In both of those systems it appears that cyclic AMP mediates pharmacologic induction of receptor display. Endotoxin induces both B- and T-cell differentiation in conjunction with cellular increases in cyclic AMP. These results were obtained in collaboration with Margaret Scheid.

As you move to more mature B cells in the lineage in association with the acquisition of a complement receptor, endotoxin becomes a polyclonal B-cell mitogen; interestingly in that context, its action seems to be mediated by cyclic GMP. Thus, it is apparent that the B cell shifts in its responsiveness. Whether the linkage of a receptor shifts to a different plasma membrane enzyme or, whether there is the acquisition of an additional functional receptor (as complement) which shifts the nature of the response, has not been studied. Other inducers have a capacity to act via more than one receptor mechanism. For example, histamine acts on two different receptors, H-1 or H-2, which are either cyclic CMP or cyclic AMP-linked; while catecholamines act via alpha or beta adrenergic receptors which are cyclic AMP or cyclic GMP-linked. Thus it is through this kind of changing pattern of responsiveness that we can accommodate that kind of cleomorphism of action that endotoxin exhibits, and can explain how it induces differentiation of lymphocytes via cyclic AMP and proliferation via cyclic GMP.

JENSEN: I think there's a consensus, Dr. Hadden, that macrophage activation is a very important mechanism for control of neoplasia. It's come to my attention that classical nonsteroidal anti-inflammatory drugs have an antimetastatic effect, and incidentally we also know that they will activate macrophages. You touched on the modulating effect of various prostaglandin metabolites. These standard anti-inflammatory drugs are known to be cyclooxygenase inhibitors. Is there any way that we can speculate today how they activate macrophages?

HADDEN: There are really several points in your question. It is new to me that cyclooxygenase inhibitors are direct activators of macrophages. Is this *in vivo?*

JENSEN: We have found macrophage activation when mice are injected with such drugs.

HADDEN: That's interesting. In our own studies of activation of macrophage *in vitro* for bactericidal activity, we saw no effect of indomethacin to activate nor to abrogate lymphokine-induced activation.

There is reason to expect that cytostatic behavior on the part of the macrophage would be negatively affected by these inhibitors. Schultz and co-workers have shown that prostaglandins inhibit the action of interferon on macrophage killing of tumor cells. It is likely that these postaglandins will have a negative effect on interferon action on natural killer cells as well.

In the intact animal there are complex interactions between the tumor and the host-immune system vis-a-vis prostaglandins. Under certain circumstances it's evident that the immune system, having reacted to a tumor's antigens and having been frustrated, attempts to turn itself off. One can see evidence of suppression in operation in a host in which obviation of that suppression by the use of indomethacin or other cyclooxygenase inhibitors could calculatedly give a positive response.

On the other hand, a number of tumors produce prostaglandins associated with suppression of the host response. In this regard, Louis Pelus has presented some very nice results. Both *in vitro* and *in vivo* he was able to show, that in the circumstances where a tumor is prostaglandin producing, inhibition of that prostaglandin production by indomethacin is associated with inhibition of tumor growth, presumably on an immunologic basis.

From what you say, and we can talk afterwards about this observation, I would conclude that activation by nonsteroidal anti-inflammatory agents probably is not a direct action, but an indirect one to relieve endogenous suppression of macrophage killing by prostaglandins. I certainly see a place for them in the immunotherapy regimen of cancer in man. It seems to me that by obviating autosuppression by the immune system or tumor-induced suppression, these agents might well complement the use of other substances to improve the efficacy of immunotherapy.

SECTION II
MEASUREMENTS OF IMMUNOLOGIC PARAMETERS

4
Measurement
and Assessment
of Immune Competency

James L. McCoy

National Toxicology Program
National Cancer Institute, Bethesda, MD

The delicate homeostatic balances controlling normal immunoregulatory processes are susceptible to strong and subtle genetic, therapeutic, and environmental factor influences that result in wide variations in the expression of immune competency ranging from depression to elevated activity. Acute and chronic dysfunctions in host immune responsiveness as a result of genetic or external insult may be expressed as a) depleted or depressed natural or specific acquired immunosurveillance leading to increased susceptibility to viral or bacterial infections or oncogenic processes or b) hypersensitivity leading to allergic responses or even possibly autoimmune processes leading to self-destruction.

In the *in vitro* measurement of immunological competency and parameters influencing it, investigators need to keep an open mind regarding results obtained and their interpretation. Experimental data may indicate a depression in immune responsiveness which might be generally assumed as detrimental to the host in certain circumstances. An example of this will be presented in this session by Drs. Cannon, Dean, and Herberman. Likewise, immune competency measurements may indicate no change in immune status of the host following some external influence, but possible autoimmune expression may occur later. Thus, extreme caution in the evaluation of experimental data and in deriving conclusions must be taken until a better understanding and acceptance of the biological relevance of

Table 1.   Desired Characteristics of Immune Competency Assays.

1. Predictors of dysfunction (Present or Future)
2. Capability of being standardized among laboratories.
3. Reproducible and rapid.
4. Easy to perform.
5. Inexpensive.
6. Miniaturized.
7. Dose responsive (reflect quantitative degree of competency).
8. Lend themselves to easily establishing baselines of normal and abnormal reactivity.
9. True predictors of changes in reactivity in longitudinal testing.
10. Ability to be used in basic mechanism studies (e.g., suppressor cell-helper cell influences).

the various permutations associated with immune depression and hypersensitivity measurements are gained.

Assays used to measure general or specific immune competence have a variety of desired characteristics. Several of these are listed in Table 1. Of prime importance is the ability of the assay to be a predictor of some dysfunction that is either about to express itself, is presently expressing itself or will express itself at a later date.

Finally, our sophistication in the *in vitro* measurement and assessment of immune competency is not yet sufficient for us to choose one particular assay that will give a reliable prediction of a biological dysfunction. It therefore appears essential today for investigators to think of possibly developing a battery of both immunological and non-immunological assays including carcinogenesis, biochemical and mutagenesis measures that can be correlated alone or together in attempts to reliably predict beneficial or pathologic conditions resulting from genetic aberrations or toxicologic insults.

5
Effects of Anti-Cancer Therapy on Various Host Defense Functions in Cancer Patients

E. M. Hersh, S. G. Murphy, Y. Z. Patt, J. U. Gutterman, D. A. Morris, C. R. Gschwind, J. Morgan, M. Adegbite, and R. Goldman

Department of Developmental Therapeutics
University of Texas System Cancer Center
M.D. Anderson Hospital and Tumor Institute, Houston, Texas

INTRODUCTION

Cancer therapy, namely surgery, radiotherapy, chemotherapy and biological therapy all have major effects on host defense mechanisms, both desired and undesirable. In an attempt to understand the disease or therapy-related alterations in host defenses and tumor host interactions in cancer, an enormous effort has been expended over the last two decades to develop quantitative and reproducible approaches to immunological evaluation in man. In addition, our basic understanding of both general and tumor-specific host defense mechanisms have improved dramatically during this time. Therefore we have available at present a broad spectrum of host defense assays for use in man through which a fairly complete profile of host defense status can be achieved. In contrast, additional mechanisms have been discovered at a fairly regular rate and much work needs to be done, particularly on more subtle alterations in apparently normal subjects.

Some of the host defense components which can now be assessed ac-

Outline 1. Host Defense Factors and Functions of Relevance to Human Cancer

LEUKOCYTE ENUMERATION	LYMPHOCYTE PROLIFERATION	CYTOKINE PRODUCTION	LEUKOCYTE EFFECTOR FUNCTIONS
Lymphocytes	PHA	MIF	Cytotoxicity
T cells	CON-A	LAI	T cell
T μ cells	PWM	MAF	NK cell
T γ cells	MLC	CSF	K cell (ADCC to CRBC)
Fc receptor	Antigens	LAF	Monocyte
B cells		Interferon	Monocyte ADCC
C' receptor		Lysozyme	Regulatory
Monocytes			Suppressor Cell
			Helper Cell

SEROLOGICAL	IN VIVO
Ig levels	DTH
Isoantibody titers	RES particle clearance
1^0 antibody response	Skin inflammatory
2^0 antibody response	response
Glycoproteins	
Macroglobulins	
C' levels	
Immune complexes	

Abbreviations: ADCC, antibody dependent cellular cytotoxicity; CSF, colony stimulating factor; CON-A, concanavalin A; CRBC, chicken red blood cells; DTH, delayed type hypersensitivity; LAF, lymphocyte activating factor; LAI, leukocyte adherence inhibition; MAF, macrophage activating factor; MIF, migration inhibitory factor; MLC, mixed lymphocyte culture; NK, natural killer; PHA, phytohemagglutinin; PWM, pokeweed mitogen; RES, reticuloendothelial system.

curately are given in Outline 1. They include: enumeration of various host defense cell populations in blood and other tissues; assessment of various host defense cell functions *in vitro* including proliferative responses and immune responses; cellular effector functions such as cytolysis, phagocytosis and intracellular killing; cellular regulatory functions such as suppressor cell activity; production of effector products such as lymphokines, lysozyme and tumor necrosis factor; and assessment of various host defense functions *in vivo* including delayed hypersensitivity, inflammatory response, reticuloendothelial system (RES) particle clearance, and the primary and secondary antibody and cell mediated immune responses. Serum levels of a variety of important molecules associated with normal or disturbed host defenses can also be assessed accurately including levels of immunoglobulin components, complement components, immune complexes, and other substances such as α_2 HS glycoprotein. Thus a fairly complete profile of host defense and its aberrations in cancer patients can be created and derangements of both a quantitative and qualitative nature can be determined. Indeed many unique abnormalities have been identified using this methodology in a variety of human cancers.

Of current interest in the cancer area is the potential role of chemical and other carcinogens in the etiology of human cancer. It has been speculated that as much as half of all human malignancy is induced by environmental carcinogens (Wynder and Mabuchi, 1972). A major question is whether these carcinogens derange host defense mechanisms throughout the body or only at the local site of malignant transformation, whether such derangements of host defense mechanisms can be detected clinically, and whether there is any causative relationship between the deranged host defenses and the development and progression of malignancy. According to Dent (1972) and others, viral carcinogenesis is immunosuppressive. Stjernsward (1965) has demonstrated that chemical carcinogens suppressed both cell-mediated and humoral immunity when given systemically in mice and that the period of immunosuppression correlated with the period of latency before the malignant tumor appears. However, if the carcinogen was administered in the form of an insoluble pellet, then the local tumor still appeared but the host was not systemically immunosuppressed (Alexander et al., 1965). These data may provide important guidelines for the study of carcinogen-associated immunosuppression in man.

MATERIALS AND METHODS

Antibody Dependent Cell Mediated Cytotoxicity (ADCC)

This assay was conducted according to the method of Poplack, et al. (1976). Human hyperimmune antiserum to type A or B human red blood cells (HRBC) was obtained from the Dade Company, and rabbit antibody to chicken red blood cells (CRBC) was obtained following three weekly IV injections of 7×10^8 CRBC. Type A and B HRBC and CRBC were obtained weekly and stored in Alsever's solution at 4°C. They were labelled fresh just before the test by incubating 10^9 cells with 100 μCi of Cr^{51} in 0.2 ml for 30 minutes at 37°C and were subsequently washed three times in 100 volumes of media. Mononuclear leukocytes were collected and separated from peripheral blood by Ficoll-Hypaque density solution centrifugation. Target cells were adjusted to concentrations of 3×10^6 per ml. Effector cells were at a concentration of 10^6 per ml. Then

0.1 ml of effector cells, 0.1 ml of target cells and 0.1 ml of a 1:10 dilution of anti-A or anti-B or a 1:1200 dilution of anti-CRBC were mixed in 12×75 ml plastic culture tubes. The experimental and control tubes were incubated 20 hours at 37°C. After incubation tubes were centrifuged at 2,000 RPM for 10 minutes and 0.6 ml of the supernatants counted in a gamma counter. Chromium release was calculated by dividing the counts per minute (CPM) in the supernatant by the CPM in the pellet $\times$ 100. The final increment of chromium release was obtained by subtracting spontaneous chromium release from the mean chromium release in experimental tubes. All reactions were conducted in triplicate.

Monocyte-Macrophage Precursors

This assay was based on the report of Currie and Headley (1977). Washed mononuclear cells were prepared at a concentration of 1×10^6/ml. Microtest II plates (with flat bottom wells) were set up with 1×10^6 mononuclear cells per well and five replicates per point. Culture volume was 0.2 ml with 50% serum. Plates were incubated for 7 days and the wells were washed gently six times with warm media at the end of the culture period. Then, 0.1 molar citric acid containing 1:2000 crystal violet was added to each well, and the plates were incubated for 30 minutes. The plates were then agitated and the released cells (detached nuclei) counted in a hemacytometer or Coulter counter. Complete release of cells from the wells by this method was confirmed by microscopy. Results were expressed as the number of adherent macrophages per ml of blood, per 10^6 mononuclear cells or per number of monocytes added to the well.

Serum Lysozyme

Serum lysozyme determinations were performed using the Worthington Diagnostics Lysozyme Reagent Set. The test is a measure of the rate at which a cell suspension of *Micrococcus lysoideikticus* is lysed. The kit contains a vial of lyophilized substrate and a vial of lysozyme standard which were reconstituted with distilled H_2O. The standard was used to prepare a standard curve for the substrate, and all subsequent determinations using that substrate were based on the curve generated. Three hundred μl of serum or standard were added to 3 ml of substrate and an absorbance reading at 500 nm was taken after a ½ minute interval and again after the three-minute interval. The difference in the OD's was computed and the amount of lysozyme present determined from the standard curve.

Lymphocyte Blastogenesis and Suppressor Cells

Mononuclear leukocytes were separated from other formed elements of defibrinated venous blood by Hypaque-Ficoll density solution centrifugation. Leukocytes were identified by light microscopy and monocytes differentiated from lymphocytes by Sudan Black staining and by nonspecific esterase staining. Leukocytes were washed and resuspended at 5×10^6 leukocytes per ml in media containing 5% fetal bovine serum.

Leukocytes were cultured in Falcon microtest plates with flat bottom wells at 1.5×10^5 cells per well in 0.2 ml of media (RPMI 1640) containing 20% serum. For the PHA (Difco), PWM (Difco), and Con-A (Pharmacia) responses, lymphocytes were cultured three days. During the last eight hours of these culture periods, lymphocytes were exposed to 1 μCi of tritiated thymidine, specific activity 1.9 Ci per mM. The cells were harvested with a MASH-II harvester and the incorporated radioactivity counted in a liquid scintillation counter as previously described by Lewinski et al. (1977). The results were recorded as net counts perminute (stimulated minus control).

Suppressor cells were measured by a co-culture technique in which 1.5×10^5 normal cells were cultured with an equal number of patient or normal cells. The latter may be irradiated with 8000r, or treated in the co-culture with 100 μg/ml of the thymic hormones, thymosin fraction V or thymic humoral factor. All other culture conditions were as described above. Suppressor cell activity was documented when normal blastogenesis was depressed by patient but not by normal cells.

RESULTS

Table 1 compares ADCC values of normal subjects and patients with various types of malignancy. The characteristics of the patient groups are described in the footnote of the table. Of considerable interest, the patients' cells were not depressed as anticipated but on the average were significantly more active than the normal control group. This was true for most but not all of the patient groups studied. Values were not elevated in breast cancer or the miscellaneous cancer groups. These observations were true for ADCC to both HRBC and CRBC.

Table 2 shows the effects of various therapeutic maneuvers on the ADCC of patients' cells to both HRBC and CRBC. Chemotherapy (de-

Table 1.   ADCC to CRBC and HRBC In Normal Subjects and Cancer Patients

SUBJECT GROUP [1]	N	ADCC TO CRBC MEAN ± SD [2]	P [3]	N	ADCC TO HRBC MEAN ± SD	P
Normal	43	23.3 ± 10.6	—	51	22.0 ± 13.3	—
Lung Cancer	24	44.0 ± 13.7	.001	27	48.3 ± 17.0	.001
Malignant Melanoma	15	32.3 ± 13.1	.02	18	31.7 ± 18.3	.02
Colon Cancer	7	48.0 ± 17.0	.001	7	45.4 ± 19.0	.001
Breast Cancer	13	30.2 ± 16.0	> .10	20	27.5 ± 16.1	> .20
Miscellaneous Cancer	13	35.5 ± 22.1	.01	14	29.3 ± 21.9	> .10
All Cancer	72	38.0 ± 17.0	.001	86	36.7 ± 19.9	.001

[1] Normal controls were hospital employees and family members of patients. Patients had stage IV disease and had previously received either surgery or local irradiation of their primary tumor site but had not received chemotherapy.
[2] Percent target cell lysis, 3:1 target effector ratio.
[3] Significance by T test compared to normal.

Table 2.   Effects of Chemotherapy and Immunotherapy on ADCC To CRBC and HRBC in Cancer Patients.

THERAPEUTIC PARAMETER	ADCC TO CRBC [1] STUDY NUMBER			ADCC TO HRBC STUDY NUMBER		
	1	2	3	1	2	3
Chemotherapy [2]	37.5 ±19.6	10.5 ± 7.6	46.8 ±15.8	33.4 ±16.9	14.4 ±17.9	50.6 ± 7.2
IV. *C. parvum* [3]	15.7 ± 6.9	46.9 ±13.0	47.9 ±21.6	34.8 ±19.8	47.3 ±15.2	53.5 ±13.2
IV MER [4]	34.4 ±17.5	40.6 ±18.4	45.4 ±20.6	24.5 ±21.5	21.6 ±11.4	29.0 ±13.2

[1] Percent target cell lysis at 3:1 target effector ratio.
[2] Ten patients with stage IV lung cancer studied 1 day before (study 1), at end of (study 2) and 9 days after (study 3) a five-day course of Florafur, Adriamycin, Cytoxan and cisplatinum chemotherapy.
[3] Twelve patients with stage IVB malignant melanoma (8) or other solid tumors (4) were studied 1 day before, 7 days after, or 14 days after the start of a 14-day course of *C. parvum,* 2 mg/m[2] IV per day.
[4] Fifteen patients were studied one day before or on days 7 and 14 of weekly IV MER (0.5 mg/m[2] on days 1, 7, and 14).

tailed in the footnote) caused a striking suppression of ADCC after only 5 days of therapy with recovery and overshoot above the baseline noted 9 days later. This suggested that the cell populations responsible for ADCC to CRBC (K cells) and HRBC (monocytes) are derived from a rapidly turning over, short-lived population of cells. In contrast to the depression of activity induced by chemotherapy, immunotherapy with intravenous methanol extraction residue of BCG (IV MER) and with IV *Corynebacterium parvum* (*C. parvum*) increased ADCC activity of peripheral blood cells significantly. The increase occurred within 4 to 7 days in the case of both IV MER and *C. parvum*. ADCC to HRBC has not been affected significantly by IV MER when examined in this way. All other increases were significant. The increased ADCC activity was observed in spite of the advanced nature of the disease in some of the patients.

Table 3 illustrates some data accumulated using the assay for adherent monocyte-macrophage precursors. Normal control and patient data are compared. It can be seen that, compared to normal, patients with a variety of different malignancies had markedly depressed numbers of adherent mononuclear cells per ml of blood. When calculated as per-number of mononuclear cells plated, this deficiency was also noted (data

Table 3.   Peripheral Blood Monocyte-Macrophage Precursors In Normal Subjects and Cancer Patients.

SUBJECT GROUP [1]	N	ADHERENT CELLS PER ML BLOOD $\times 10^4$		
		MEAN	MEDIAN	P [2]
Normal	83	17.9	14.8	—
Melanoma	44	4.5	3.1	.0001
Breast Cancer	23	1.9	1.5	.0001
Lung Cancer	18	8.1	1.5	.01
Colon Cancer	9	7.1	7.5	.05
Sarcoma	4	10.2	6.3	NS
Leukemia	27	6.9	1.7	.0001
All Patients	125	5.4	2.5	.0001

[1] Normals were hospital employees, patients had stage IV disease with no prior history of chemotherapy except 27 melanoma patients were stage III NED, 2 breast cancer patients were stage II NED, 9 lung cancer patients were stage III and 6 colon patients were Dukes' C. The leukemia patients were mainly AML, had received chemotherapy, and had no circulating leukemic cells.
[2] Compared to normal by the Mann Whitney U Test.

Table 4. Effects of IV *C. Parvum* and IV MER Immunotherapy on the Peripheral Blood Levels of Monocyte Macrophage Precursors.

THERAPEUTIC PARAMETER	STUDY NUMBER		
	1	2	3
IV. *C. parvum*	6.4	7.5	11.4 [3]
	±5.8	± 7.5	±11.7
IV MER	3.6	12.5	13.4
	±6.1	±12.9	±12.7

[1] Same patient groups and study intervals as in table 2.
[2] Adherent monocyte-macrophage precursors per ml blood $\times$ 10^4.
[3] Significance by Wilcoxon signed rank test: study 2 vs 1: not significant, study 3 vs 1 p $<$.05.
[4] Significance by Wilcoxon signed rank test: study 2 vs 1: p $<$.05, study 3 vs 1 p$<$.05.

not shown). Only in lung cancer was there a clear-cut relationship to the stage of disease with patients in Stage IV showing lower values than patients in Stage III (data not shown). Thus a striking deficiency of these cells in cancer patients has been defined.

Immunotherapy with IV MER or with IV *C. parvum* definitely boosted this activity (Table 4). Boosting of the numbers of adherent cells per ml of blood or per number plated was slow in patients receiving *C. parvum* (sometimes requiring more than a month, but was often seen after the first dose of IV MER). After initial boosting by MER, repeated doses tended to maintain the activity at an elevated level rather than cause a progressive increase in activity.

Table 5 shows the serum lysozyme levels of normal subjects and patients with various histologic types of malignancy. The patient groups on the average were all within the normal range except for lung cancer (Stages III and IV) which was significantly increased. However, within each patient group there were at least a few patients whose serum lysozyme was above the upper limit of normal and a few whose values were below the lower limit of normal. Table 6 shows the effects of IV MER immunotherapy on the serum lysozyme level. This was significantly boosted, often after only one injection. *C. parvum* was not studied for its effects on serum lysozyme.

Suppressor cell activity was evaluated by a co-culture system utilizing equal mixtures of patient and normal cells stimulated with mitogens. Suppressor cell activity was found in about 70% of 35 patients with

Table 5.   Serum Lysozyme Levels in Normal Subjects and in Cancer Patients.

SUBJECT GROUP	n [1]	MEAN	MEDIAN	COMPARISON TO NORMAL (P)[2]
Normal	58	6.1	5.8	—
Melanoma	96	6.0	6.2	.76
Breast Cancer	122	6.5	5.9	.19
Lung Cancer	98	10.4	8.3	<.0001
Colon Cancer	21	5.4	5.0	.28
Leukemia	54	8.0	6.0	.67
All Patients	391	7.5	6.6	.028 [3]

[1] Serum lysozyme measured in μg/ml of serum.
[2] Statistical comparison done by Mann Whitney U test.
[3] With lung cancer patients excluded P = .49.

various types of advanced malignancy (Table 7). There was an excellent correlation between suppressor cell activity and immunodeficiency but only a non-significant correlation between suppressor cell activity and a history of prior chemotherapy (Table 8).

DISCUSSION

Chemical carcinogenesis is a major problem in human health. Data of Wynder and Mabuchi (1972) suggest that as much as 50% of human malignant disease may be caused by environmental factors. It is well established that the systemic administration of carcinogens in large doses

Table 6.   Effects of Intravenous Mer Therapy on the Serum Lysozyme Level.

PARAMETER	STUDY NUMBER		
	1	2	3
Mean	7.6	10.8	11.4
± SD	±3.1	± 4.9	± 4.9
Median	7.5	10.2	9.5
No. showing increase	—	10	10

Note: Same patient group and interval as shown in Tables 2 and 4. Serum lysozyme measured in μg/ml of serum. Significance calculated by Wilcoxon signed rank test. Fifteen patients studied. Studies 2 and 3 significantly greater than study 1, p <.05.

Table 7. Suppressor Cell Activity Detected by Mitogen Stimulation of Lymphocytes in Co-Culture.

MALIGNANCY [1]	n	SUPPRESSOR CELL [2] FOR PROLIFERATIVE RESPONSE [3] TO	
		PHA	CON-A
Lung Cancer	21	15(71)[4]	13(62)
Acute Leukemia	7	4(57)	5(71)
Miscellaneous Solid Tumors	7	6(86)	7(100)

[1] Patients with lung cancer and miscellaneous solid tumors had disseminated disease and 12/28 had previously received chemotherapy. Patients with leukemia had all received chemotherapy and had no circulating leukemia cells.

[2] Suppressor cell activity defined as a 3–fold reduction in normal cells' blastogenic response by added patient cells.

[3] Proliferative responses to PHA and Con-A are measured by H^3 thymidine incorporation. Cells are cultured separately and also co-cultured in equal numbers.

[4] Number (percent) patients showing suppressor activity when their cells are added to normal cells.

is immunosuppressive for animals (Stjernsward 1965), that the concurrent administration of immunosuppressive drugs can increase the rate of tumor formation and growth in carcinogen treated animals (Bourgoin et al., 1972) and that immunotherapy with BCG can reduce or delay tumor appearance (Zwilling et al., 1977). Grubbs (1977) has shown that retinoids (which have potent immunostimulating effects) also have this capacity, but their action is at least in part independent of the host de-

Table 8. Correlation Between Suppressor Cell Activity and Patient Status.

CATEGORY	NUMBER STUDIED	SUPPRESSOR CELL PRESENT FOR	
		PHA RESPONSE	CON-A RESPONSE
Immunocompetent	11	4	4
Immunodeficient	23	17	21
No prior chemotherapy	15	9	8
Prior chemotherapy	19	12	17

Note: Suppressor cell activity more prevalent in immunodeficient than immunocompetent patients, p = .50 (PHA), p < .01 (CON-A). Chemotherapy vs no prior chemotherapy, not significantly different regarding suppressor cell activity.

fense system since they can reverse malignant transformation of cell lines *in vitro*. Finally host defence mechanisms are known to decline in patients with progressive malignancy (Hersh, 1976). It has been speculated by Burnet (1971), although not proven, that a failure of one or more host defense mechanisms is responsible for the development and/or progression of malignancy in man (Burnet, 1971). This intriguing idea has been the subject of considerable controversy (Melief and Schwartz, 1975).

For the above outlined reasons it seems appropriate to propose that intensive immunological evaluation be conducted in individuals exposed to environmental carcinogens. The possibility exists that immunodeficiency (or some other abnormality of host defense) might define systemically exposed subjects or a population at risk of subsequent tumor development.

On the other hand, one might argue that this would be of little value. First the immunosuppressive doses of carcinogens used in animals are far higher than anticipated human exposure. Second there is immunological recovery at the time of appearance of overt malignancy in some of the animal models. Indeed in a recent study of asbestos workers we were unable to find a defect in lymphocyte number and function once other factors such as race were taken into account (Morris, unpublished). However, it does seem worthwhile to consider studies at least in subjects with a high degree of exposure.

In this paper we have shown data on five approaches to host defense evaluation which may be of interest in such studies. Measurement of K cells, of monocytes with ADCC activity, of the numbers of monocyte or macrophage precursors in the peripheral blood, of serum lysozyme and or suppressor cells should be considered as assays which can reflect changes induced by carcinogens or other host defense modifying factors.

In the current study we report data on these assays in cancer patients. ADCC to both HRBC and CRBC and serum lysozyme were normal in the majority of patients. However, they were rapidly depressed by chemotherapy and boosted by immunotherapy. Suppressor cell activity was present in most patients who manifested immune deficiency by conventional assays. We propose these assays as sensitive adjuncts to other approaches to host defense evaluation. Certainly at this point, since almost nothing is known about how or which host defenses are altered by carcinogens, the most broadly based assay approach must be taken.

REFERENCES

Alexander, P., Delorme, E. J., Hamilton, L. D., et al.: Effect of nucleic acids from immune lymphocytes on rat sarcomata. *Nature, 213:*569 (1967).
Bourgoin, J. J., Cueff, J., Bailly, C., et al.: Incidence of nephroblastomas in the

Sprague Dawley Rat immunodepressed with ALS. Bull. Cancer (Paris), *59*:429 (1972).

Burnet, F. M.: Immunological surveillance in neoplasia. Transplant Rev., *7*:3 (1971).

Currie, G. A., and Headley, D. W.: Monocytes and macrophages in malignant melanoma. I. Peripheral blood macrophage precursors. Brit. J. Cancer, *36*:1 (1977).

Dent, P. B.: Immunodepression by oncogenic viruses. Prog. Med. Virol., *14*:1 (1972).

Grubbs, C. J., Moon, R. C., Squire, R. A., et al.: 13-cis-retinoic acid: Inhibition of bladder carcinogenesis induced in rats by N-butyl-N- (4-hydroxybutyl) nitrosamine. Science, *198*:743 (1977).

Hersh, E. M., Mavligit, G. M., and Gutterman, J. U.: Immunodeficiency in cancer and the importance of immune evaluation of the cancer patient. Med- Clin. North Amer., *60*:623 (1976).

Lewinski, U., Mavligit, G. M., Gutterman, J. U., et al.: Interaction between repeated skin tests with recall antigens and temporal fluctuations of *in vitro* lymphocyte blastogenesis in cancer patients. Clin. Immunol. and Immunopath., *7*:77 (1977).

Melief, C. J. M., and Schwartz, R. S.: Immunocompetence and malignancy. In: Cancer, A Comprehensive Treatise. F. F. Becker (ed.), Plenum Press, New York, 1975.

Poplack, D. O., Bonnard, G. D., Holinian, B. J., et al.: Monocyte mediated antibody dependent cellular cytotoxicity: A clinical test of monocyte function. Blood, *48*:809 (1976).

Stjernsward, J.: Immunosuppressive effect of 3-methyl cholanthrene: Antibody formation at the cellular level and reaction against weakly antigenic homografts. J. Natl. Cancer Inst., *35*:885 (1965).

Wynder, E. L., and Mabuchi, K.: Etiological and preventive aspects of human cancer. Preventive Med. 1:300 (1972).

Zwilling, B. S., Springer, S. T., and Kaufman, D. G.: Effect of systemic administration of BCG cell walls on bronchogenic carcinoma in hamsters. J. Natl. Cancer Inst., *58*:1473 (1977).

ACKNOWLEDGMENTS

Supported by Grant CA–05831 and Contract N01–CB–33888 from the National Cancer Institute. Dr. Murphy is a Leukemia Society of America scholar.

DISCUSSION

BOORMAN: How does your monocyte adherence assay for macrophage progenitors in the peripheral blood compare with the other clonal assays in semisolid media for macrophage granuloycte progenitors (CFU-C assays)? A second question is: Are you monitoring bone marrow in these patients for progenitor cells?

HERSH: In hairy-cell leukemia there seems to be a correlation between the number of granulocytic-macrophagic colonies, or lack of them, and the various monocyte parameter deficiencies that we've observed. We have not studied this in the spectrum of other cancer patients so we do not know whether there is a correlation in these also. I think it is a very important point. We have not monitored the progenitor cells in the bone marrow of patients receiving various modalities of immunotherapy. The only thing that I can say in this regard is that MER is the most potent *in vitro* inducer of colony-stimulating activity that Spitzer, Verma, and our colleagues at M. D. Anderson Hospital have identified. This was a motivation for us to explore MER therapy in patients with bone marrow failure.

HELLMAN: In your assay I noticed that basically there were times when you saw appreciable depression, which suggests that a single assay of a patient using all parameters is really not very satisfactory. In other words, one has to follow this over a long-term basis. Also, is there a clinical rationale for some of the suppressions that you see?

HERSH: Suppression is a critically important factor. Holland and Bekesi have observed that there is immunosuppression as measured by the PHA response in patients receiving MER intradermally. If MER is stopped, there is recovery. In animal systems, the microbial adjuvants have been demonstrated to induce suppressor cells. Indeed this can be reversed with indomethacin. So I think this is very important and we are currently beginning to investigate this question in our patients.

One of the problems that the clinical immunologist faces is that the immunological or host-defense reactivity of man, measured by whatever parameter selected, is highly variable. It is essential to do concurrent controls. In our Phase I studies of immunotherapeutic agents, we are now testing a concurrent normal control subject—the same subject each time. We also try to do a frozen-control standard. As an example of this approach, a cooperative lung cancer study group (six institutions) is performing immunological monitoring of lung cancer patients receiving immunotherapy. In comparing one laboratory with another the data were not consistent until a frozen standard was used. Dr. R. Oldham's group has demonstrated that this really makes a difference and allows data from several labs to be related to each other. When the data were normalized, all investigators' data were the same. So I think this approach is needed to iron out this tremendous day-to-day variability that we encounter in our immunological activity.

SIGEL: In your restoration of response in blastogensis using normal monocytes, how much of the restorative action was due to the need for normal monocytes and how much was due to the presence of the alloantigen in the system?

HERSH: It wasn't at all due to the presence of alloantigen. We harvest these cultures at 48 hours, and the contribution of the MLC-type response is minimal at that time. That question is also applicable to our co-culture suppressor cell assay, where the same information holds true.

SIGEL: So the magic number is 48 hours to be able to dissect the phenomenon? Second, a perennial question: There was one patient you told us about who showed a good correlation clinically with the restoration of her responses. How often do you see such a correlation in your patients on immunotherapy?

HERSH: In our patients who were getting BCG by scarification and in our patients getting subcutaneous *C. parvum*, the answer is virtually never. This was one of the big disappointments that we experienced: BCG boosted delayed hypersensitivity but that didn't correlate at all with what we saw clinically. Almost all patients converted to PPD positive, even patients with advanced disease. With the current studies it's really too early to comment. We are just getting into the intravenous purified adjuvants. At least I think we now have methods to do a dose-response study, so we could develop a biologically relevant immunotherapeutic dose.

HADDEN: A brief methodological question. You described the reciprocal relationship of cell concentration to cytocidal activity for the two kinds of ADCC. I didn't understand that.

HERSH: I'm sorry, I didn't make that clear. The rising curve was the numbers of cells lysed with increasing numbers of cells added. The declining curve was the percent target-cell lysis. We use a 3-to-1 target effector ratio because that is the point at which the maximum number of cells is lysed as you add increasing numbers of targets to a fixed number of effectors. It happens that it comes out around 20 percent. I think most people who have studied ADCC have conducted this kind of manipulation to determine the optimal ratios for study.

MAO: Your results concerning the activity of lysozyme in the serum or tumor cells may be affected by the treatment. I wonder if you measured the change of lysozyme activities during pretreatment, treatment, and post-treatment periods? Did you stop treatment for some time and measure the lysozome activity again to see if the activity was restored? Also, does the treatment have a permanent effect on the lysozyme?

HERSH: Are you referring to chemotherapy?

MAO: Yes.

HERSH: We have not yet studied patients receiving chemotherapy. The patients that I described were those who had received either surgery or radiation for their primary tumor and were now canidates for post surgical adjuvant treatment. They had not yet received chemotherapy.

MAO: One more question along the same line: Did you measure the activity of the lysozymes in terms of total lysozyme activity or did you consider it as the activity of any individual isomer of lysozyme?

HERSH: No. We simply use the Worthington Biochemical's kit which measures lysis of *micrococcus lysoideikticus* in a spectrophotometer. I think that lsozymes may be particularly interesting, at least in lung cancer patients, where we have fairly clear-cut evidence that the serum lysozyme level is elevated. It would also be of interest in patients receiving experimental immunotherapy and in animals receiving immunotherapy where there might be some clue as to the source of this lysozyme. My assumption is that it's coming from activated macrophages.

McCOY: One final comment before we move on. I think one of the major aspects of Dr. Hersh's work, which he emphasized but that I want to stress further, is the measurement of monocyte function. It is well known today that monocytes are important accessory cells in cell-mediated immune reactions. Monocyte function is one of the key starting points in the immune process. Dr. Hersh showed very clearly that many of his patients are immunologically depressed and many of them have abnormal monocyte functions, which may account for much of the depression as he stated.

The dichotomy in this finding, which possibly will come out in tomorrow's session is: Why do these patients have a dysfunction in monocyte function and still have suppressor-cell activity?

6
Assessment of Immune Parameters of Transplant Recipients on Immunosuppressive Therapy

Ronald H. Kerman and Barry D. Kahan

Division of Organ Transplantation, Department of Surgery,
The University of Texas Medical School at Houston

INTRODUCTION

The major cause of rejection of renal allografts is recipient sensitization toward foreign histocompatibility antigens, in man coded for by multiple gene loci on the sixth chromosome (Guttman, 1979). The presently identified genetic loci influencing allograft survival include the HLA A, B, C, and DRW series of antigens (serologically detected) and the HLA D antigen (cellularly detected). Matching for HLA antigens in living related-donor transplants is useful because of inheritance of the entire chromosomal region within families; compatibility markedly improves graft survival. Matching recipients of cadaveric-donor transplants by HLA A and B loci is less useful: the relation is unclear to graft survival (Terasaki et al., 1978; Opelz and Terasaki, 1976; Williams, 1979; Mittal et al., 1975). Recent reports suggest that matching for DRW alleles may influence cadaveric graft survival (Ting and Morris, 1978; Persijn et al., 1978).

Variables other than HLA matching may determine allograft success: 1) specific host anti-donor reactivity toward disparate antigens, and 2) recipient immunocompetence. Immunological investigations can determine the existence of recipient anti-donor presensitization towards disparate donor antigenic factors. These procedures should be performed to expose pre-existing host immunity since the secondary reactions are not readily controlled by existing immunosuppressive agents and lead to early graft loss. Procedures detecting host presensitization against donor disparate antigens include both humoral and cellular immune assays. Humoral studies include detection of complement dependent antibody (CDA) by visual (dye exclusion) or radionuclide (^{51}Cr release) methods and of lymphocyte-dependent antibody (LDA) by radionuclide release in the presence of normal effector K cells. Cellular assays include detection of T cell lymphocyte-mediated cytotoxicity (LMC) and the antibody-dependent cell-mediated cytotoxicity (ADCC) effector (K) cell reactivity (both by a radionuclide release assay).

We have recently reviewed our experience using specific host anti-donor assays to predict early rejection with graft loss (Kerman and Kahan, in press, 1979). Specific anti-donor cross-match procedures are critical prior to renal allografting to reveal host presensitization and to circumvent early graft loss: pre-transplant positive LDA, LMC, ADCC or CDA tests correlated with the occurrence of accelerated rejection episodes and graft loss. However, these tests failed to predict rejection episodes when used after transplantation to monitor specific anti-donor immune reactivity.

Correlation of Pre-Transplant Non-Specific Immunocompetence and Prolonged Allograft Survival

Of the many factors other than histocompatibility which influence the outcome of cadaveric allograft survival, the level of recipient immunocompetence may be the most important. Thus, strong immune responders would be predicted to have a poorer chance of one year graft survival independent of the degree of HLA compatibility (Kerman and Kahan, in press, 1979; Kerman et al., 1977; Rolley et al., 1978; Wilson and Kirkpatrick, 1964; Kerman et al., 1979). We have developed a pre-transplant battery of non-specific immunologic tests to identify weak responders likely to have prolonged graft survival. The battery includes: enumeration of total and active T rosette forming cells (T-RFC); spontaneous blastogenesis; mixed lymphocyte culture to a stimulation panel of three to five unrelated donors; lymphocyte response to mitogens; and cutaneous hypersensitivity to five microbial antigens and to dinitrochlorbenzene. The duration of cadaveric allograft survival in chronic renal failure patients correlated with values below the median in percent of active T-RFC, in cpm of ^{3}H-thymidine incorporated during spontaneous blastogenesis or during panel mixed lymphocyte culture and to a negative recall response to microbial antigens eliciting cutaneous hypersensitivity.

METHODS

Briefly, peripheral blood lymphocytes (PBL) are separated on a Ficoll-Hypaque gradient, washed in Dulbecco's phosphate buffered saline (PBS), pH 7.3 and brought to a final concentration of 2×10^6 PBL/ml in PBS. For the *total T-RFC* assay, 0.25 ml (5×10^5 PBL) are mixed with 0.25 ml of 0.5% washed unsensitized sheep red blood cells (SRBC), centrifuged at 200 x g for 5 minutes at room temperature, and then incubated in an ice-water bath (4–8°C) for 60 minutes. After the cell pellets are gently resuspended, a drop of the suspension is placed onto a hemacytometer. The number of rosettes (three or more SRBC surrounding a lymphocyte) are counted. All tests are performed in duplicate; 200 or more PBL are counted to determine the percentage of total T-RFC. For the *active T-RFC* 0.25 ml (5×10^5 PBL) are mixed with 0. 25 ml of 0.5% washed unsensitized SRBC and centrifuged at 200 x g for 5 minutes at room temperature. Cell pellets are gently resuspended and the active T-RFC counted immediately (without a 60 minute 4–8°C ice-water incubation). For the *in vitro* studies of PBML stimulation with *PHA, Con A, PWM* or *alloantigen stimulation* in a *panel MLR,* PBL are isolated and brought to a concentration of 1×10^6 PBL/ml. For the assays 1×10^5 PBL in media (RPMI-1640, glutamine, pen/strep, Hepes, and 15% inact. AB plasma) are seeded into microtiter plate wells and incubated with either three concentrations of each mitogen or with 1×10^5 donor panel stimulation cells (previously inactivated with mitomycin-C) in triplicate in a humidified chamber containing 95% air and 5% CO_2 at 37°C for 96 hours. The lymphocyte response to stimulation is determined by measuring the incorporation of ^{3}H-thymidine in DNA. Eighteen to twenty-four hours prior to harvesting the cultures 1 μCi of ^{3}H-thymidine (specific activity 48 Ci/mM, ICN) is added to each well. Incubations are terminated using a MASH harvester; ^{3}H-thymidine incorporation is measured by liquid scintillation counting. Results are expressed as counts per minute (cpm). *Spontaneous blastogenesis* (SB) is performed in triplicate by adding 50 μl of ^{3}H-thymidine (Sp. activity 48 Ci/mM) to 50 μl of heparinized whole blood diluted with 200 μl of media. The mixture is incubated for two hours at 37°C in a 5% CO_2 incubator prior to harvesting using a MASH unit. The filter strips are dried and counted in a liquid scintillation system.

Skin test antigen responses are elicited by intradermal inoculation of 0.1 ml of dermatophytin (1:30), dermatophytin-0 (1:100) (Hollister-

Steir Labs), Streptokinase-Streptodornase (50 units SK, Lederle Labs), mumps (Eli Lilly and Co.) and intermediate strength tuberculin antigen (Parke, Davis and Co.). Reactions are measured at right angles (mm) at 24 and 48 hours for the average dimension of induration and erythema. Induration greater than 5 mm is considered positive. DNCB was used as a non-specific measure of leukocyte mobilization by observing the spontaneous flare reaction which occurred at the application site. Doses were 2,000 μg to the upper arm and 50 μg to the forearm. A flare after 14 days was scored 4+, at the 2,000 μg site only, 3+ at the 50μg site only. If neither site developed a flare after 14 days, a challenge of 50 μg was applied to the opposite forearm. A cutaneous hypersensitivity reaction at this new site within 48 hours was scored as 2+. An equivocal reaction which required biopsy for confirmation counted 1+ if the histological features of delayed cutaneous hypersensitivity were seen. In practice, reactions of 4+ or 3+ were considered normal and positive; below these values, abnormal or negative to DNCB without further testing (Kerman et al., 1979; Kerman and Stefani, 1976).

The median values for the pre-transplant immunological assessment among 41 cadaveric renal allograft recipients were: 55% total T-RFC, 34% active T-RFC, 12,079 cpm spontaneous blastogenesis, 21,470 cpm (or 5.7 stimulation ratio) on panel MLC response; 103,725 cpm response to PHA, 77,030 cpm response to Con A and 134,249 cpm response to PWM. Patients were considered postive responders if they reacted to 1 or more microbial antigens or positively to DNCB. Prolonged graft survival correlated with patients having pre-transplant values below the group median for three of the four *in vitro* immune assessment tests: active T-RFC less than 34% ($p<0.05$); *in vitro* lymphocyte spontaneous blastogenesis less than 12,079 cpm ($p<0.01$); panel MLC response less than 21,470 cpm ($p<0.01$) and negative response to all microbial skin test antigens ($p<0.04$) (Table 1). De novo response to DNCB, % total T-RFC, as well as lymphocyte response upon stimulation with mitogens were not prognostic of graft survival.

Patients with strong pre-transplant immune response in the four relevant tests displayed an earlier onset of rejection, reduced mean survival time (MST) and requirement for large steroid doses to dampen rejection events (Table 2).

Correlation of Non-Specific Immune Assays with Impending or Ongoing Rejection Episodes

Tissue typing and crossmatching procedures attempt to minimize donor histoincompatibility and avert grafting into pre-sensitized hosts. Since

Table 1. Mean Survival Time of 41 Cadaveric Renal Allografts Based on Pre-Transplant Non-Specific Immune Assessment.

	MST (DAYS)[1]		P VALUE [2]
% Active T-RFC	<34%[3] (20)	>34% (20)	
	228 ± 68	100 ± 69	<0.05
Spontaneous Blastogenesis	<12,079 cpm[3] (20)	>12,079 cpm (20)	
	255 ± 36	70 ± 61	<0.01
Panel Mixed Lymphocyte	<21,470 cpm[3] (20)	>21,470 cpm (20)	
Reaction	255 ± 47	78 ± 51	<0.01
Microbial Skin Test	Anergic (18)	Positive[4] (23)[5]	
Antigens	239 ± 42	115 ± 41	<0.04

[1] Mean survival time in days ± standard deviation
[2] Data analyzed by the two-tailed Wilcoxon test
[3] Median value for the test
[4] Positive response to one or more microbial skin test antigens
[5] ( ) Indicates number of patients in group

the signs, symptoms and laboratory evidences of rejection are late events, immunological evidences of a primary immune response may alert the clinician, thereby affording the possibility for prompt initiation of immuno-suppressive therapy to minimize tissue damage. As stated above host specific anti-donor immune testing after transplantation did not predict or correlate within 5 days significantly with clinical rejection episodes (Kerman and Kahan, in press, 1979). The apparent lack of correlation

Table 2. Cadaveric Graft Survival Based on Pre-Transplant Immune Response.[a, b]

	WEAK IMMUNE RESPONSE [c]	STRONG IMMUNE RESPONSE	P VALUE[d]
1) Mean Survival Time (Days)	386 ± 78	111 ± 86	<0.01
2) No. Rejection Episodes			
(First 30 Days)	1.1 ± 0.4	1.5 ± 0.28	N.S.
3) Day of Rejection Onset	17 ± 4.9	8.5 ± 7.0	<0.05
4) Mean Grams Solu-Medrol/PT			
(First 30 Days)	4.45 ± 1.05	6.65 ± 2.6	<0.05

[a] No significant differences in HLA mismatches between groups
[2] Data analyzed by the two-tailed Wilcoxon test
[c] Weak Responses: <34% A-TRFC; (−) Skin Tests; Low Spontaneous Blastogenesis; Low Panel MLC
[d] Two-tailed Wilcoxon Test

between tests reflecting anti-donor reactivity and allograft rejection may relate to: 1) the present assays do not reflect reactivity toward antigenic systems critical to allograft survival; 2) relevant determinants not being expressed on lymphocytes, the target utilized in the donor-specific assays; 3) depletion of the vectors of anti-donor immune activity from the peripheral blood due to sequestration in the allograft; and finally 4) limitations of the present *in vitro* technology to mimic *in vivo* conditions during allograft rejection.

On the other hand, measurement of the percent active T-RFC and spontaneous blastogenesis, two non-specific immune parameters, was more predictive or confirmatory of rejection episodes following allografting (Kerman et al., 1979). Presumably, the non-specific assays reflect fluxes in populations responsive to end organ attack or to lymphokines or mediators of allograft rejection. These indicators may be independent of the mechanism of rejection and of the target of the immune response. Since non-specific assays demand only simple technology, are reproducible, and permit daily measurements, they are presently more useful in monitoring allograft recipients than specific host anti-donor assays.

Two non-specific assays appear to detect emerging host reactivity: enumeration of the active T-RFC and measurement of spontaneous blastogenesis (Kerman et al., 1979; Kerman and Geis, 1978; Kerman and Geis, 1976; Hersh et al., 1971; Morris et al., 1978). Since cellular allograft rejection is probably mediated by T cells, numerous investigators have monitored their numbers (Kerman and Geis, 1978; Kerman and Geis, 1976; d'Apice and Morris, 1974; Buckingham et al., 1977). Two T cell populations can be identified based upon their differential ability to bind SRBC in rosette configurations (Fudenberg et al., 1975; Wybran and Fudenberg, 1973; Kerman et al., 1976). Total T-rosette forming cells (T-RFC) are enumerated after incubation of PBL and SRBC in an ice-water bath for at least one hour. The total T-RFC presumably represents all T cells in the peripheral blood. A second population, termed the active T-RFC (A-T RFC) is detected by rosette formation immediately after incubation of PBL and SRBC. A-T RFC has been proposed to be a subpopulation of the total T-RFC with surveillance properties more closely reflecting cell-mediated immune events than the total T-RFC (Kerman and Stefani, 1976; Kerman and Geis, 1978; Fudenberg et al., 1975; Wybran and Fudenberg, 1973).

There have been contradictory reports of the diagnostic value of the total T-RFC after renal transplantation. Thomas et al., (1976) claimed a good correlation between high levels of total T-RFC and acute rejection episodes: greater than 80% of recipients demonstrating acute rejection had a total T-RFC level above 20% of normal (360 T-RFC/mm^3). In contrast, the majority of patients not having acute rejection appeared to have total T-RFC levels below 20%. They claimed that when the total T-RFC levels were maintained below 20% in the early post-cadaveric transplant period, acute rejection was a rare event. In 85% of cases they found the onset of acute rejection to be heralded by a rise in the level of total T-RFC. However, T cell levels also rose above 20 percent in the absence of acute rejection, especially after the first transplant month. Buckingham et al. (1977) failed to confirm these findings.

An evaluation of total T and active T-RFC levels in transplant recipients by Kerman and Geis (1976, 1978) demontrated no association between rejection episodes and total T-RFC, but a good correlation with a decreased percentage of active T-RFC. The absolute numbers of either T cell population did not discriminate rejection, but rather the important index was the degree of change. In a recent report applying the same tests at an entirely different transplant center, Kerman et al. (1979) confirmed the diagnostic value of serial monitoring of active T-RFC in renal allograft recipients. Clinically apparent rejection episodes were always associated with decreased active T-RFC. Episodes of decreased active T-RFC, which were not associated with clinically apparent rejection episodes, and might therefore have been interpreted as false positive reactions, were usually associated with increased spontaneous blastogenesis and impaired renal handling of radionuclides, two sensitive measures of modest, subclinical events. All patients subsequently experienced clinically evident rejection episodes within 5-10 days.

The non-specific active T-RFC assay is easy to perform on a daily basis, since it does not require donor cells or large volumes of recipient blood. The decrease in active T-RFC prior to the onset of a clinically detected rejection episode presumably reflects specific host anti-donor T cell immune sensitization, leading to the release of lymphokines which attract and hold T cells in the attack on the end organ. Alternatively, donor alloantigens may activate T-RFC, causing increased expression or activity of the T-RFC receptor and resulting in active emigration of these cells from the peripheral blood to recognize and attack the renal allograft (Kerman et al., 1978).

The spontaneous blastogenic activity (SB) of peripheral blood mononuclear cells from renal allograft recipients presumably reflects the presence of circulating blastoid cells possibly due to an *in vivo* MLR response upon allogeneic stimulation. Transformed blasts capable of incorporating thymidine appear in the lymph draining transplanted kidneys (Hamburger et al., 1971). Significant increases in DNA or RNA synthesis occur prior to, or concomitant with, clinical signs of rejection in both renal and cardiac transplantation (Hersh et al., 1971; Morris et al., 1978). The studies presented herein confirm the prognostic value of the spontaneous blastogenesis test (Kerman et al., 1979).

The two non-specific immune monitoring assays, active T-RFC and SB, were used to monitor patients thrice weekly after renal allotransplantation . The immune parameters were correlated with: 1) glomerular and tabular function tests and 2) serial measurements of kidney function by radionuclide studies of glomerular function utilizing ^{99m}Tc-DTPA and of tabular function with ^{131}Hippuran. The radionuclide studies were processed using an MDS-Trinary 32 K computer and graded on a scale of 30 to yield ratios of kidney/aorta (normal = 5, score = .08), kidney/background DTPA concentration ratios (normal = 5, score = 3.0), DTPA bladder appearance time (normal = 5.0, score = <4.49 minutes), hippuran kidney/background ratio (normal = 5, score = <4.49 minutes) and peak hippuran renogram (normal = 5, score = <4.49 minutes). Immunological and radionuclide studies were performed and interpreted blindly by individuals unaware of the patient's clinical course.

The following sequence of events was consisently observed in 63 acute cellular rejection episodes (no hyperacute rejections occurred) displayed by 47 renal allograft recipients during their first 30 postoperative days: 1) an initial immediate increase in SB and decrease in active T-RFC following transplantation surgery; 2) an increase in SB prior to (76%) or at the same time (24%) as clinical evidences of rejection; 3) a decrease in active T-RFC concomitant with or shortly after increased SB; 4) a decrease in SB and increase in active T-RFC with resolution or rejection. Clinically apparent rejection episodes were significantly associated (p<0.01) with abnormal radionuclide studies of kidney function, that is, a 5–6 point (or 25%) decrease in the combined computer analysed scores. The results of the immunological and radionuclide monitoring displayed an excellent correlation (p<0.001) with graft rejection.

During the first 30 post-operative days of 47 renal allograft recipients who experienced 63 acute rejection episodes, there occurred 121 immune events (increased SB and decreased active T-RFC) and 102 abnormal (decreased) radionuclide scans (Table 3). There were 63 immune events and 58 cases of decreased radionuclide scans, that is, 5 rejection episodes occurred in the absence of a prior decreased radionuclide scan (Table 3, Line 1). The 58 remaining immune events, which occurred in the absence of clinical rejection, were associated with impaired renal function by the radionuclide scan in 44 cases (Table 3, Line 2). There were 14 remain-

Table 3. Immunologic and Radionuclide Results of 63 Treated Rejection Episodes during the First 30 Post-Operative Days in 47 Non-ATG Treated Patients.

	CONCOMITANT FINDINGS			
	↓ % ACTIVE T-RFC	↑ SPONTANEOUS BLASTOGENESIS	↓ RADIONUCLIDE SCANS	CLINICAL REJECTION
Line 1	63	63	58	63
Line 2	58	58	44	0
Line 3	14 [a]	14 [a]	0	0
Line 4	4 [b]	4 [b]	0	0

[a] 14/121 = 11.5% false positive immune events
[b] 14 Extra A T-RFC and spontaneous blastogenesis less 10 infection related events = 4
4/121 = 3.3% false positive immune events

ing extra immune events in the absence of either clinical rejection or an impaired radionuclide scan (Table 3, Line 3). That these 14 episodes do not represent an 11.5% rate of false positive results was concluded from documentation of ten infectious episodes occurring at these times. Thus 10 of the 14 paradoxical immune events may have possibly been due to infection. Thus, the false positive rate is 3.3% (4/121; Table 3, Line 4).

The application of serial immune monitoring with these two non-specific assays and radionuclide scanning is illustrated in Figure 1. Figure 1 shows the immunologic monitoring data following transplantation of a cadaveric kidney HLA-A3, -; B12, BW35; CW4, -, into a 33 year-old recipient (HLA-A29, A31; B12, BW35, CW4, -) with renal failure due to chronic pyelonephritis in crossed ectopic kidneys. Following a modest rejection reaction at day 6 clinically associated with 1) significantly reduced creatinine clearance, 2) change in albumin clearance and 3) significant hypertension and also as evidenced by a change in both immune and radionuclide parameters there was return of graft function. At day 13 increased spontaneous blastogenesis was accompanied by decreased active T-RFC and a subsequent decline in handling of radionuclides on day 19 all unassociated with significant clinical changes except for increased hypertension on day 18. This triad might have been a premonition of a clinical rejection episode. Although there was a modest decrease in radionuclide handling by the kidney on day 25, accompanied by changes in immune parameters, significant chemical and clinical signs of rejection (decreased creatinine clearance, increased albumin clearance and significant hypertension) were not evident until day 28 when therapy was instituted

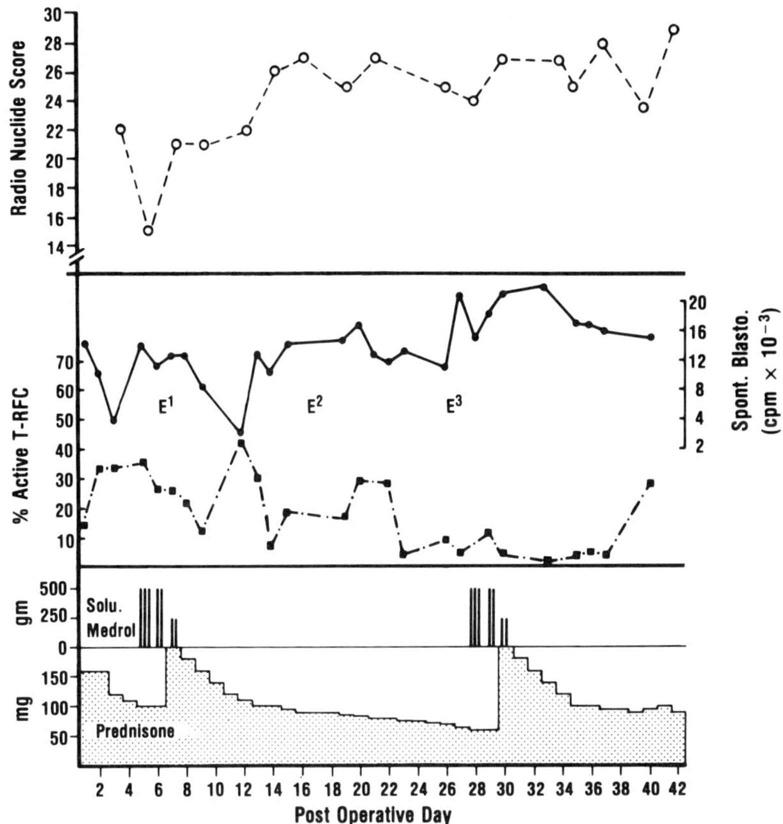

Figure 1. Serial immunological monitoring data of renal transplant no. 24.

with prompt restoration of renal function and resolution of the immune parameters.

These data suggest that alterations in two non-specific immune assays, when coupled with computerized radionuclide scans, afford early indices of rejection. Immune events always occurred prior to clinical detection of rejection. Resolution of the active T-RFC fall prior to institution of additional immunosuppressive therapy, may be due to 1) internal homeostatic regulation, such as spontaneous activation of suppressor cells; 2) entrapment in the organ followed by a second wave of release of additional cells; 3) a possible cellular role of the active T-RFC to activate other T cell subpopulations or antibody production leading to subsequent attack on the end organ; or 4) effects of humoral antibody or chemotactic factors on cellular homing or traffic patterns. The trigger and the control of these T cell fluxes is unclear.

CONCLUSION

Immunological monitoring has evoked considerable interest as an early diagnostic key to the events leading to allograft rejection. Presumably, sophisticated analysis should reveal and dissect the antigenic determinants eliciting alloimmunity. However, since rejection is mediated by a complex interplay of cellular and humoral effector mechanisms, it is unlikely that any single test will provide the crucial data in every case. Indeed, the failure of available techniques to detect alloimmune reactions precipitating clinical rejection underlines the limited utility of tissue typing for HLA-A and B antigens. It is uncertain whether matching for the DRW antigens, which may represent the serologically identified analog of the HLA-D locus, will improve cadaveric allograft survival. Of potentially great import is the application of non-specific immune evaluation of potential allograft recipients prior to transplantation. Preliminary data suggest that intrinsic immune competence may be an important determinant of graft outcome. Patients with weak immune responsiveness as determined by low numbers of active T-RFC, anergy to microbial skin test antigens, low spontaneous blastogenesis and poor response to allogeneic stimulation from a panel of unrelated lymphocytes displayed prolonged graft survival compared to strong responders.

One cannot be assured of compatibility based upon present typing techniques. A pre-transplant cross-match assessing specific host anti-donor reactivity must be performed to detect potential presensitization. We recommend a battery of LDA, CDA, LMC and K cell assays using recipient materials directed against ^{51}Cr-labelled donor targets, in addition to the visual cross-match technique. Patients with positive pre-transplant reactivity experienced accelerated or early acute rejection and a high incidence of graft loss. However, this battery of assays may not delineate recipient pre-sensitization against all relevant antigens, since it is only directed against determinants represented on peripheral blood lymphocytes, and does not reflect potentially important determinants on kidney or endothelial cells.

Since the major cause of renal allograft loss is rejection, immunological monitoring assays may be important probes to detect emerging recipient sensitization and afford indices for prompt therapy. Immune reactions against donor lymphocytes in CDA, LDA, LMC or K cell assays do not correlate with clinically defined rejection episodes. Indeed, documented episodes were not accompanied by demonstrable immunity, presumably due to 1) use of inappropriate target cells (i.e., lymphocytes) as target antigens; 2) infrequency of testing; or 3) compartmentalization of recipient elements into the allograft and therefore inaccessible in the peripheral blood. Since the relevant antigens or immune reactions mediating rejection are variable and not well understood, it presently appears more feasible to monitor non-specific cellular assays. Combined alterations in two tests, the percent active T-RFC and spontaneous blastogenesis, correlate with renal functional changes be it subclinically as altered handling of radionuclides or clinically as rejection. Furthermore, when alterations in the two non-specific immune assays were combined with changes in the computerized radionuclide tests, one obtained a more reliable index to diagnose rejection than that afforded by the presently available donor-specific assays. The present success of non-specific methods should only be regarded as an impetus for dissection of the actual antigen provoking renal allograft immunity, in order to obtain scientific and diagnostic skills to detect the evolution of specific host immunity.

REFERENCES

Guttman, R., N.: Eng. J. Med., *301*:975 (1979).

Terasaki, P. I., Opelz, G. and Mickey, M. R.: Transplant. Proc., *10*:417 (1978).

Opelz, G. and Terasaki, P. I.: Transplantation, *21*:483 (1976).

Williams, G. M.: Transplant. Proc. *11*:4 (1979).

Mittal, K. K., Kahan, B. D. and Bergan, J. J.: Transplantation, *19*:410 (1975).

Ting, A., and Morris, P. J.: Lancet, *1*:575 (1978).

Persijn, G. G., Gabb, B. W., van Leeuwen, A. et al.: Lancet, *1*:1278 (1978).

Kerman, R. and Kahan, B. D.: In, *Current Trends in Histocompatibility,* Reisfeld, R. and Ferrone, S., Eds. Plenum Press, 1979 (in press).

Kerman, R. H., Ing, T. S., Hano, J. E. and Geis, W. P.: Surgery, *82*:607 (1977).

Rolley, R. T., Widman, D. G., Parks, L. C., Sterioff, S. and Williams, G. M.: Transplant. Proc., *10*:505 (1978).

Wilson, W. E. C. and Kirkpatrick, C. H.: In, *Experience in Renal Transplantation* T. Starzl, ed. W. B. Saunders, New York, pp. 239, 1964.

Kerman, R. H., Floyd, M., Conner, W., McConnell, B. J., McConnell, R., Van Buren, C. T. and Kahan, B. D.: Transplant Proc., *11*:1229 (1979).

Kerman, R. and Stefani, S.: In, *Neoplasms Immunity: Mechanisms,* R. G. Crispen, ed., University of Illinois Press, p. 109 (1976).

Kerman, R. H. and Geis, W. P.: Transplant Proc., *10*:633 (1978).

Kerman, R. H. and Geis, W. P.: Surgery, *79*:398 (1976).

Hersh, E. M., Butler, W. T., Rossen, R., Morgan, R. O. and Suki, W. J.: J. Immunol. *107*:571 (1971).

Morris, R. E., Dong, E., Struthers, C. M., Griepp, R. B. and Stinson, E. B.: Transplant. Proc., *10*:585 (1978).

d'Apice, A. J. and Morris, P. J.: Transplantation, *18*:20 (1974).
Buckingham, J. M., Ritts, R. E., Woods, J. E. and Ilstrup, D. M.: Mayo Clin. Proc., *52*:101 (1977).
Fudenberg, H. H., Wybran, J. and Robbins, O.: New Engl. J. Med.: *292*:475 (1975).
Wybran, J. and Fudenberg, H. H.: N. Engl. J. Med., *288*:1072 (1973).
Kerman, R., Smith, R., Ezdinli, E. and Stefani, S.: Immunol. Comm., *5*:685 (1976).
Thomas, F., Lee, H. M., Wolf, J. S., Mendez-Piron, G., and Thomas, J.: Surgery, *79*:408 (1976).
Kerman, R. H., Roesler, H. and Kahan, B. D.: Fed. Proc., *37*:1686 (1978)
Hamburger, J., Dimitriu, A., Bankir, L. and Crosnier, J.: Nature, *232*:633 (1971).

DISCUSSION

HERSH: It's interesting that I have to come two-and-a-half thousand miles to find out what's happening 150 yards away! Have you done a logistic regression analysis on the four-parameter data? That has been extremely useful in immunological studies and other clinical studies of cancer patients and is necessary to identify the prognostic values of greatest relevance.

KERMAN: The data that I'm showing now are the result of our first analysis done about 6 months ago on the first half of our patients who were non-ATG treated. At that point there seemingly was no delineation in terms of importance of one parameter over another. I think it was a matter of small numbers, when we broke them up. But we now have over 120 transplants and I'm preparing to re-do the analysis of the approximately 80 to 90 non-ATG treated patients. Hopefully, we can then get some idea about the hierarchy of parameters.

HERSH: I have two more brief questions. First, I take it you have not yet started a protocol for the prophylactic treatment of the rejection episodes that you diagnose immunologically? Second, I know you also have a keen interest in malignant disease and I was wondering whether you have any data applying these immunological assays to immunological staging of cancer patients?

KERMAN: The answer to the first question is no, we have not. In answer to your second question, I do have data from some work done about three years ago in lung cancer patients with inoperable disease who were treated by conventional radiation therapy alone, or with radiation and BCG in combination. In measuring the percentage of active T-cell, prior to the institution of therapy, those patients with high percentages of active T-cell could be predicted to live longer than those with low percentages; in addition, those patients who converted from low to high, following the institution of therapy as opposed to those who did not change from low to high, had prolonged survival and that included the BCG conversions. So it was seemingly prognostic. I don't want to emphasize this too strongly, because I think the study needs to be repeated with more patients. We studied about 40 patients.

HADDEN: If your false positives represent infectious episodes, how could you decide to treat rejection prophylactically in the absence of alteration of renal function?

KERMAN: In transplant patients, when rejection episodes occur, they are diagnosed clinically vis-a-vis weight gain, BUN, creatinine, clearance, and temperature, and sometimes the intuition of the attending surgeon. They are treated with pulses of solu-medrol (500 mg $\times$ 2 for days; 250 mg c $\times$ 2 for one day; et cetera). You may end up giving an accumulation of 5 or 6 grams of solu-medrol in a two- to three- week period of time. If we immune monitored and saw an increase in blastogenesis and a decrement in active T-cells, we would pulse with a dose of solu-medrol 500 mg $\times$ 2, or with a dose smaller than that. We would continue to do this until we saw resolution of the immune event, regardless of the presence of clinical signs of rejection. The immune event that preceded diagnosed rejection was potentially the leading edge of the rejection reaction albeit subclinical, i.e., insufficient accumulated kidney damage. If we shut that immune response off, we could potentially halt accumulated kidney damage; or at least see a smaller immune event, encounter less kidney damage, and be required to give less steroid. We therefore, could stop the steroid pulsing based on the resolution of the immune event; but not necessarily that based on the resolution of chemistry factors.

In terms of infections, we have an infectious disease consultant on daily rounds with us. There were some 60 different infections in these patients. Many were associated with rejection; many occurred with declining radionuclide parameters. Once again, we encountered kidney function decrement; however, ten incidents occurred in the absence of rejection or change in radionuclide parameters, i.e., independent of kidney function. Thus, these ten incidents were clearly caused by the infection. Now, if we consider 10 percent false positive due to infection episodes, verified by the infectious disease consultants we would stop pulsing with solu-medrol.

YUNIS: I was curious about the data on correlation of immune vigor before transplantation when you assess nonspecific parameters. Were those data collected from patients who received transplants from cadavers or living donors?

KERMAN: We get them from both. The data presented here are reflective of cadaveric transplants.

YUNIS: What happens in patients with living-donor transplants? Do you find infections?

KERMAN: Yes.

YUNIS: Have you analyzed the data for haploidentical donors?

KERMAN: We had four antigen matches.

YUNIS: For haploid?

KERMAN: The data are essentially identical. There were slight changes in terms of survival time, but, as I stated, the data were essentially identical. This is very interesting because, as you know, haploid identical transplants essentially do as well as cadaveric ones at one year.

YUNIS: So you would predict, then, that if you assessed immune vigor in cadaver transplantation and tried to correlate HLA by matching the different numbers of antigens, there might be correlation in one group, let's say in the less vigorous immune group rather than in the one that has immune vigor. Do you think the discrepancy might be related to the matching?

KERMAN: No, in the patients with values above the median of a parameter in each of the groups, when we put strong and weak responders in whatever parameter we are looking at, there was no HLA mismatch difference. We looked at this but I didn't mention it. If you look at active T-cells above and below the median, the low T-cell, pre-transplant recipients had better graft survival. There was no difference in HLA-B mismatch between either group. So it was not dependent on the matching. I apologize for not stating that before.

YUNIS: And my last question is that as you know, some people claim that transfusions are important in this kind of situation. Is it possible that the lower immune vigor group had received more transfusions?

KERMAN: Yes, it's entirely possible. At this point I cannot answer this very important question on the influence of transfusions because we have no data on the patients' transfusion history.

McCOY: I'll just make one final comment. Dr. Kerman indicated that there seems to be no correlation between specific *in vitro* assay monitoring and the *in vivo* transplant graft acceptance or rejection. I think this raises the very important issue of how well these assays are standardized in your laboratory, to the point that you can say with confidence: We can measure a specific phenomenon, whether the response is against a recall antigen or HLA antigens. I think it would be unfortunate to leave the audience with an impression that specific monitors are not relevant. Would you like to comment on this?

KERMAN: My point on that is the following: At least in renal transplant, where we think there is a defined antigen, i.e., HLA, we use donor lymphoid cells as targets for *in vivo* testing of specific anti-donor reactivity. We find that only half of the time there is a correlation of a positive *in vitro* kill with clinical rejection. This suggests that you've got sensitivity and the patient is killing his kidney clinically. The other half of the time, however, there is a positive or negative *in vitro* response in the face of a contrary negative or positive clinical response.

I think this is because 1) we are looking for immune elements in the peripheral blood that may not be there because they are on the kidney, therefore we get a clinical reaction with a negative *in vitro* assay; or 2) we are looking for an *in vitro* assay, presumably against the defined antigens. In fact, however, the *in vitro* reaction has no relationship to *in vivo* rejection; that's why we don't get good correlation of *in vitro* reaction with rejection.

The carry-over of this is that it's very hard to identify specific antigens, whether you're talking about tumors or transplants, and I think it is better if you can use nonspecific assays where you do not have to ask the question: Do I have defined antigenic moiety that I can look at *in vitro* as a predictor or as a serial monitor?

7
Lymphoproliferative Responses to Alloantigens by Postoperative Patients with Stage I Lung and Breast Cancer and Their Application to Prognosis

Grace B. Cannon
Jack H. Dean
Ronald B. Herberman

*Department of Immunology, Litton Bionetics, Inc.,
Kensington, MD
Immunology Section/Environmental Biology Branch,
National Institute of Environmental Health Science,
Research Triangle Park, NC
Laboratory of Immunodiagnosis, National Cancer Institute,
National Institutes of Health, Bethesda, MD*

INTRODUCTION

In cancer of the breast, lung, and other neoplastic diseases in which the primary tumor can be removed by surgery, the probability of developing recurrent disease is appreciable and variable. Clinical and pathological staging have been utilized to assess prognosis in order to assist in further therapy decisions. In breast cancer, other prognostic variables have been combined with the clinical and pathological prognostic variables in an attempt to improve predictions concerning the course of the disease (Cooperative Breast Cancer Study Group, 1978; Kister et al., 1979; Cooke

98

et al., 1979). However, even with improved staging only 43% of Stage I lung cancer patients remain free of disease at 2 years after surgery and 30% appear to be cured following surgical resection of all detectable tumor (Mountain et al., 1974). The long-term outlook for breast cancer is also grave in that only 74% of Stage I patients survive for 5 years and 45% of Stage 2 patients survive for 5 years (Brinkley and Haybittle, 1975) and the cure rate for all cases at 20 years is only 16-30% (Adair et al., 1974).

In the present study, we have evaluated the application of an assay of immune competence to prognosis in Stage I lung cancer patients and patients with resectable breast cancer. It has previously been shown that some lung cancer patients have depressed lymphoproliferative responses to various stimuli (Ducos et al., 1970; Rees et al., 1975; Han and Takita, 1972; Catalona, Sample and Cretien, 1973; Dean et al., 1977, 1979). In breast cancer patients, the pretreatment lymphoproliferative response has been depressed less frequently (Stein et al., 1976; Teasdale et al., 1979). A study was initiated in 1974 to test lung and breast cancer patients with immune competence assays in the postoperative period (at least one week and usually by two months following surgery) and prior to any other form of therapy. We have recently analyzed these results relative to the present disease states of the patients and have found that the immune competence of these patients as measured by their lymphoproliferative response to allogeneic peripheral blood mononuclear cells in a one-way mixed leukocyte culture (MLC) was related to their subsequent disease-free interval (Cannon et al., 1979). The standardization of our assay with the relative proliferation index (RPI) (Dean et al., 1977) was important in quantitation of the patients' responses.

MATERIALS AND METHODS

Ficoll-Hypaque separated peripheral blood mononuclear leukocytes (PBML) from 35 lung cancer patients from the Medical University of South Carolina (MUSC), the National Naval Medical Center, Portsmouth Naval Hospital and Walter Reed Army Medical Center and 95 breast cancer patients from MUSC and the George Washington University Hospital were tested in a microculture LP assay as previously described in detail (Dean et al., 1977). All of the lung cancer patients were classified as having Stage I disease and the breast cancer patients all had resectable disease and most had radical mastectomy. Staging in lung cancer was based on the pathology report, using the information on tumor size and lymph node involvement which was obtained at surgery and by histopathologic examination, according to established guidelines (Harmer, 1978). Patients with all histological types of lung cancer except small cell carcinoma were included in the study. Patients with a history of any other form of cancer, including previous breast cancer or bilateral breast cancer were excluded from the analysis.

The breast cancer patients were classified into two groups based on the presence or absence of axillary lymph node metastases as this has proven to be the single most useful prognostic factor in patients with invasive cancer (Cooperative Breast Cancer Study Group, 1978; Kister et al., 1979). Information on the nodal status was obtained from pathology reports on each patient and the patients were classified as having negative nodes (57 patients) or positive nodes (38 patients) based on these reports. All tests were performed prior to clinical evidence of tumor recurrence and the majority of patients were tested within the first 2 months following surgery. None of the lung cancer patients received any other form of therapy prior to disease recurrence. All of the breast cancer patients were tested prior to any other form of therapy, but many subsequently received radiation or chemotherapy. To ensure that the time at which the initial LP test was performed did not bias the results, the time of the test rather than the time of surgery was used as the starting point of the life tables. Data analyzed with the surgery date as the starting point showed the same pattern of results as the time of test as the starting point, but the actual length of time between the test and recurrence is evident when the test is used as the starting point (time 0).

The PBML were tested for LP responses to alloantigens, using mitomycin-C (MMC)-treated cryopreserved allogeneic PBML from a standard pool of six leukophoresis donors in one-way mixed culture (MLC) (Dean et al., 1977). MLC cultures were terminated on day 7 following a 6-hour pulse with 1 μCi of tritiated thymidine (^{3}H-TdR; New England Nuclear, Boston, MA; specific activity 6.7 Ci/mmole).

LP responses in the MLC were expressed as a relative proliferation index (RPI) (Dean et al., 1977), which was calculated as follows:

$$\frac{\text{nCPM of test individual}}{\substack{\text{Mean nCPM of normal individuals} \\ (\geqslant 3) \text{ tested simultaneously}}}$$

with nCPM = counts per minute (CPM) of PBML incubated with stimulant minus CPM of PBML incubated alone. Most (90%) of the normal individuals used in these tests were less than forty years old. However, Dean et al., (1977) have shown that the median RPI for normal donors in older age groups was also very close to 1.0.

Cutoff values were set at the lowest tenth percentile of RPI of a large number of normal donors and any response falling below this tenth percentile cutoff in MLC ($\geq$ .50) was considered depressed.

Each patient was classified as normal or depressed in their MLC response according to the results of the initial test following surgery.

Disease-free distributions by the Kaplan-Meier product-limit estimate were performed with the BMDPIL program, to evaluate the effect of the clinical variables (BMDPIL, 1977). Patients were classified in this program into a relevant number of mutually exclusive categories and the length of the disease-free intervals following the time of the test was compared (among these categories). Disease-free statistics were computed based on individual survival time free of disease. Persons entered the study at different times over a 4-year period and were on study for different lengths of time. An attempt was made to use as much of the available data as possible, so the study period was not restricted. Thus, all patients were lost to study by recurrence or were censored (i.e., their time on study was less than the time interval for which disease-free survival statistics were calculated).

Tests of significance were made by the Breslow (generalized Wilcoxon) and Mantel-Cox (chi-square) methods. In the results, p values obtained with both methods are given. The first computes the rank order significance of length of disease-free intervals between the test groups. Using the rank order rather than the actual disease-free interval minimizes the effect of long-term survivors, or conversely weights earlier events more heavily. The second test, Mantel-Cox, is a calculation of the departure of the distribution of events from what would be expected if there were no effect due to the ascribed categories, summed overall by a chi-square procedure.

Many comparisons were made with this program. The categories used to analyze the effect of immunologic response was depressed (RPI $\leq$ .50) MLC, compared to normal (RPI $>$ .50) MLC. Separately, patients were divided into either $T_1N_0M_0$ or $T_2N_0M_0$ and $T_1N_1M_0$ for lung cancer and into positive or negative axillary breast cancer nodes.

RESULTS

Lung Cancer

Incidence of depression in MLC response relative to disease recurrence

The LP response in MLC was used to determine the incidence of immune depression among these post-surgical Stage I lung cancer patients. Twelve of thirty-five (34%) patients were depressed (MLC RPI $\leq$ .50). During

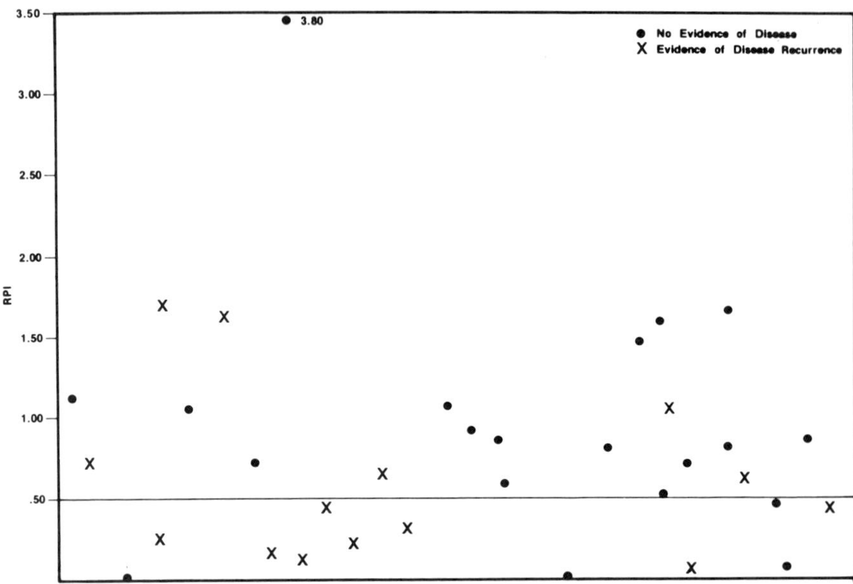

Figure 1.   Scattergram of relative proliferation indices of 35 post surgical Stage I lung cancer patients.

the course of our study, twelve patients have been demonstrated to have clinical evidence of disease recurrence. Eight of the patients with disease recurrence had been depressed in the MLC response post surgery and prior to clinical evidence of disease recurrence (Figure 1).

Relationship between LP response and disease-free interval

To determine the usefulness of the test for prognosis, the lung cancer patients were separated into two groups based on the normal versus depressed MLC response. The disease-free interval of the normal LP responders was significantly longer than the disease-free interval of the patients depressed in MLC, $p = .0019, .0012$ (Figure 2). The time interval between the test and recurrence is shown and ranged from 65 days to 690 days. All four patients in the depressed LP groups who have remained without evidence of disease have been followed for less than two years since their test. In contrast, eight of seventeen of the apparently disease-free normal LP responders have been followed for more than 2 years since their tests. Four of the six patients in the normal LP group who

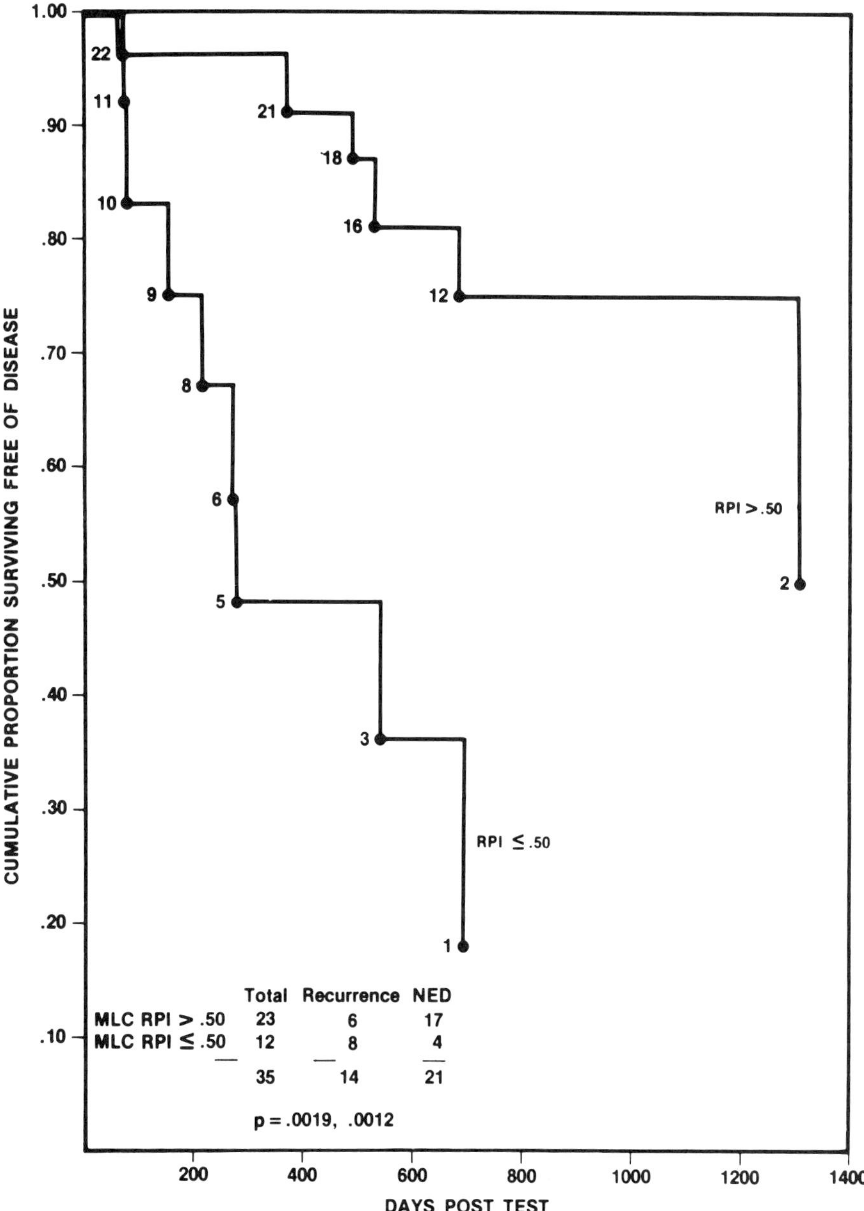

Figure 2. Recurrence time in days in Stage I lung cancer patients with normal proliferative responses to alloantigen (MLC RPI > .50) and patients with depressed proliferative response to alloantigen (MLC RPI < .50). Numbers on graph refer to actual number of patients remaining disease-free at the corresponding time points. The first p value was calculated by the Breslow (generalized Wilcoxon) method and the second p value by the Mantel-cox (chi-square) method as described in Materials and Methods.

103

developed recurrent disease had epidermoid carcinomas and three were female. In fact, the incidence of disease associated depression was higher in the males $(7/10)$ than in the females $(\frac{1}{4})$.

Relationship between pathologic classifications and disease-free interval

When these same patients were subdivided according to the TNM classification, the disease-free interval was longer for the patients in the $T_1N_0M_0$ category than the combined $T_2N_0M_0$ and $T_1N_1M_0$ patients, but not significantly, p = .73, .48 (Figure 3).

When the histological type was used to classify these same patients, the mean disease-free interval of the epidermoid patients was slightly longer than that of the adenocarcinoma patients. The shortest disease-free interval was in the combined anaplastic, alveolar category. However, these disease-free intervals were not significantly different as is shown in the Kaplan-Meier plot, p = .51, .38 (Figure 4).

Relationship between LP response and disease-free interval for patients with a particular pathological category

It was of interest to determine whether MLC responses have prognostic value for patients with the same pathological stage of disease. Five of 17 patients with $T_1N_0M_0$ disease developed clinical evidence of recurrent disease and four had a depressed response in MLC. The patients depressed in MLC had a significantly shorter disease-free interval than the normal responders, p = .006, .005. Thus, the immunological test could identify a subset of patients with increased risk of recurrence, among a group of patients considered to have early, localized disease.

Twelve of eighteen patients who were classified as $T_2N_0M_0$ or $T_1N_1M_0$ were normal in their MLC response. They had a longer disease-free interval than the patients depressed in MLC but not to a significant degree, p = .13, .14.

Twenty of the patients had epidermoid lung cancer. Eleven of the fifteen patients with normal MLC remained disease-free as compared to only two of five of the patients depressed in MLC; the disease-free intervals of the two groups differed, but not significantly, p = .09, .08.

Among the fifteen patients in the study with other histologic types of lung cancer, those depressed in MLC had a significantly shorter disease-free interval than the normal responders, p = .013, .008. Five of seven of the LP depressed patients developed disease recurrence as compared to two of eight of the normal responders.

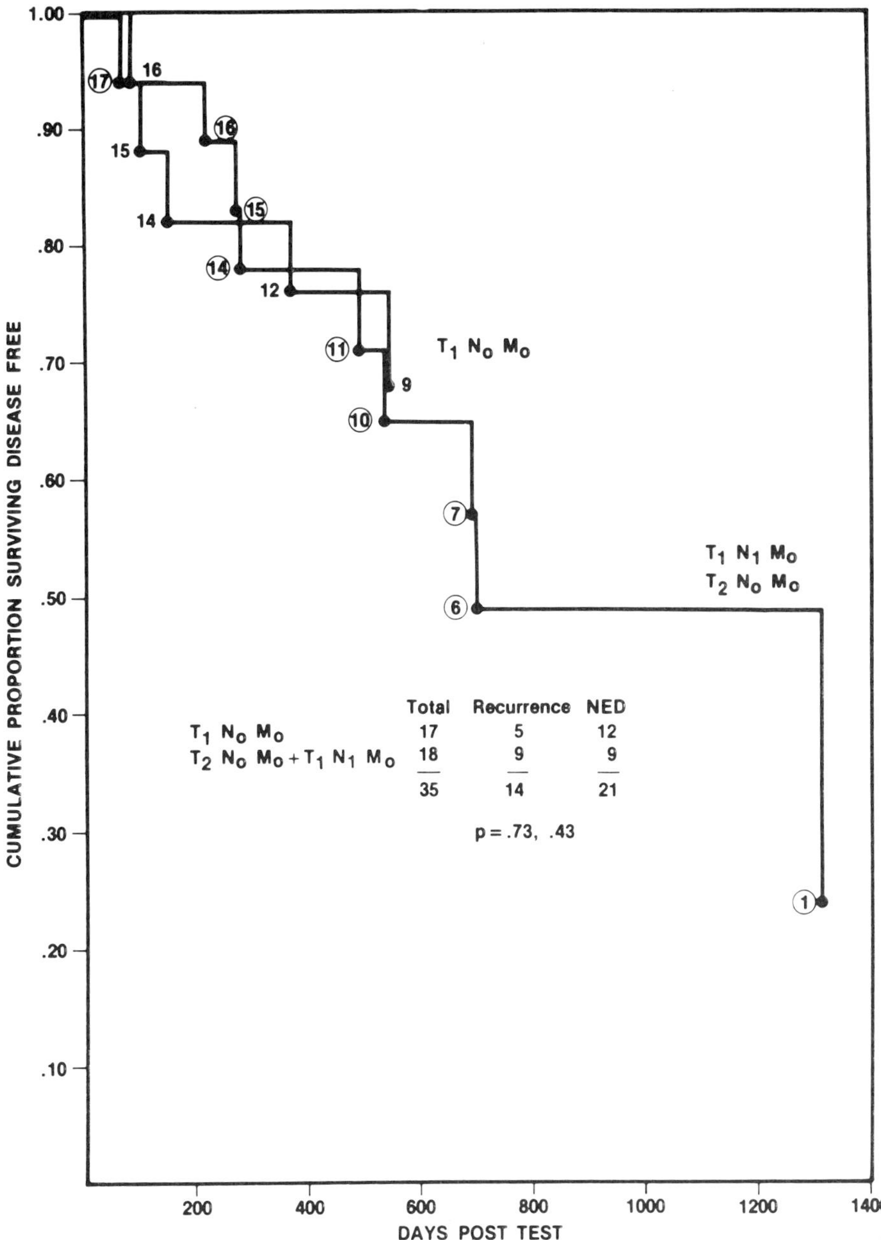

Figure 3. Recurrence time in days in the same Stage I lung cancer patients as in Figure 2, but according to TNM classification, $T_1 N_0 M_0$ and $T_1 N_1 M_0$ and $T_2 N_0 M_0$ combined.

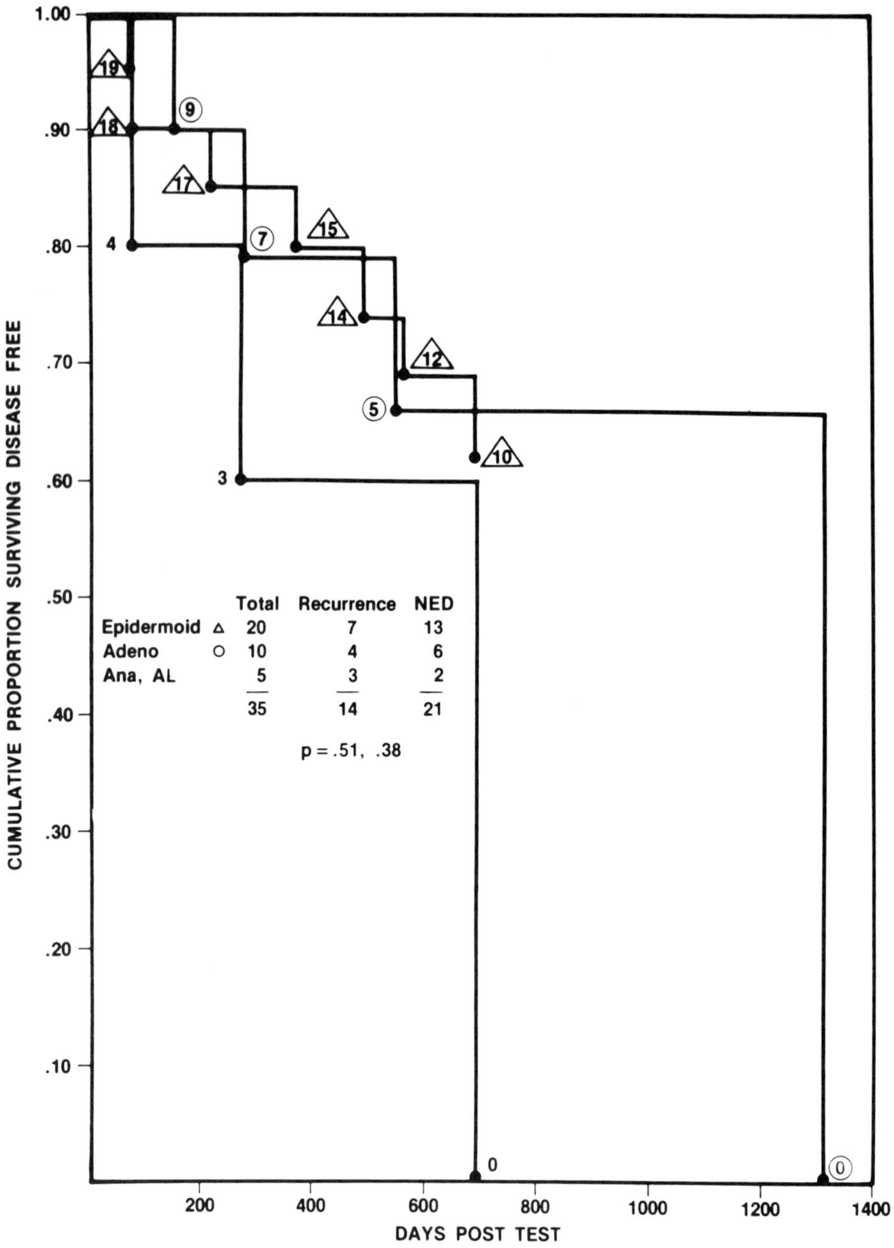

Figure 4. Recurrence time in days in the same Stage I lung cancer patients as in Figures 2 and 3, but according to histological type, epidermoid, adenocarcinoma and anaplastic and alveolar combined.

Breast Cancer

*Relationship between depression in MLC response
and disease recurrence*

The incidence of depressed MLC responses among the post-surgical breast cancer patients (23 of 93 or 23%) was less than that of the lung cancer patients. Twelve of fifty-seven (21%) patients without nodal involvement and eleven of thirty-eight (29%) patients with nodal involvement were depressed in MLC. Unexpectedly, breast cancer patients with depressed MLC had a low incidence of recurrent disease (1/23) (Figure 5), in contrast to the association of depressed MLC and disease recurrence in lung cancer. Twenty-four of the twenty-five breast cancer patients that developed clinical evidence of disease recurrence had a normal MLC response in their early post-surgical test.

To determine the value of the test for prognosis, the breast cancer patients were divided into two groups relative to their normal or depressed MLC response. The disease-free interval of the depressed LP responders was significantly longer than the disease-free interval of the

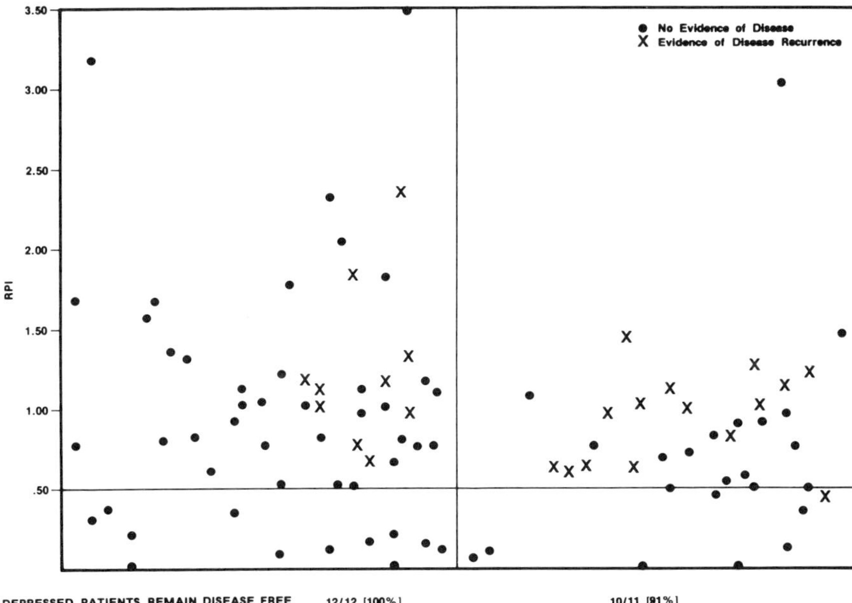

Figure 5. Scattergram of relative proliferation indices of 57 post surgical breast cancer patients with negative nodes on the left and 38 post surgical breast cancer patients with lymph node metastases on the right.

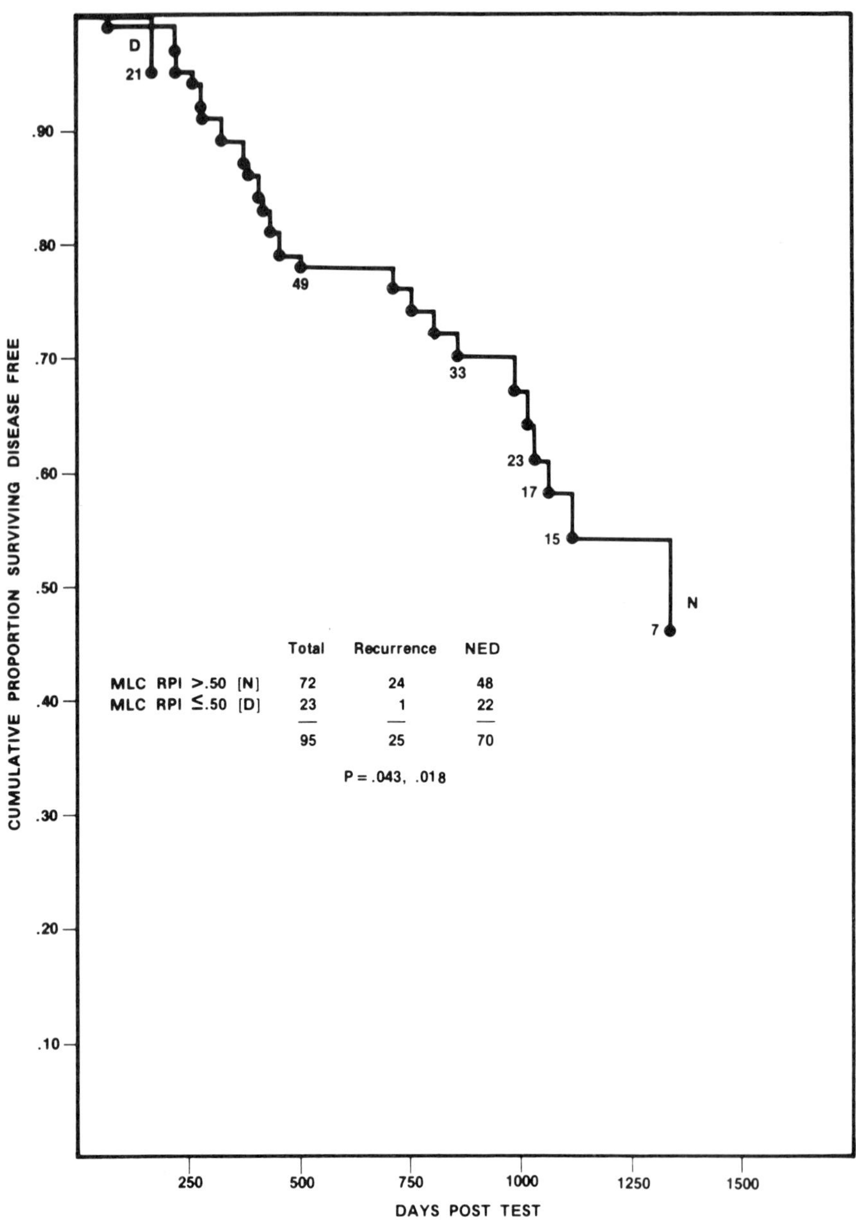

Figure 6. Recurrence time in days in resectable breast cancer patients with normal proliferative response to alloantigens (MLC RPI > .50) and patients with depressed proliferative response to alloantigens (MLC RPI < .50). Numbers on the graph refer to actual number of patients remaining disease-free at the corresponding time points.

patients normal in MLC, p = .043, .018 (Figure 6). The time interval between the test and recurrence ranged from 178 days (four and one half months) to 1020 days (thirty-three months). Seven of twenty-two (32%) LP depressed patients have been followed for more than three years since their test and have remained free of clinical evidence of disease, as have thirteen of forty-eight normal responders.

Relationship between pathological classifications and disease-free interval

When these breast cancer patients were categorized according to presence or absence of metastases in their axillary lymph nodes, the disease-free interval was longer for the patients with negative nodes than those with positive nodes, but not significantly, p = .110, .063 (Figure 7).

Relationship between LP response and disease-free intervals for within a particular pathological category

It was of interest to determine whether MLC responsiveness had prognostic value for patients within a particular pathological stage of disease. Fifty-seven of the breast cancer patients had no detectable evidence of tumor metastases in their lymph nodes according to their pathology report and the majority of them had at least ten nodes examined. All of the patients who developed clinical evidence of disease recurrence had a normal response in MLC. In contrast, none of the patients with depressed MLC responses have developed disease recurrence. Although this conforms to the same pattern as the overall group of breast cancer patients, in the smaller number of Stage I patients the normal MLC responders did not differ significantly from the MLC depressed patients, p = .112, .100. Approximately twenty-five percent of the normal responders in each group who remain disease-free have been followed for more than three years.

A high proportion (14/15) of these patients identified by their pathology to have lymph node metastases and who developed disease recurrence had a normal MLC response. Only one of eleven patients with depressed MLC developed recurrent disease. The difference in disease-free interval between the two groups approached significance, p = .149, .064. Only four of the thirteen patients (4/13, 31%) with the normal MLC response and no evidence of disease recurrence had been followed for more than three years as compared to four of ten (40%) of the depressed patients who remain disease-free. Thus, the follow-up time may

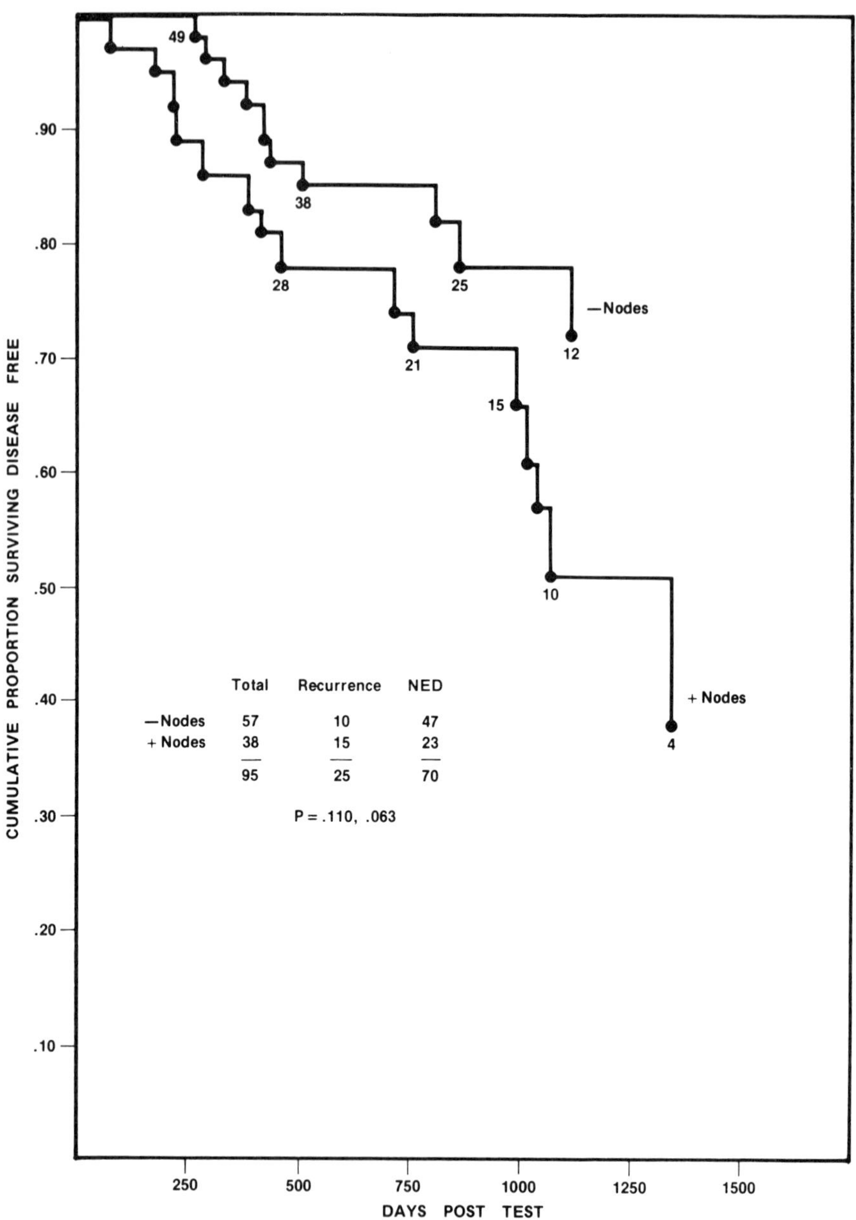

Figure 7.   Recurrence time in days in the same breast cancer patients as in Figure 6, but according to the presence (+ nodes) or absence (− nodes) of metastases in their axillary lymph nodes.

not be adequate to detect significantly disease associated immune responses within two pathological categories of breast cancer patients.

Relationship between MLC responsiveness and lymphoproliferative response to autologous tumor

Although MLC responsiveness provides some indication of cellular immune competence, lymphoproliferative responses to autologous tumor antigen would seem more relevant to host resistance against development of recurrent disease. We therefore evaluated the relationship of the response in MLC to the response of autologous hypotonic extracts of tumors. In lung cancer, there was a positive correlation of the patients' responses to the two stimulators (Figure 8). However, most of the breast cancer patients responded much more in MLC than to the autologous extract. By Spearman's rank correlation coefficient, the simultaneous responses of the lung cancer patients were significantly correlated ($p < .05$, $r = +.56$) and the breast cancer patients simultaneous responses were minimally correlated ($r = +.04$). In lung cancer, four of seven patients who were tested with both stimulants and who showed evidence of disease recurrence were depressed to both stimulants ($< 10,000$ CPM). In breast cancer, it appears that the particularly poor prognostic group is that of patients who have the ability to respond normally in MLC but are unreactive to the tumor extract.

DISCUSSION

Depressed lymphoproliferative responses have been described in many studies of cancer patients (Ducos et al., 1970; Rees et al., 1975; Han and Takita, 1972; Catalona, Sample and Chretien, 1973; Dean et al., 1977; Liebler et al., 1977; Dalbow et al., 1977; Dean et al., 1978; Hersh and Oppenheim, 1965; Cohen et al., 1973; Graze, Perlin and Royston, 1976; Faquet, 1975; Mellstedt and Holm, 1973; King et al., 1976; Matchett, Huang and Kremer, 1973; Garrloch, Good and Gatti, 1970; McKhann et al., 1975; Golub, O'Connell and Morton, 1974; Whittaker, Rees and Clark, 1971; Weese et al., 1977). However, it is unclear from most studies how frequently depression occurs in patients with early stages of disease and whether depressed reactivity correlates with prognosis. The present study has evaluated the prognostic usefulness of MLC responsiveness in patients with resected primary lung and breast cancer. For immunologic tests to aid clinicians in their evaluation and care of cancer patients, it is important that they be able to categorize patients

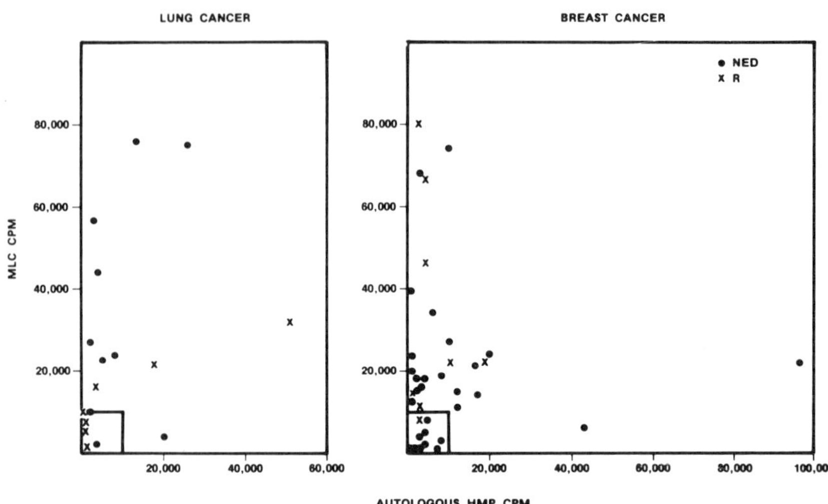

Figure 8.   Correlation graph of the proliferative response in MLC and to autologous tumor hypotonic membrane preparations (HMP) in simultaneous tests of lung and breast cancer patients.

beyond the point presently available. For this reason, we studied whether MLC reactivity could identify good and poor prognosis patients within groups in which all evident disease has been removed. The tests were performed early so that their subsequent usefulness could be evaluated. The time immediately following surgery was found to be superior to that before surgery (Cannon et al., unpublished observations). The MLC reactivity in this early post-operative period seems most predictive of subsequent detectable recurrence and may reflect important T-cell-mediated defense mechanisms operative at a particularly critical time for the host, when the operative stress and removal of the primary tumor may have altered the host-tumor balance or when tumor cells released during surgery are in the circulation or are as yet not established as metastatic foci.

To explain the apparent paradox of an association of immune depression with poor prognosis in lung cancer and with favorable prognosis in breast cancer, it is worthwhile to consider the elegant studies of immunologic responsiveness and neoplasia in mice and to consider the type of cellular immune function that the MLC is measuring.

The MLC measures recognition by T-cells of alloantigens determined by the major histocompatibility complex and present on the lymphocyte surface membrane. It appears that a subpopulation of T-cells is involved in this reaction, with some cells undergoing a proliferative response and others developing into cytotoxic effector cells (Bach, 1974). Recent studies have indicated that recognition of a wide variety of foreign antigens, including tumor antigens, is influenced to a large extent by parallel recognition of antigens of the major histocompatibility complex (Zinkernagel et al., 1978; Gooding, 1976).

In some tumor systems, particularly those induced by viruses, T-cell competence appears to be critical for effective resistance against tumor growth (Law, 1966). Neonatal thymectomy or other procedures producing depression or elimination of T-cell function have been associated with increased incidence of such tumors. The observations in patients with lung cancer would be consistent with such experimental data, since a significantly higher incidence of recurrent disease was seen in patients with depression in one measure of T-cell competence.

The critical protective role for T-cells has not been seen in a variety of other experimental tumor systems. Of particular possible relevance to our observations of the association of a low MLC and a low incidence of disease recurrence in breast cancer patients, neonatal thymectomy of C3H mice, which normally have a high incidence of spontaneous mammary tumors, resulted in a lower frequency of tumors and an increased latent period (Martinez, 1964). This, in both mouse and human breast cancer, functional integrity of some subpopulations of T-cells may actually contribute to enhanced tumor growth. Along this line, Small (1977) has shown that one subpopulation of T-cells is responsible for inhibition of growth of a transplantable tumor and another T-cell subpopulation acts as supressors of effective host resistance. In that tumor system, partial ablation of T-cell function reduced suppressor T-cell activity and led to reduced tumor growth. In breast cancer patients, maintenance of normal reactivity in MLC may reflect or correlate with functionally active suppressor T-cells, which interfere with effective defense against development of recurrent disease. Lack of lymphoproliferative response to autologous tumor antigens, in the presence of normal reactivity in MLC, may be a good indicator of this unfavorable balance. Clearly, more studies are needed to explore the mechanisms underlying these intriguing correlations in breast cancer patients.

Regardless of the immunologic mechanisms responsible for the correlations between MLC reactivity and prognosis, this study has demonstrated that measurement of this function may have important practical value in the management of patients with resectable lung and breast cancer. One test performed during the early postoperative period appeared to be a better discriminator of prognosis than were TNM classification, nodal involvement or histological type of tumor. Of particular importance, MLC reactivity appeared to subdivide otherwise indistinguishable patients with local disease, into patients with high or low risk of developing recurrent disease. If this discriminatory ability of the MLC is confirmed in further prospective studies, this procedure may allow better staging of patients and identification of high risk patients who might be candidates for adjunctive chemotherapy or immunotherapy.

It should be noted that some particular aspects of the methodology used for our measurements of MLC reactivity may have been of critical importance for generating data with this degree of discrimination. A rather large pool of cryopreserved allogeneic leukocytes was used as stimulant, which probably provided a more standard degree of stimulation than the more usual one-way MLC with one allogeneic donor. Furthermore, calculation of the relative proliferation index probably contributed to less variation among assays (Dean et al., 1977) and permitted better discrimination between normal and low reactors.

CONCLUSIONS

Thirty-five Stage I lung cancer patients and ninety-five resectable breast cancer patients were tested in the early postoperative period to assess lymphoproliferative responses. Depressed lymphocyte proliferation (LP) responses to alloantigens in one-way mixed leukocyte culture (MLC), expressed as the relative proliferation index (RPI), were associated with a significantly shorter disease-free interval in Stage I lung cancer and a significantly longer disease-free interval in resectable breast cancer. In this group of patients, a single MLC test performed during the early postoperative period appeared to be a better discriminator of prognosis than were TNM classification, nodal involvement or histological type of tumors. The lymphoproliferative response in MLC was significantly correlated to the lympoproliferative response to autologous tumor hypotonic membrane preparations in lung cancer and not in breast cancer. Patients who developed recurrent breast cancer had a normal blastogenic response in MLC and minimal response to their autologous tumor.

ACKNOWLEDGMENTS

The authors are indebted to Ms. Frances LeSane, Ms. Brenda Baumgardner and Ms. Connie Leonard for technical assistance, to Ms. Joyce Siwarski and Ms. Marion Keels for collection of the clinical information; to Ms. Carolyn Fox for preparing the manuscript; and to Mrs. Connie LeBash for preparation of the figures. The authors wish to thank Drs. J. Reid, E. Perlin, C. Miller, R. Bradham, E. Parker, W. Cain, H. Gregorie, J. Hawk, J. Stallworth, M. Lipton, R. Cathcart, D. Appleby, P. O'Brien and N. Walsh for supplying patient blood and follow-up information on the patients included in the study.

REFERENCES

Adair, F., Berg, J., Joulbert, L., Robbins, G. F.: Long-term follow-up of breast cancer patients: The 30-year report. Cancer, *33*:1145–1150 (1974).

Bach, F. H.: Normal histocompatibility antigens as a model for tumors. Amer. J. Clin. Path., *62*:173–183 (1974).

BMDPIL, The Life Table and Survival Functions, Health Sciences Computing Facility, University of California, Los Angeles (1977).

Brinkley, D. and Haybittle, J. L.: The curability of breast cancer. Lancet *2*:95–97 (1975).

Cannon, G. B., Dean, J. H., Herberman, R. B., Perlin, E., Reid, J., Miller, C. and Lang, N. P.: Association of depressed postoperative lymphoproliferative responses to alloantigens with poor prognosis in patients with Stage I lung cancer. Int. J. Cancer, (in press) (1980).

Catalona, W. J., Sample, W. F. and Chretien, P. B.: Lymphocyte reactivity in cancer patients: Correlation with tumor histology and clinical stage. Cancer, *31*:65–71 (1973).

Cohen, L. and Howe, M.: Syngenism between subpopulations of thymus derived cell mediating the proliferative and effector phases of the mixed lymphocyte reaction. PNAS, *70*,2707–2710 (1973).

Cohen, G., Douglas, S. D., Konig, E. and Brittinger, G.: *In vitro* lymphocyte response to phytohemagglutinin and pokeweed mitogen in Hodgkin's disease. An electron microscope and function study. Cancer, *31*:1946–1953 (1973).

Cooke, L., Howe, D., Shields, R., Maynard, P. and Griffiths, K.: Estrogen receptors and prognosis in early breast cancer. Lancet, *31*:1946–1953 (1979).

Cooperative Breast Cancer Study Group. Identification of breast cancer patients with high risk of early recurrence after radical mastectomy. II. Clinical and Pathological Correlations. Cancer, *42*:2809–2826 (1978).

Dean, J. H., Connor, R., Herberman, R. B., Silva, J., McCoy, J. L. and Oldham, R. K.: The relative proliferation index as a more sensitive parameter for evaluating lymphoproliferative responses of cancer patients to mitogens and alloantigens. Int. J. Cancer, *20*:359–370 (1977).

Dean, J. H., McCoy, J. L., Cannon, G. B., Connor, R. J., Weese, J., Oldham, R. K. and Herberman, R. B.: Lymphocyte proliferation responses of patients with carcinoma of breast or lung to mitogens, alloantigens and tumor-associated antigens. Proc. Third. Int. Symp. on Detection and Prevention of Cancer, pp. 525–546 (1978).

Dean, J. H., Cannon, G. B., Jerrells, T. R., McCoy, J. L and Herberman, R. B.: Sensitive measurements of immunocompetence and anti-tumor reactivity in lung cancer patients and possible mechanisms of immunosuppression. Proc. Chicago Symposium.

Ducos, J., Mingueres, J., Columbies, P., Kessous, A. and Poujoullet, N.: Lymphocyte response to PHA in patients with lung cancer. Lancet, *1*:1111–1112 (1970).

Faquet, G. G.: Quantitation of immunocompetence of Hodgkin's disease. J. Clin. Invest., *56*:951–957 (1970).

Garrloch, D. B., Good, R. A. and Gatti, R. A.: Lymphocyte responses to PHA in patients with non-lymphoid tumors. Lancet, *1*:618 (1970).

Golub, S. H., O'Connell, T. X. and Morton, D. L.: Correlation of *in vivo* and *in vitro* assays of immunocompetence in cancer patients. Cancer Res., *34*:1833–1837 (1974).

Gooding, L. R.: Expression of early fetal antigens on transformed mouse cells. Cancer Res., *36*:3499–3502 (1976).

Graze, P. R., Perlin, E. and Royston, I.: *In vitro* lymphocyte dysfunction in Hodgkin's disease. J. Natl. Cancer Inst., *56*:239–243 (1976).

Han, T. and Takita, H.: Impaired lymphocyte responses to allogeneic cultured lymphoid cells in patients with lung cancer. N. Engl. J. Med., *286*:605–606 (1972).

Harmer, M. H. (Editor): TNM classification of malignant tumors. Int. Union Against Cancer, pp. 4–45 (1978).

Hersh, E. M. and Oppenheim, J. J.: Impaired *in vitro* lymphocyte transformation in Hodgkin's disease. N. Engl. J. Med., *273*:1006–1012 (1965).

King, G. W., Yanes, B., Hurtubise, P. E., Balcerzak, S. P. and Lobuglio, A. F.: Immune function of successfully treated lymphoma patients. J. Clin. Invest., *57*: 1451–1460 (1976).

Kister, S., Aroesty, J., Rogers, W., Huber, C., Willis, K., Shagola, G. and Lincoln, T.: An analysis of predictor variables for adjuvant treatment of breast cancer. Cancer Chemotherapy Pharmacology, *2*:147–158 (1979).

Law, L. W.: Studies of thymic function with emphasis on the role of the thymus on oncogenesis. Cancer Res., *26*:551–574 (1966).

Liebler, G. A., Concannon, J. P., Magovern, G. L., Dalbow, M. H. and Hodgson, S. E.: Immunoprofile studies for patients with bronchongenic carcinoma. I. Correlation of pretherapy studies with survival. J. Thor. Cardiovas. Surg., *74*:295–302 (1977).

Martinez, C.: Effect of early thymectomy on development of mammary tumors in mice. Nature, *203*:1188 (1964).

Matchett, K. M., Huang, A. T. and Kremer, W. B.: Impaired lymphocyte transformation in Hodgkin's disease. Evidence for depletion of circulating T-lymphocytes. J. Clin. Invest., *52*:1908–1917 (1973).

McKhann, G. F., Slade, M. S., Gunnarsson, A. and Burk, M. W.: Lymphocyte responsiveness in cancer and transplantation. Transplant. Proc.,*7*:287–290 (1975)

Mellstedt, H. and Holm, G.: *In vitro* studies of lymphocytes from patients with plasma cell myeloma. I. Stimulation by mitogens and cytotoxic activities. Clin. Exp. Immunol., *15*:309–320 (1973).

Mountain, C. F., Cores, D. T. and Anderson, W. A. D.: A system of the clinical staging of lung cancer. Ther. Nucl. Med., *120*:130–138 (1974).

Rees, J. C., Rossio, J. L., Wilson, H. G., Minton, J. P. and Dodd, M. C.: Cellular immunity in neoplasia. Antigen and mitogen responses in patients with bronchiogenic carcinoma. Cancer, *36*:2010–2015 (1975).

Small, M.: Characteristics of the immature cells involved in T-cell mediated enhancement of syngenesis tumor growth. Journal of Immunol., *118*:1517–1523 (1977).

Stein, J. A., Adler, A., Ben Efraim, S. and Maor, M.: Immunocompetence, immunosuppression and human breast cancer. Cancer, *38*:1171–1187 (1976).

Teasdale, C., Hillyard, J. W., Webster, D. J. T., Bollon, P. M. and Huges, L. F.: Pretreatment general immune competence and prognosis in breast cancer. A prospective 2-year follow-up. European Journal of Cancer, *15*:975 (1979).
Weese, J. L., Oldham, R. K., Tormey, D. C., Barlock, A. L., Moreales, A., Cohen, M. H., Alford, T. C., Shorb, P. E., Tsangaris, N. T., West, W. H., Cannon, G. B., Dean, J. H., Djeu, J., McCoy, J. L. and Herberman, R. B.: Immunologic monitoring in carcinoma of the breast. Surg. Gynec. Obst.,*145*:209–218 (1977).
Whittaker, M. G., Rees, K. and Clark, C. G.: Reduced lymphocyte transformation in breast cancer. Lancet, *1*:892–893 (1971).
Zinkernagel, R. M., Callahan, C. N., Klein, J. and Dennert, G.: Cytotoxic T-cells learn specificity for self H-2 during differentiation in the thymus. Nature, *271*: 251–253 (1978).

DISCUSSION

HERSH: I think that the question of the depression associated with surgery in studies like this is very important. Several studies done over the years have shown that immune depression after surgery can last a fairly long time. You have shown us data for breast cancer. In lung cancer patients did you have the opportunity to do both pre- and postsurgery studies, and was there a relationship between the degree of depression induced by surgery? In other words, the sensitivity, if you will, of the immune system and the subsequent prognosis?

Also, in the breast cancer patients, did any receive adjuvant therapy after surgery, and did that relate to the results in any way?

CANNON: In the lung cancer patients, we tested very few both before and after surgery and so I really can't relate it. We tested only four and I just don't think it's meaningful.

We have not specifically studied the effect of surgery, but certainly these tests were done quite soon after surgery and could well be associated with surgery but, we have centered our study on the fact that they were associated with a subsequent disease status.

In reply to your question: Did they receive adjuvant therapy? Most of these breast cancer patients were from the Medical University of South Carolina. All had received radiation; very few had received adjuvant chemotherapy. This study was started in 1974.

KERMAN: Did all patients in the lung cancer study receive the same treatment?

CANNON: They all had surgery. Some had pneumonectomy, some lobectomy, but none received subsequent therapy. Some of the patients were part of a BCG study but the ones we presented today did not receive BCG.

KERMAN: Several years ago I was involved in a study of patients with inoperable lung cancer who had received radiation therapy. In that study we investigated the percentage of active T-cells. The high responders showed prolonged survival compared with the negative responders; this included patients with both locally advanced or metastatic disease. I can corroborate that your survival time by clinical staging was meaningless. It was the same in our study. At that time we tried to convince the radiation therapist to give these patients curative courses of therapy. We suggested palliative treatment, rather than 4,000, 5,000 or 6,000 rads for the patients with locally advanced disease, who were low responders. Have you requested the surgeons to treat patients with more aggressive therapy for positive responders and less aggressive therapy for low responders?

CANNON: We have done immunotherapy on another group of patients, and I think it's possible that this may apply to that group, but so few of them have relapsed that I cannot make any conclusions and, unfortunately, we tested only a few of them prior to the initiation of immunotherapy.

KERMAN: Do you show conversions with immunotherapy on the low responders?

CANNON: I do not know because it is difficult to interpret the effects of the immunotherapy. We are performing a very extensive study of that right now, because we have found great fluctuations with immunotherapy, and we feel that it's important to evaluate this by using the person as his own control. We think one has to look at what the pre-immunotherapy level was, very carefully, before one can interpret the results with immunotherapy and ascribe the results as due to the immunotherapy.

8
Investigation of the Immunobiological Effects of Polybrominated Biphenyls in Michigan Farmers

J. George Bekesi, Henry Anderson, Julia P. Roboz, and Irving J. Selikoff

Department of Neoplastic Diseases and Environmental Sciences Laboratory, Mount Sinai School of Medicine, New York, New York

INTRODUCTION

A commercial preparation containing polybrominated biphenyls (PBB) was inadvertently used in place of magnesium oxide in the preparation of a special feed supplement for lactating cows (Carter, 1976; Dunckel, 1975). The contaminating PBB preparation was identified as Firemaster FF-1, a flame retardant manufactured by the Michigan Chemical Company (Sundstrom et al., 1976). The contaminated feed supplement contained an estimated PBB level of 4,000 to 13,500 ppm (Kay, 1977). Adverse effects of PBB on animals were first reported by Jackson and Halbert in 1974, noting that the contaminated feed caused anorexia and a 40% drop in milk production of cows within a few weeks. Although the supplemented feed was removed within 16 days, milk production failed to return and the weight loss of the herd continued. A portion of the herd developed hematomas, abscesses, abnormal hoof growth, alopecia, thickening of skin; wasting and death occurred within six months to 24 of the group of 400 exposed cows (Jackson and Halbert, 1974; Humphrey

"

and Hayner, 1974). Similar observations were made on a number of 6-18 month old heifers and bulls. Some of the animals appeared to have atrophied testicles and abnormal semen showing no spermatozoal motility, with numerous headless and tailless spermatozoa (Jackson and Halbert, 1974). In total, during 1973 and 1974 more than 500 Michigan dairy herds and poultry farms were quarantined and over 30,000 cattle and 1.5 million chickens died or had to be destroyed (Carter, 1976; Dunckel, 1975; Jackson and Halbert, 1974).

Dairy products containing PBB (beef, poultry, eggs, milk, cheese, butter) were widely consumed in Michigan until 1978 (Carter, 1976; Dunckel, 1975; Jackson and Lambert, 1974, Anderson et al., 1978; Lilis et al., 1978). PBB was subsequently found in the serum and/or adipose tissues of dairy farm residents, workers employed by the Michigan Chemical Co., as well as in many urban Michigan residents (Humphrey and Hayner, 1974; Anderson et al., 1978; Lilis et al., 1978; Wolf et al., 1978; Bekesi et al., 1978).

Experimental data suggest that polybrominated biphenyls, which are similar to polychlorinated biphenyls, are fat-soluble and are stored in the thymus, liver, brain and adipose tissues, and persist in those tissues for very long periods of time (Fries and Marrow, 1975; Guttenmann and Lisk, 1975; Erney 1975; Fehringer, 1975). Because of toxicity and lack of active metabolism of halogenated biphenyls, there has been concern over the short- and long-term health consequences in exposed Michigan residents (Anderson et al., 1978; Lilis et al., 1978; Wolf et al., 1978; Lee et al., 1975; Sleight and Sanger, 1976; Lee et al., 1975; Farber and Baker, 1975; Moore et al., 1976; Kimbrough et al., 1978).

We have previously reported functional abnormalities in the peripheral blood lymphocytes of Michigan dairy farmers who consumed contaminated food (Bekesi et al., 1978, 1979a, 1979b). Abnormalities included a decrease in the numbers and percentages of T-lymphocytes, increase in lymphocytes with no detectable surface markers ("null cells"), and impaired lymphocyte functions. There was no consistent correlation found between PBB concentration in the plasma and immune dysfunction (Bekesi et al., 1978).

In a recent report by Roboz et al. (1980) it is indicated that there is higher concentration of the most abundant hexaisomer (2,2',4,4',5'5' hexabromobiphenyl) on the surface membrane of white blood cells and erythrocytes as compared to plasma. The β lipoprotein fraction appears to be the major protein carrier in the plasma and there is a strong suggestion of correlation between the high PBB content in white cells and β

lipoprotein fraction, and the decreased immunological functions found in the PBL of the PBB-exposed subjects.

Data reported here represent a brief summary of our findings obtained from PBB-exposed subjects in Michigan (Bekesi et al., 1978, 1979a, 1979b; Roboz et al., 1980).

Subject Population

Two groups of subjects were examined: a.) 45 adult dairy farm residents, from quarantined and nonquarantined farms, who have eaten PBB-contaminated food for a period of 3 months to 4 years; b.) 46 Wisconsin dairy farmers and members of their families who did not eat PBB-contaminated food. In addition, the lymphocyte functions of the survey team members participating in this study were also examined. Table 1 summarizes the major characteristics of the two study groups. Approximately equal numbers of males and females were examined in the study. However, the mean age of the PBB-exposed individuals was lower than that of the control population.

EXAMINATION OF POSSIBLE ADVERSE EFFECTS OF TRANSPORTATION ON THE LYMPHOCYTE FUNCTION

The question immediately arose: to what extent, if at all, transportation of blood specimens might alter the functional integrity of peripheral blood lymphocytes. All blood samples were carried on the plane journey from Wisconsin and Michigan to the Mount Sinai School of Medicine in New

Table 1.

	WISCONSIN DAIRY FARM RESIDENTS	PBB EXPOSED MICHIGAN FARM RESIDENTS
Number of Subjects	46	45
Males	30	25
Females	16	20
Mean Age	45.0 ± 9.5	35 ± 12.8
WBC	6.5 ± 0.2	7.1 ± 2.2
Lymphocytes	32.4 ± 7.9	32.7 ± 4.6

Approximately equal number of males and females were examined in the study. However, the mean age of the PBB-exposed individuals was younger than the control population.

Table 2.   Effect of Transportation on the Lymphocyte Function.

	FRESHLY DRAWN BLOOD *			18 HRS AFTER BLOOD SAMPLES WERE DRAWN AIRPLANE TRANSPORTATION †		
	SUBJECTS			SUBJECTS		
WBC $\times$ $10^3/\mu l$	7.21	6.85	7.62	7.30	6.71	7.78
% Lymphocytes	34	30	35	35	31	33
T-cells						
%	77	72	68	76	74	70
Absolute no./μl	1888	1479	1814	1942	1539	1797
B-cells						
%	18	24	21	17	22	20
Absolute no./μl	441	493	560	434	458	513
PHA						
Maximum stimulation c.p.m. $\times$ 10^3	101.6	103.7	91.3	97.3	102.1	93.7

* Blood specimens were used for assays 60 minutes after blood was drawn.
† Blood samples were hand carried from Wisconsin to New York and tested 16 hours after blood was drawn.

York City. Similarly, control blood samples were obtained from personnel participating in the field study, and were sent along with the test subjects' blood specimens. The summary of our findings is shown in Table 2 and indicates that transportation of blood specimens at room temperature in the original plastic syringe did not alter the function and number of lymphocytes as compared to freshly drawn and processed blood specimens.

IN VIVO IMMUNOLOGICAL ASSESSMENT OF IMMUNOCOMPETENCE OF PBB-EXPOSED MICHIGAN FARM RESIDENTS

The *in vivo* cell-mediated immunity of 45 PBB-exposed Michigan dairy farm residents and 46 Wisconsin dairy farm control subjects who had not eaten PBB-contaminated food was measured by the delayed cutaneous hypersensitivity response to PPD, mumps, Candida, varidase and dermatophytin. The recall antigens were applied in the volar forearm by intradermal inoculation with a 27-gauge needle in a volume of 0.1 ml. Delayed cutaneous hypersensitivity response to antigens was read after 48 hours. Skin test was considered positive if the perpendicular bisector diameter of induration was $\geq$ 5mm. Data obtained from these *in vivo*

Table 3.   Delayed Hypersensitivity Response to Recall Antigens in Wisconsin and PBB Exposed Michigan Dairy Farm Residents.

RECALL ANTIGENS	WISCONSIN (CONTROL)	MICHIGAN (PBB EXPOSED)
PPD	8.7	0
Mumps	63.0	68.9
Candida	26.0	80.0
Varidase	50.0	77.8
Dermatophytin	41.3	17.8
No. of Subjects Tested	46	45

Skin test diameter at 48 hrs. $\geq$ 5 mm.

tests are presented in Tables 5 and 6. They show that 43 of 46 tested individuals in the control group responded to at least one recall antigen. In general, these subjects showed reactivity particularly to mumps, varidase and dermatophytin. There were 4 individuals of 46 who showed positive PPD reaction, but none in the PBB-exposed group (Table 5). Contrariwise, of the Michigan farm residents, sharing similar work and living conditions but who had eaten PBB-contaminated food for 3 months

Table 4.   Comparison of DCH Response to Five Recall Antigens.*

RESPONSE TO NO. OF RECALL ANTIGENS	% OF INDIVIDUALS RESPONDING	
	WISCONSIN (CONTROL)	MICHIGAN (PBB EXPOSED)
0	6.5	17.8
1	13.0	15.6
2	21.7	15.6
3	39.0	33.3
4	19.6	8.9
5		
No. of Subjects Tested	46	45

* Recall Antigens used: PPD, Mumps, Candida, Varidase, Dermatophytin Skin test diameter at 48 hrs. $\geq$ 5mm

Table 5.   Comparison of T-Lymphocyte Subpopulation and Function in the PBL of Wisconsin Versus the PBB Exposed Michigan Dairy Farm Residents.

| SUBJECTS | T-LYMPHOCYTES [1] [2] | | MITOGENS FOR T-CELLS [2] | | PROLIFERATIVE T-CELL [2] RESPONSE |
| | | | PHA | CONA | |
	%	ABSOLUTE NUMBER	MAX. STIM. C.P.M.	MAX. STIM. C.P.M.	MAX. STIM. C.P.M.
Wisconsion Dairy Farm	71.0	1,473 *	97,662	96,662	38,172
residents N = 46	±2.1	±63	±2,693	±3,151	±1,209
PBB-Exposed Michigan dairy farm residents					
a) with normal T-cell	60.0	1,341	92,272	94,634	28,248
function N-27	±1.8	±79	±2,231	±4,502	±2,072
b) with decreased	43.7 *	917 *	28,457%	36,117	10,147 *
T-cell function N-18	±4.1	±119	±3,406	±2,694	±317

[1] Spontaneous E-rosette-forming PBL's at 4°C with sheep red blood cells.
[2] Data are means ± standard error
* Statistical significance (Student's T-test) between maximum lymphoblastogenesis of Wisconsin farm residents and that of Michigan dairy farm residents p < .001

Table 6. **B-Lymphocyte Subpopulation and Function in the PBL of Wisconsin Versus the PBB Exposed Dairy Farm Residents.**

| SUBJECTS | TOTAL NUMBER OF MONONUCLEAR CELLS [1] PER mm^3 | B-LYMPHOCYTES [1] | | B-LYMPHOCYTE RESPONSE [1] |
		% [2]	ABSOLUTE [2] NUMBER	PWM MAX. STIM. C.P.M.
Wisconsin Dairy Farm	2,103	23.1	487	90,636
Residents N = 46	±149	±1.1	±29	±3,406
PBB-Exposed Michigan				
dairy farm residents:				
a.) with normal T-cell	2,214	21.4	467	93,199
function N = 27	±162	±1.3	±34	±7,412
b.) with decreased T-cell	2,098	15.8	331	39,159
function N = 18	±150	±1.4	±32	±3,537 p < .001

[1] Data are means ± Standard error
[2] Binding of PBL's with EAC

to 4 years, 8 (17.8%) of 45 were completely anergic to each of the recall antigens (Table 6). All of the 37 tested subjects in this group showed an increase in sensitivity and heightened response to Candida and varidase. However, the heightened response to these two antigens, was in most cases accompanied by a decline in number of T-cell subpopulation and function in the peripheral blood lymphocytes.

Preparation of Peripheral Blood Lymphocytes for the in Vitro Immunodiagnostic Tests

Peripheral blood (50 ml) was taken by venipuncture in a plastic syringe containing preservative-free heparin. The blood samples were hand carried at room temperature from Michigan and Wisconsin to New York City. In addition, control blood samples were sent along with the study samples from both Wisconsin and Michigan to investigate possible side effects of the plane journey on the specimens. Peripheral blood lymphocytes (PBL) were isolated and purified from blood by Ficoll-Hypaque sedimentation 12 to 18 hours after the blood was drawn. After separation, the lymphocytes were located at the interface of the gradient, washed three times with RPMI 1640 medium supplemented with 20% heat deactivated autologous plasma.

Quantification of Different Lymphocyte Subpopulations

Quantification of T- and B-lymphocytes was carried out by the method of Wybran and Fudenberg (1972) and Nussenzweig (1974) respectively. Lymphocytes with three or more E or EAC rosettes were considered to be positive. The percentage and number of PBL's without characteristic membrane markers was calculated by subtracting from the percentage or total number of mononuclear cells the percentage or absolute number of E plus EAC rosette-forming lymphocytes. Tables 5 and 6 show that the median value for Wisconsin farm residents' mononuclear cells is 2,103; 71% E-rosetting PBL, with 1,473 as the absolute number of T-lymphocytes; 23.1% EAC-rosetting PBL, with 487 as the absolute number of B-lymphocytes. Deviation from the normal range in both percent and absolute number of T-lymphocytes was observed in 18 out of 45 examined Michigan farm residents who had eaten PBB-contaminated food for a period of 3 months to 4 years (Table 5). There was no change, however, in the total number of mononuclear cells and only marginal decrease in B-lymphocyte subpopulation as compared to values obtained from the Wisconsin farm residents (Table 6). The most tangible change observed in the PBL of the PBB-exposed Michigan residents was the marked dominance of lymphocytes without any detectable membrane markers ("null cells") (Figure 1). This marked shift may be due to a defect in the maturation process of T-lymphocytes and/or to the selective binding of PBB to the surface membrane, thus masking the receptor sites in the T-lymphocytes.

Lymphocyte Function: Mitogens and Antigens

Lymphocyte blastogenesis for PBL was determined by selected mitogens: phytohemagglutinin (PHA) and Concanavalin A (ConA) for T-cells and pokeweed mitogen for B-cells. 100,000 purified PBL's were cultured in each of the five replicate wells of the Falcon microplates with RPMI-1640 medium supplemented with 20 percent heat-inactivated autologous plasma in the presence of high purity PHA (Burroughs Wellcome), ConA (Sigma Co.) or PWM (Gibco). Maximum stimulation occurred at 0.15 μg/well for PHA, 5 μg/well for ConA and 30μg/well for PWM. Lymphocyte blasto-

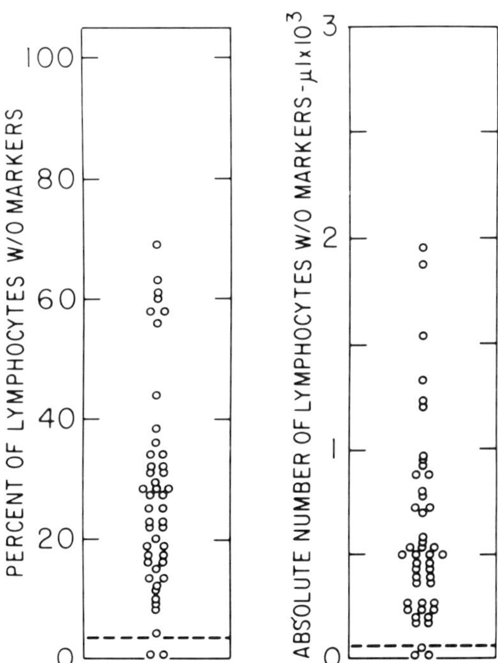

Figure 1   Increased percent and absolute number of "Null Cells" in PBB-exposed Michigan dairy farm residents

genesis was determined by measuring the level of DNA synthesis upon addition of 1 μCi of [³H] thymidine (New England Nuclear Co.) to each well 18 hours prior to termination of the culture. The amount of [³H] thymidine incorporated was determined in a Packard liquid scintillation spectrometer. One-way mixed leukocyte cultures were performed as follows: Stimulating PBL's from six different donors were incubated with mitomycin C (25 μg/ml of 2×10^6 cells in suspension) for 20 minutes at 37°C; cells were washed, then 2×10^5 were distributed in each of the replicate wells of the Falcon microplates containing 10^5 responding lymphocytes per well in RPMI-1640 medium supplemented with 20 % heat-inactivated autologous plasma. After 96 hours of incubation 1 μCi of [³H] thymidine was added to each well. Cultures were harvested 18 hours later with the addition of an excess of cold thymidine. Tables 5 and 6 summarize the maximum stimulation induced by PHA, ConA and PWM as well as the proliferative T-cell response to PBL obtained from Wisconsin and PBB-exposed Michigan dairy farm residents. The mean values of maximum stimulation of PBL obtained from Wisconsin farm residents were 97,662 c.p.m. for PHA, 96,662 c.p.m. for ConA, 90,636 for PWM and 38,172 c.p.m. for the proliferative T-cell response to alloantigens (Tables 5 and 6). Significant deviation from these values was apparent in at least 18 individuals in the Michigan group. In most cases, the decreased response to T-cell mitogens and decreased proliferative T-cell response was accompanied by a proportionately lower percentage and number of T-lymphocytes. However, in a few Michigan subjects the decreased response to T-cell mitogens occurred despite a normal range of lymphocytes, indicating a possible impairment in the function of T-lymphocytes. There was no apparent reduction of B-lymphocyte subpopulation in the PBL of Michigan farm residents who had eaten PBB-contaminated food. The PBL of a group of these subjects responded poorly to PWM. This decrease in response may reflect a.) a functional defect of B-cells and/or b.) a reduced helper T-cell subpopulation (Table 6). The lower proliferative T-lymphocyte response confirms and further extends our observations, made with all three mitogens, that immunocompetence of at least 30 percent of the Michigan dairy farm residents is at least partially impaired due to a reduction in their lymphocyte function as compared to control subjects in Wisconsin.

Distribution of Immunological Changes According to Family Units

The above described data were obtained from Michigan and Wisconsin dairy farm families. This allowed us to examine the possibility of genetic determinants which might affect the integrity of lymphocyte function in the

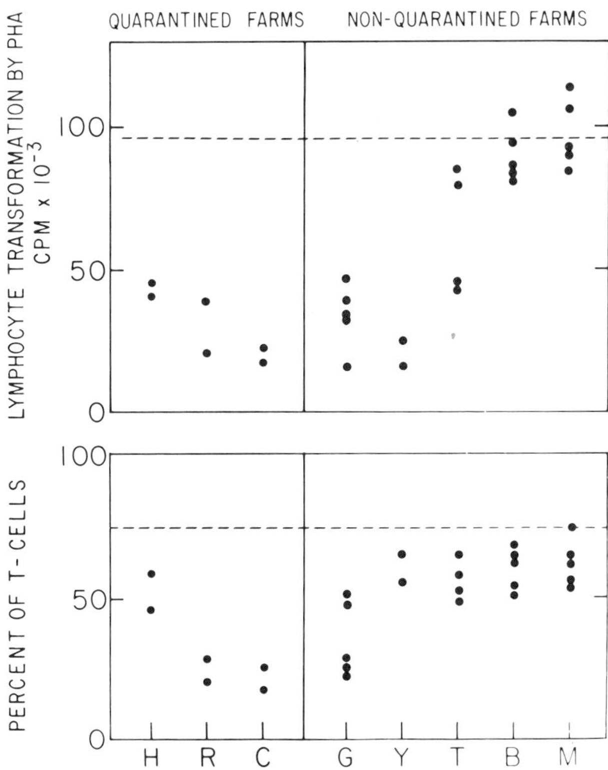

Figure 2   Lymphocyte function of peripheral blood lymphocytes in quarantined and nonquarantined Michigan farm residents who ate food containing PBBs.

PBB-exposed population. Figure 2 shows the cell-mediated immunity as measured by PHA-induced lymphocyte blastogenesis and the T-lymphocyte subpopulation in the PBL of three quarantined and five nonquarantined family units of PBB-exposed Michigan farm residents. Results presented in Figure 2 appear to indicate that the changes in lymphocyte function observed tend to affect families as a unit and appear to be independent of exposed individuals' age or sex. This diminishes the possibility of genetic predisposition and correlates well with the magnitude of PBB exposure from the common dietary sources of the affected families.

CONCLUSION

In 1973 Firemaster FF-1, a flame retardant containing polybrominated biphenyls, was accidentally mixed into cattle feed. Dairy products from contaminated animals (beef, poultry, eggs, milk, cheese, butter) were widely consumed in Michigan until 1978. The presence of PBB has been confirmed in human blood, fat and breast milk. Subsequently we observed functional abnormalities in the peripheral blood lymphocytes of Michigan dairy farmers who consumed contaminated food. Abnormalities included decreased numbers of T-lymphocytes with a concomitant increase of lymphocytes with no detectable surface markers ("null cells"). Significant reduction of immune function was noted in about 30% of the Michigan farm residents who had eaten food containing PBB. In some cases the impaired lymphocyte response can be attributed to decreased number of functional T-lymphocytes.

The immunological dysfunction detected among PBB-exposed subjects tended to affect families as a unit and was independent of age or sex, thus excluding the possibility of genetic predisposition.

ACKNOWLEDGMENTS

The cooperation of Drs. K. Rosenmann, M. S. Wolff and Wm. Rom is greatfully acknowledged. Thanks are also due to Rogena Brown, Frances Camper, Susan S. Gillman, Shirely Levine, Angeles Mison, Frances Perez and Robert Suzuki for technical assistance. We also gratefully acknowledge the excellent help and cooperation of the Marshfield Medical Foundation, Marshfield Medical Clinic in the course of our Wisconsin clinical field survey.

This research was supported by Center Grant for the National Institute of Environmental Health Sciences, ES00928 and by Contract N01–ES–9–0004.

REFERENCES

Anderson, H. A. R., Lilis, R., Selikoff, I. J.: Unanticipated prevalence of symptoms among dairy farmers in Michigan and Wisconsin. Environ. Health Perspect., *23*: 217 (1978).

Bekesi, J. G., Holland, J. F., Anderson, H. A., Fischbein, A. S., Rom, W., Wolff, M. S., Selikoff, I. J.: Lymphocyte function of Michigan dairy farmers exposed to poly-brominated biphenyls. Science, *199*:1207 (1978).

Bekesi, J. G., Anderson, H. A., Roboz, J. P., Roboz, J., Fischbein, A., Selikoff, I. J., Holland, J. F.: Immunological dysfunction among PBB-exposed Michigan dairy farmers. N.Y. Acad. Sci., *320*:717 (1979a).

Bakesi, J. G., Roboz, J., Anderson, A. H., Roboz, J. P., Fischbein, A. S., Selikoff, I. J., Holland, J. F.: Impaired immune function and identification of polybrominated biphenyls (PBB's) in blood compartments of exposed Michigan dairy farmers and chemical workers. Drug. and Chem. Toxicol., *2*:179 (1979b).

Carter, L. J.: Michigan's PBB incident: chemical mix-up leads to disaster. Science, *192*:240 (1976).

Dunckel, A. E.: An updating on the polybrominated biphenyl disaster in Michigan. J. Am. Vet. Med. Assoc., *167*:838 (1975).

Erney, M. J.: Confirmation of PBB residues in foods and dairy products, using ultraviolet irradiation-gas: Liquid chromatographic technique. J. Assoc. Off. Anal. Chem., *58*:1202 (1975).

Farber, T. M., Baker, A.: Microsomal enzyme induction by hexabromobiphenyl. Toxicol. Appl. Pharmacol., *29*:102 (1974).

Fehringer, V. N.: Determination of polybrominated biphenyl residues in dairy products. J. Assoc. Off. Anal. Chem. *58*:978 (1975).

Fries, F. G., Marrow, G. S.: Excretion of polybrominated biphenyls into the milk of cows. J. Dairy Science, *58*:6 (1975).

Gutenmann, W. H., Lisk, D. J.: Tissue storage and excretion in milk of polybrominated biphenyls in ruminants. J. Agric. Food. Chem., *23*:1005 (1975).

Humphrey, H. E. B., Hayner, N. S.: Polybrominated biphenyls; an agricultural incident and its consequences. An epidemiological investigation of human exposure. Michigan Department of Health, Lansing, Michigan, 1974.

Jackson, T. F., Halbert, F. L.: A toxic syndrome associated with the feeding of polybrominated biphenyls-contaminated concentrate to dairy cattle. J. Am. Vet. Med. Assoc., *165*:437 (1974).

Kay, K.: Polybrominated biphenyls (PBB) environmental contamination in Michigan, 1973–1976. Envir. Res., *13*:74 (1977).

Kimbrough, R. D., Burse, V. W., Liddle, J. A.: Persistent liver lesions in rats after a single oral dose of brominated biphenyls (FireMaster FF-1) and concomitant PBB tissue levels. Environ. Health. Perspect, *23*:265 (1978).

Lee, K. P. *et al.*: Octabromobiphenyl-induced ultrastructural changes in rat liver. Arch. Environ. Health, *30*:465 (1975).

Lee, K. P., Hebert, R. R., Sherman, H., Aftosmis, J. F., Waritz, R. S.: Bromine tissue residue and hepatotoxic effects of octabromobiphenyls in rats. Toxicol. Appl. Pharmacol., *34*:115 (1975).

Lilis, *et al.*: Comparison of findings among residents on Michigan dairy farms and consumers of produce purchased from these farms. Environ. Health. Perspect., *23*:105 (1978).

Moore, R. W., Danna, G., Aust, S. D.: Induction of drug metabolizing enzymes in rats nursing from mothers fed polybrominated biphenyls. Fed. Proc., *35*:709 (1976).

Nussenzweig, V. N. Receptors for immune complexes on lymphocytes. Adv. Immunol., *19*:217 (1974).

Roboz, J., Suzuki, R. K., Bekesi, J. G., Holland, J. F., Selikoff, I. J.: Mass spectrometric identification and quantification of polybrominated biphenyls in blood compartments of Michigan chemical workers. J. Env. Path. Toxicol., *3*:151 (1980).

Sleight, S. D., Sanger, V. L.: Pathologic features of polybrominated biphenyl toxicosis in the rat and guinea pig. J. Am. Vet. Med. Assoc., *169*:1231 (1976).

Sundstrom, G., Hutzinger, O., Safe, S.: Environmental chemistry of flame retardants: Part II. Identification of 2,2',4,4',5,5'-hexabromobiphenyl as the major component of flame retardant Firemaster BP-6. Chemosphere (CMSHAF, 5:11, 1976).

Wolff, M. S., Aubrey, B., Camper, F., Haymes, N.: Relation of DDE and PBB serum levels in farm residents, consumers, and Michigan chemical corporation employees. Environ. Health Perspect. *23*:177 (1978).

Wolff, M. S., Haymes, N., Anderson, H. A., Selikoff, I. J.: Family clustering of PBB and DDE values among Michigan dairy farmers. Environ. Health Perspect., *23*:315 (1978).

Wybran, J., Carr, M. C., Fudenberg, H. H.: The human rosette-forming cell as a marker of a population of thymus-derived cells. J. Clin. Invest., *51*:2537 (1972).

DISCUSSION

McCOY: Thank you, Dr. Bekesi. I would like to open the discussion by asking a few questions. First, are these studies being continued? Are you longitudinally monitoring the individuals who were exposed? What do you think is the real significance of this work? If you have depressed levels, is this meaningful or not? I know there has been another report by Landrigan et al. (Ann. N.Y. Acad. Sci. *320*:284, 1979) of immunological studies of these PCB-exposed individuals. These studies reported no depression with these same people, apparently, or at least with a comparable group of PCB-exposed individuals. Are the differences in your findings and theirs the results of a difference in the test times following exposure? When exactly did you test these patients versus their exposure?

BEKESI: Question number one: Indeed, due to the good offices of NIEHS, a comprehensive program is under way in which we are monitoring the correlation of PBB level, for its immunological significance. We are aware of efforts by other groups in this area. Indeed I had the privilege of reading the preprint of an article from one group and I can only say that essentially they reproduce our results; they have not presented their raw data.

Second, I think you are all aware that collecting blood in a glass vacuum container is not the best way to collect and store a blood specimen for lymphocyte study because some cells definitely adhere.

Third, I think that in this day and age we ought to use purified mitogens. I am referring here to PHA.

McCOY: I think you are saying that the assays may not be totally standardized yet. Is that what you are inferring?

BEKESI: This is not a new assay. It's a routine assay at Mt. Sinai. Every blood sample coming in for testing is collected and hand-carried back on an airplane. We perform all assays within 18 hours after the blood sample has been drawn. However, we have found no difference between testing specimens after transportation or 13 minutes after collection at Mt. Sinai.

McCOY: The critical point I want to get across is that in a study such as this it is important logistically to set the study up properly initially and to use standardized assays. If one has most of the problems worked out—and obviously you do, by having the advantage of an ongoing program with a large number of cancer patients—one is in a strong position to readily apply a particular technology to this type of problem.

I would also like to ask whether there were any immunologic studies done on the cows prior to their destruction?

BEKESI: Unfortunately, Dr. Selikoff will not be able to come here today to present a more detailed study on asbestosis, malignant mesothelioma, and the role and usefulness of immunological testing.

To answer your second question: I was asked by the veterinarian from Chicago to perform identical assays, on ten animals. We found, in contrast to humans, the presence of a serum factor.

SIGEL: That is a very fascinating report, Dr. Bekesi, and I would like to address one question that was raised by our chairman earlier about the long persistence, in view of the short-life of some cells. I was wondering first of all if you were able to transfer this inhibitory action to normal cells, either by serum or by lymphocytes of the affected people, to see if there is any sort of transfer mechanism which would explain how one can expect these people to go on for 20 years manifesting suppressed immune responses, even though the affected cells are presumably removed by natural mechanisms?

Second, a related point: Do the cells that are affected act as suppressor cells in any sort of a way?

BEKESI: These are studies which are being actively pursued presently; we are looking at two aspects. One, where we know definitely that the chemical agent is on the cell surface, we tried to dislodge it and to look at whether the removal of this molecule can reverse the phenomena.

The second aspect of our work in progress is to look at the effects of some of these chemicals on animals, particularly mice, which have been chronically infected with virus which produces leukemia.

KATELEY: I wonder if you referred to Dr. Joseph Silva's studies that were recently reported (J. Reticuloendothel. Soc.). Had you made any attempt to do a double-blind study with Dr. Silva in the 50 or 60 PBB-exposed and non-exposed individuals? You mentioned that your assays aren't standardized; have you both had the opportunity to study the same specimens?

BEKESI: In answer to this: At a congressional hearing about one-and-a-half years ago I offered to transfer the technology from our laboratory either by training people, or by going out and performing this study. We do cooperate with Dr. Noel Rose at Wayne State University.

KATELEY: Dr. Rose and I have discussed this very problem closely.

As of this past September, he has not been involved in any immunological studies in PBB-exposed Michigan residents.

The next question concerns the follow-up testing of the 45 patients that you reported in Science. Have these individuals been studied a second time and, if there are preliminary results, what are they?

BEKESI: That study is ongoing. Some of the 45 patients have been admitted to our clinical center because of fever and failure to respond to antibiotics. There is no apparent change in their immune status as compared with the original observation. Some of these individuals also show deficiency in the ability of their serum to promote opsonization, that is, to fight infections. This correlates well with their health status and our earlier findings.

KATELEY: So you think there is a complement-mediated event that may be different?

BEKESI: We have not seen any dysfunction as far as the complement levels are concerned. Please take note this relatively large heterocyclic molecule, as any chemical agent, persists in the hepatic tissue. Thus, these individuals also show elevated liver enzyme function similar to that seen in cancer patients receiving chemotherapy.

KATELY: Just one final comment. Dr. McCoy asked about the cattle studies. I have performed such studies in both low-level and high-level PBB-exposed animals. From these studies, it doesn't appear there are quantitative or functional lymphocyte deficiences, even in animals which are anorexic and moribund. There might be some neutrophil defect in these animals; however, whether these defects are, directly or indirectly, the influence of PBB on neutrophils is under investigation.

CANNON: Was the incidence of depression which you observed to PHA similar in males and females exposed to the chemical?

BEKESI: We have invited these individuals as a family unit, some families with 6 or 7 members; some families, 2 members. The family as a unit, undoubtedly with similar eating habits, moved together; no difference in sex or age was noted.

McCOY: Let me ask two final questions. First, you described two people who worked in a factory in production of this material, who showed depressed immunologic values. You also made the statement that some of the exposed individuals had spiked fevers, and so forth. Have you seen any toxicologic effects, or have toxicologic effects been observed with factory workers?

Second, have those two factory workers who showed a depression shown any toxicologic symptoms in any way?

BEKESI: The chemical workers, as I said, are those with direct exposure. Farmers have indirect exposure. That is, they received the bio-concentrate of the material. We only recently had access to the chemical workers, because the company has been dissolved and it is not easy to track down the workers. The neurological symptoms found in the chemical workers are noteworthy and so are the results of sperm studies.

9
The Potential of High Resolution Protein Mapping as A Method of Monitoring the Human Immune System

N. L. Anderson and N. G. Anderson

*Molecular Anatomy Program, Division of Biological
and Medical Research, Argonne National Laboratory,
Argonne, Illinois*

INTRODUCTION

Immunology traditionally deals with complex cellular systems and hetero-
geneous mixtures of effector molecules (primarily antibodies). Some sense
has emerged from this chaos through the use of functional assays (cell
proliferation, killing, etc., or antigen-antibody reactions). Such an approach however naturally leaves a great deal undiscovered since the
assays are simple and the assayed objects are complex. In this chapter we
describe some experimental approaches to immunological problems using
high-resolution two-dimensional electrophoresis (O'Farrell, 1975; Anderson and Anderson, 1978a, b), a method that can resovle thousands of
proteins and can thus begin to treat immunological entities at their appropriate level of complexity. In addition, we discuss the possible application of this work to the problem of monitoring events in the individual
human immune system.

MATERIALS AND METHODS

The two-dimensional electrophoretic method used here is based on that
of O'Farrell (1975), and consists of isoelectric focusing in 9 M urea, 2%

136

NP-40 followed by sodium dodecyl sulfate gradient gel electrophoresis. Equipment developed in this laboratory (termed the ISO-DALT system; Anderson and Anderson [1978a, b]) enables large numbers ($\sim$ 100/day) of analyses to be performed and standarized (Anderson and Anderson, 1979; Anderson and Hickman, 1979). The method is denaturing in both dimensions and hence protein activity is generally lost upon analysis.

Lymphocytes are prepared using Ficol-Paque gradients (Pharmacia) and are radioactively labeled by incubation with ^{35}S methionine in methionine-free (RPMI 1640 medium with or without 10% fetal calf serum). Serum immunoglobulins are prepared using protein A Sepharose microcolumns (Pearson and Anderson, 1980) and human urinary proteins by established concentration procedures (Anderson et al., 1979a, b).

Two-Dimensional Analysis of Human Lymphocytes

The two-dimensional pattern of human peripheral blood lymphocytes is shown in Figure 1. Although several hundred protein spots are visible, many more are revealed in longer autoradiographic exposures. How can such data be dealt with in the absence of knowledge as to the names and functions of these molecules? In our view (Anderson and Anderson, 1979; Anderson et al., 1979c), the problem may best be attacked by accumulating the following sorts of information on all the spots: (1) cytoplasmic localization (i.e., is the protein located mainly in the nucleus, plasma membrane cytoskeleton, etc.?); (2) chemical characteristics (i.e., is the protein phosphorylated or glycosylated?; what is its amino acid composition?); and (3) genetic and control properties (what chromosome bears the gene in question?; is this protein specific to the lymphocyte—or one type of lymphocyte?; what other proteins are coregulated with this one?; what is the lifetime of this protein's mRNA?). All of this information and quite a bit more can be obtained from experiments in which cells or extracts from them are analyzed on 2-D gels. The strength of the gel-based approach is that information on many spots can be obtained simultaneously. Once the groundwork is done, interesting questions can be posed as to the function of selected proteins: what does it mean, for instance, when a protein is found to be (a) unique to lymphocytes, (b) polymorphic, (c) located mainly in the nucleus, (d) produced from a very short-lived messenger RNA, and (e) phosphorylated only when cells are exposed to a tumor promoter? Obviously, a satisfactory explanation of function requires much more than this, but at least this approach provides some objective basis for choosing proteins for detailed study. As biochemistry now stands, it is generally only those proteins detectable in

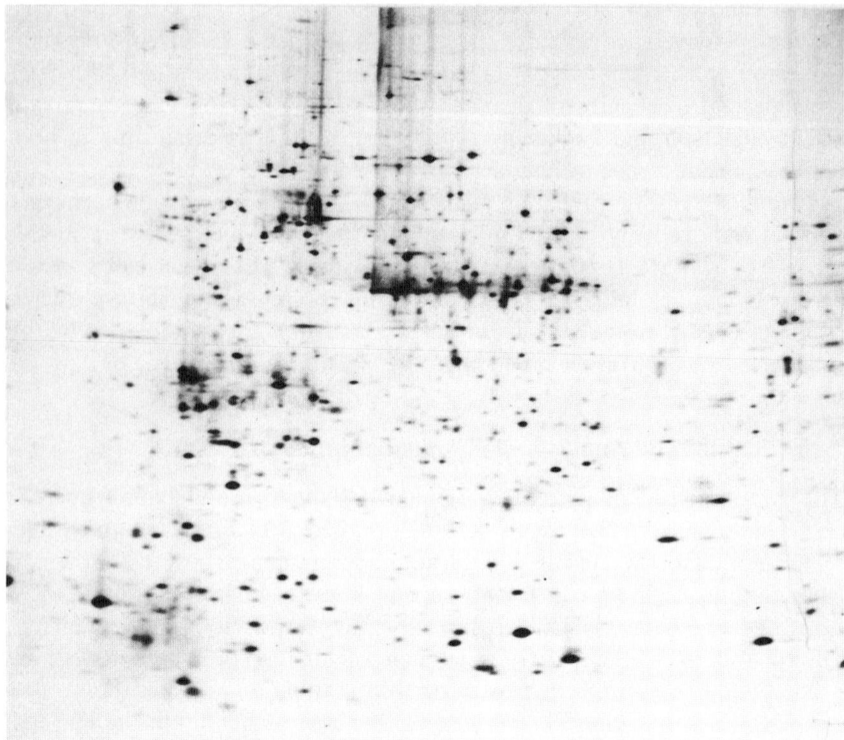

Figure 1. Short exposure autoradiograph of a two-dimensional analysis of normal human peripheral blood lymphocytes labeled for 24 hr *in vitro* with ^{35}S methionine. So far, only thirteen spots have been identified with known proteins (N. L. Anderson, unpublished results). Iso-electric focusing dimension is horizontal, acid end to the left (Anderson and Hickman, 1979), and SDS electrophoresis proceeds downwards (high molecular weight at the top).

some preconceived assay of function that can be investigated. Clearly, this is unsatisfactory in view of the fact that only 1-2% of the human proteins (excluding immunoglobulins) have so far been named or thought of.

A systematic 2-D gel study of lymphocytes has at least two applications in the area of immune system monitoring. First is the obvious desirability of looking for associations between particular genotypes and various immune dysfunctions. An interesting lymphocyte polymorphic system is shown in Figure 2; the protein involved is of unknown function. Since the

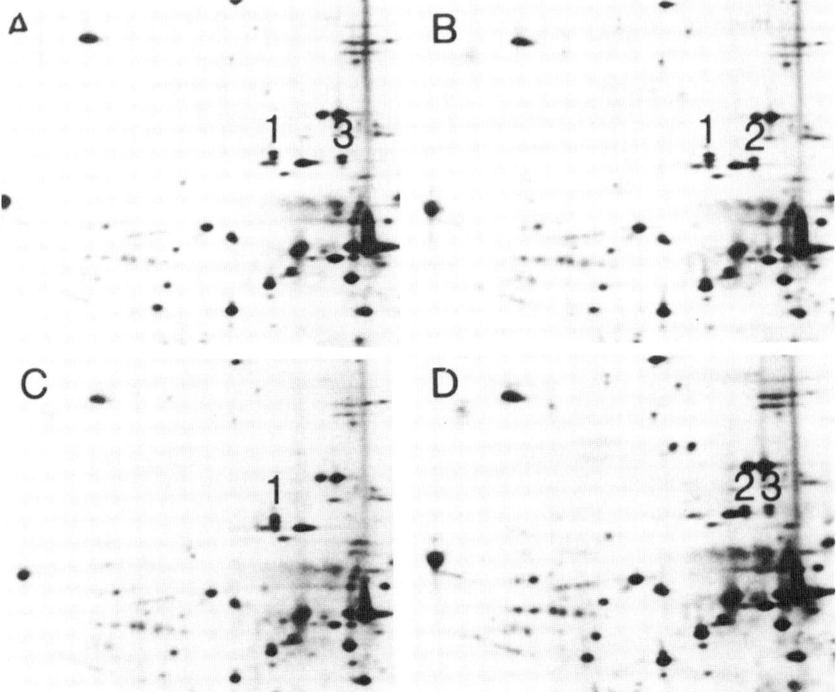

Figure 2. A small section from two-dimensional separations of methionine-labeled lymphocytes from four individuals (the section is equivalent to part of the upper left quadrant of Fig. 1). Numbers indicate positions of three allelic forms of an unknown protein. A, B, C, D. are mother, father, son, and daughter, respectively, and show segregation of the various alleles (From Anderson et al., 1980c, with permission of the publisher).

horizontal (isoelectric focusing) positions of protein spots are very sensitive to small charge changes (generally 0.1 charge), one can assume that approximately one third of the possible amino acid substitutions would lead to detectable spot shifts. So far it appears that the number of polymorphic proteins in nucleated cells is much lower than would be expected from serum protein genetics; although this leaves few "nonhistocompatibility" polymorphisms to study, it makes the job of recognizing rare variants and new mutations much easier. A second application involves examining the protein pattern of lymphocytes (prepared as before directly from fresh blood) as an indication of their functional status *in vivo*. We have found evidence that stimulation with concanavalin A, exposure to certain tumor promoters, etc. causes different distinctive changes in the pattern of newly synthesized lymphocyte proteins. These observations suggest that some nongenetic abnormalities in the patterns of lymphocytes from various individuals can ultimately be interpreted as indications of the functional state of these cells *in vivo*.

Two-Dimensional Mapping of Serum Immunoglobulins

Figure 3 shows the antibody light chain regions of two-dimensional gels of serum Ig from a number of individual BALB/c mice. The patterns are extremely similar, sharing approximately 79-80% of the spots. The result is slightly surprising in view of the notable heterogeneity of most antibody responses, but the similarities can be regarded as the predominant expression of a certain set of germ-line genes in "nonimmunized" inbred animals. Typical patterns of human Ig show much greater heterogeneity, as expected in outbred individuals, and almost no distinct light chain spots can be resolved on gels of the type used in Figure 3 ($7'' \times 7''$ gels). By running larger, higher resolution gels, some distinct spots can be seen (particularly in the serum of cancer patients; Figure 4). Each small, well-resolved spot is likely to be the light chain product (either κ or λ) of a single clone of B-cells. The rate of increase of the amount of each spot with time is probably a reasonable measure of the rate of growth of the associated clone, and hence a measure of the "strength" of one particular antibody response. Unfortunately, it would be quite difficult to determine what antigens correspond to each of the various antibody molecules produced; due to genetic heterogeneity, each human immune system would probably be a unique case. What may be of interest, however, is the ability to study the rate of appearance and disappearance of a substantial number of clonal products in a given individual (patient). This could give a much broader picture of humoral immune competence than a test of response to one or a few common antigens. Ultimately, it might be possible to monitor a person's exposure to strong antigens by comparing the Ig light chain micropatterns from serum samples obtained at, for instance, yearly intervals. Initial studies to examine this possibility are now under way.

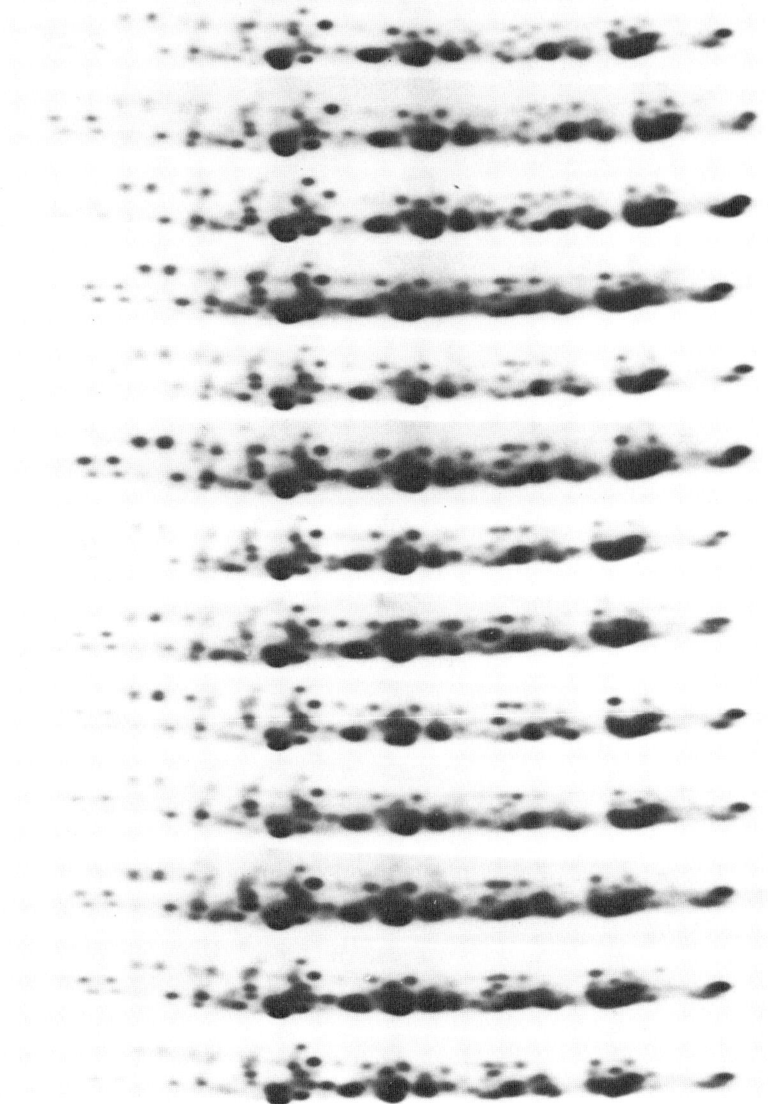

Figure 3. Light chain regions of two-dimensional separations of serum Ig from a number of nonimmunized BALB/c mice. Approximately 70-80% of the 70 or so visible spots are common to most of the individual mice.

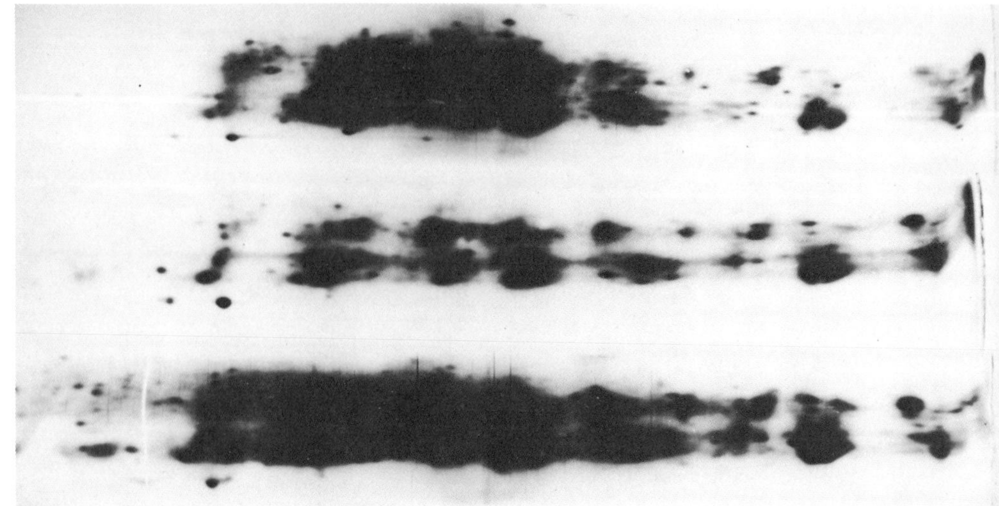

Figure 4. Light chain regions of three two-dimensional separations of serum Ig from two cancer patients (the middle gel is a lower protein loading from the same patient as shown in the bottom panel). Although most of the light chains remain unresolved, number of clonal products (different in the two individuals) are nevertheless visible. These gels were 12" x12" in size (almost twice as large in each dimension as standard gels).

Two-Dimensional Analysis of Urinary Proteins

A great variety of proteins is excreted in small amounts even by normal people, and many diseases (particularly those of the kidney) lead to dramatic increases in the excretion of some of these or of different, normally absent, polypeptides (Anderson et al., 1979a, b). Since the kidney passes small, nonserum proteins rather freely, it is expected that many molecules indicative of specific damage to a variety of organs can be detected in the urine simply as a result of leakage from affected cells. This situation makes possible two interesting approaches to the monitoring of immune function. First, it may enable accurate assessment of damage to transplanted organs caused by the host immune system. If rejection episodes are indeed characterized by a rather abrupt rise in cell damage in the organ, then it could be quite useful to be able to follow the release of proteins specific to these cells into the blood and finally the urine.

Second, it is possible to examine proteins synthesized by immune cells which themselves appear in the urine. Bence-Jones proteins are an obvious example. Even in this case, however, two-dimensional analysis (Figure 5) indicates that in addition to the overwhelming amount of the clonal light chain, there are detectable amounts of many other abnormal molecules present.

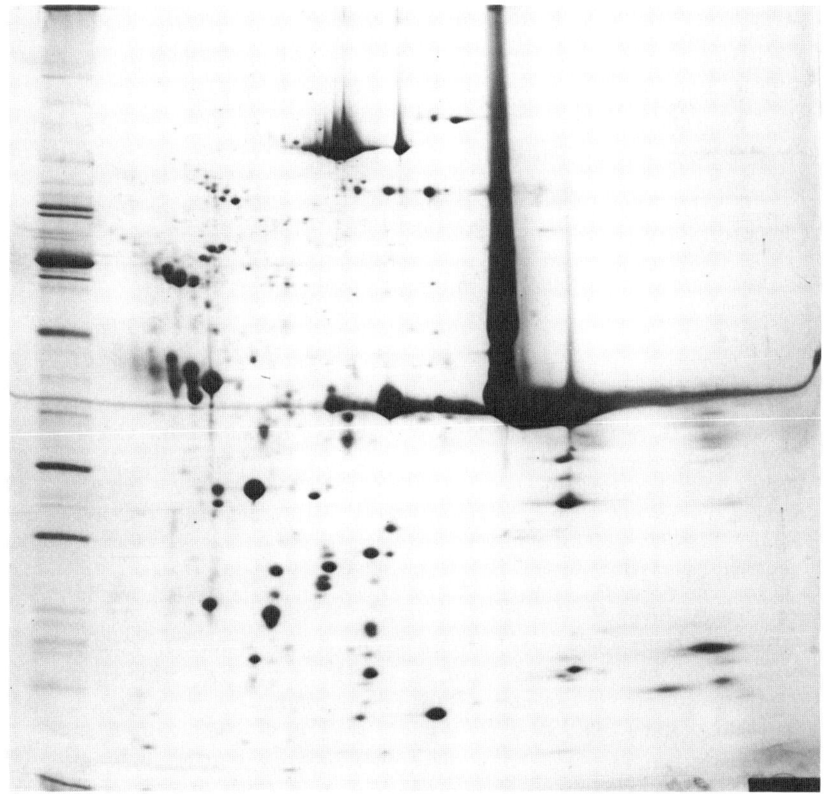

Figure 5. Two-dimensional separation of urinary proteins from a patient with a myeloma producing a λ-type Bence-Jones protein. The heavily overloaded protein spot about halfway down and to the right of center is the λ chain. Many of the smaller spots below this and to the left are additional abnormal spots, perhaps also produced by the myeloma cells.

CONCLUSIONS

The principal point to be made is that the complexity of the immune system (or indeed any cell or organism) is far greater than the resolving power of any of the conventional methods of studying it. Two-dimensional gel electrophoresis is the first method of sufficient resolving power to be able to catalog the cells' primary functional parts (the proteins) more or less to completion, and therefore to enable a rational search for the most important and interesting parts. It seems clear that the true molecular basis for many diseases and abnormalities (especially those due to genetic factors) will be open to elucidation only when we possess such a complete catalog of the proteins, heavily annotated with chemical and functional characteristics. Almost as a by-product of this work, we expect to find a substantial, we hope diagnostically useful, set of molecular indicators of pathologic cellular states.

ACKNOWLEDGMENTS

This work is supported by the U.S. Department of Energy under contract No. W–31–109–ENG–38.

REFERENCES

Anderson, N. G. and Anderson, N. L.: Analytical Techniques for Cell Fractions. XXI. Two-Dimensional Analysis of Serum and Tissue Proteins: Multiple Isoelectric Focusing. Anal Biochem., *85*:331-340 (1978a).

Anderson, N. L. and Anderson, N. G.: Analytical Techniques for Cell Fractions. XXII. Two-Dimensional Analysis of Serum and Tissue Proteins: Multiple Gradient-Slab Gel Electrophoresis. Anal. Biochem., *85*:341-354 (1978b).

Anderson, N. G. and Anderson, N. L.: Molecular Anatomy. Behring Inst. Mitt., *63*:169-210 (1979).

Anderson N G.. Anderson N., L., Tollaksen, S. L., Hahn, H., Giere, F., and Edwards, J.: Analytical Techniques for Cell Fractions. XXV. Concentration and Two-Dimensional Electrophoretic Analysis of Human Urinary Proteins. Anal. Biochem., *95*:48-61 (1979a).

Anderson, N. G., Anderson, N. L., and Tollaksen, S. L.: Proteins of Human Urine. I. Concentration and Analysis by Two-Dimensional Electrophoresis. Clin. Chem., *25*:1199-1210 (1979b).

Anderson, N. L., Edwards, J. J., Giometti, C. S., Willard, K. E., Tollaksen, S. L., Nance, S. L., Hickman, B. J., Taylor, J., Coulter, B., Scandora, A., and Anderson, N. G.: High Resolution Two-Dimensional Electrophoretic Mapping of Human Proteins, In Proceedings of Electrophoresis '79, B. Radola, ed., W. deGruyter, in press (1980c).

Anderson, N. L. and Hickman, B. J.: Analytical techniques for Cell Fractions. XXIV. Isoelectric Point Standards for Two-Dimensional Electrophoresis. Anal. Biochem., *93*:312-320 (1979).

O'Farrell, P. H.: High Resolution Two-Dimensional Electrophoresis of Proteins, J. Biol. Chem., *250*:4007-4021 (1975).

Pearson, T. and Anderson, L.: Analytical Techniques for Cell Fractions. XXVIII. Dissection of Complex Antigenic Mixtures Using Monoclonal Antibodies and Two-Dimensional Gel Electrophoresis. Anal. Biochem. (1980) in press.

ACKNOWLEDGMENTS

The submitted manuscript has been authored by a contractor of the U.S. Government under contract No. W–31–109–ENG–38. Accordingly, the U.S. Government retains a nonexclusive, royalty-free license to publish or reproduce the published form of this contribution, or allow others to do so, for U.S. Government purposes.

DISCUSSION

HADDEN: I would like to comment on this elegant and futuristic presentation. In addition to generating a static repertoire of lymphocyte structural proteins, it seems to me that one of the strongest contributions that might be made with this technology involves the development of a dynamic repertoire. We know from the work of Edward Johnson in Vincent Alfrey's laboratory that there are a number of nuclear acidic proteins, which are phosphorylated within minutes of mitogen action. With us, Dr. Johnson extended this observation to hormone action. These changes occur within minutes—so that one doesn't have the problems of changes of structural proteins related to proliferation. One can study protein modifications with phosphorylation that would indicate which ones might be regulatory proteins. Within the context of T-lymphocyte secretion, we know that there is a plethora of lymphokines, the identities of which are just beginning to be perceived on a biochemical basis that are secreted during one or another form of activation. The analysis of secreted labeled extracellular proteins would give another reference profile for meaningful lymphocyte proteins which would be easily distinguished from structural proteins. I think this technology offers great potential for analyzing lymphocytes.

ANDERSON: Well, you're 100 percent correct! I neglected to mention that our actual current experimental program includes a serious effort to try to find as many chemical substances as possible which have effects on the pattern of protein synthesis in leukocytes. There are several bizarre things which I hope a pharmacologist will explain to me some day. Number one: It's extremely difficult to find compounds which affect gene expression. There is an infinite number of ways to kill cells, but there is almost no way to actually switch on a gene in them. If you think about it, there should be compounds which make every cell in your body turn red, because they accidentally turn on the hemoglobin genes—one of the globin genes. Apparently, there aren't.

Now there is, of course, the case of DMSO and erythroleukemia cells. There are all kinds of ways of making a cell fall over a differentiational event that it was about to do anyway. But there are very few ways of actually getting in and putting a wrench in the mechanisms of gene regulation and making a change.

The first thing we are trying to do is to make a catalogue of all of the ways that one can cause changes in gene expression; either differentiational or simply regulatory, and then to try all possible permutations of those in an attempt to get an idea of how many separate mechanisms there are that are doing this work. The kinases are a good one. That's why I was asking you about the phorbal esters, because those things apparently do things to proteins in lymphocytes that you just wouldn't believe. They make kinase stimulation look like a sort of trivial event.

HADDEN: If I might follow up on my comment; with the 100 percent rating, it's hard to stop! I only wish you were reviewing my NIH grant proposal! Using similar technologies we hope to approach the action of the thymic hormones. Considered within the context of differentiation, these hormones, of which there are several, offer the possibility indeed of picking out specific gene products related to the ontogeny of T-lymphocytes.

ANDERSON: I won't go so far as to say that it can't fail, but it will certainly work!

MAO: I was very much impressed by your presentation. I thought that your presentation perhaps offers a brand new approach in this area. Did you consider, or do you propose to consider, the use of some other conventional immunoassay methods or will you consider the use of a very sensitive method, such as RIA, immunofluorescence assay, or rosette technique in order to compare your work materials and approaches with the antisera produced against serum constituents, Jones' protein, or any other kind of proteins which may be available to you? If you don't have the antisera, you can make it in your own laboratory. And if you want to make an antiserum against a chemical compound, you make the hapten antibody out of it so that you can make a comparison study such as I mentioned moments ago. I do think that it is essential in this case.

ANDERSON: Yes. It's absolutely essential to try to identify, to start with, as many of these spots as we can. One of those is beta-2 micro-globulin. There's band across the middle right by actin that contains most of the HLA molecules; that's most of the genetic difference between people. Clearly one wants to identify all the spots which are known, and those are the spots for which one potentially could do radioimmunoassays, spots for which antibodies are available.

The point is that beta-2 microglobulin just doesn't include very many proteins; the second point is that it doesn't necessarily include the best proteins to be looking at. It includes the proteins which are easy to isolate intact, which is a vast minority of proteins; also it includes proteins that one can get from people who you believe have produced pure antibodies or pure proteins. We try to do this to the extent that we can, but the main point is to do the analysis from an objective point of view, where one does not start out prejudiced in favor of ornithine decarboxylase, just because you read in a paper somewhere that it has something to do with something! We start with a spot, and when we find a spot which is interesting, we say, "We had better cut out this spot. We had better make an antibody to it, eventually a monoclonal antibody, and then start looking, using fluorscence microscopy, exactly where that antigen is produced and ultimately use it as a diagnostic tool if possible."

MAO: One more question: I wonder if you are trying to make this new approach only for qualitative data or for both qualitative and quantitative measurements in your studies?

ANDERSON: At the moment it's qualitative because the computer systems are not finished; but ultimately it's quantitative, more or less, for all of the spots.

For instance, during the cell cycle there are not vast qualitative changes in the proteins being synthesized—at least in HELA cells or WI-38, all you really see are quantitative changes in the phosphorylation of particular proteins, or in the rate of synthesis of other particular proteins. So there are some processes which do not yield gigantic changes. On the other hand, if one starts sticking viruses into cells, or hitting them with Concanavalin A or something like that, one can get fairly substantial changes in gene expression. That's easier to find by eye!

As a last note, it just occurred to me to contradict one thing in what was said by the gentleman who was 100 percent correct [Hadden], and it is that this is not exactly futuristic, as he implied. There are a number of people around the world working on systems like this. I think once the systems are fully functional, it will be quite easy to arrange to pump a lot of experimental material through them and to collate results fairly quickly. Looking at 500 proteins and finding out how each of them varies as a function of anything, from the concentration of magnesium to erythropoetin, or anything else you care to name, is pretty quick business, once it gets going.

SECTION III
EXPERIMENTAL CHANGES IN IMMUNOLOGIC PARAMETERS FOLLOWING EXPOSURE TO ENVIRONMENTAL AGENTS

10
Experimental Changes in Immunologic Parameters Following Exposure to Environmental Agents

Chairman: John A. Moore

This session will be devoted to papers describing the application of immunology assays to the study of chemically induced alterations of immune responses. I think the major area of immunotoxocity assessment we must begin to focus on is the only reason we do immunology tests from a toxicologic standpoint: species extrapolation to man. We will hear this morning that a variety of chemicals may have some particular effect on the immune system of certain rodents; however these are all experimental pieces of information. Important though they are, we still must demonstrate a parallel in man.

This may be a function of dose. I think principally what we are seeing right now is that we just haven't done clinical studies on groups with the kind of chemical exposures necessary to see if immunosuppression commonly exists in exposed populations. Dr. Bekesi's studies begin to approach this problem with preliminary sucess.

The other point I want to make is that the National Toxicology Program, which was initiated just about a year ago as a DHEW effort, has determined that immunology is an area that needs to be assessed. Studies are being initiated in order to see if one can come up with an adequate data base to reach a determination as to the proper role of immunologic assessment in a toxicologic evaluation of a chemical. We hope that this goes in a sequenced process and that we can: (1) come up with a battery of tests that one can use, which is modest, but will provide the necessary data; and (2) through the testing of chemicals, we might be able to get insight as to when, during a toxicological characterization of a chemical, one should suspect or look for an immunologic effect. I'm not convinced that one should look at each and every compund using a battery of immunologic tests. To do that certainly implies a significant increase of expense for toxicologic evaluation. As we test more chemicals of various classes we might be able to draw enough data together to suggest that certain chemical classes indeed should always be looked at because of structure-activity relationships.

The National Toxicology Program is in essence in the stage of methods development and validation in experimental animals. Hopefully, somewhere down the road we can also get into a validation exercise that carries the connotation: How does it extrapolate to man?

11
Immunological Alterations in Mice Following Acute Exposure to Diethylstilbestrol

Michael I. Luster
Gary A. Boorman, Jack H. Dean, Lela D. Lawson,
Ralph Wilson and Joel K. Haseman

*Laboratory of Environmental Chemistry, Environmental Biology
and Biometry Branches, National Institute of Environmental
Health Sciences, Research Triangle Park, North Carolina*

INTRODUCTION

Diethylstilbestrol (DES) is a synthetic nonsteroidal compound possessing estrogenic activity. Following its synthesis by Dodds (1938) it has been extensively employed as a theraputic agent in humans (rev. by McLachlan and Dixon, 1976) as well as a growth-promoting agent in sheep and cattle (rev. by McMartin et al., 1978). While DES is no longer used in the treatment of threatened abortions, it is currently administered to women for hormonal replacement, as estrogen replacement in gonadal dysgenesis and as a contraceptive, the so called "morning after" treatment. Furthermore, DES is employed theraputically in men for treatment of prostatic cancer. There have been several incidents of workers in chemical plants and feed lot areas inadvertently exposed to relatively high doses of DES with some of the male workers exhibiting hypospermia, loss of libido and gynecomastia (rev. by McMartin et al., 1978). Some of the toxicological effects attributed to DES in humans include an association with cardiovascular disease (Bailer and Byar, 1976), breast tumors in men (IARL, 1979) and mixed adenosquamous carcinomas of the uterus (endometrium) in young women (Cutler, et al., 1972). The most publicized effect attributed to DES is an increased incidence of latent clear-cell adenocarcinoma of the vagina in young women exposed to DES *in utero* (Herbst, 1971).

153

From an immunological standpoint, glucocorticoid induced immune alterations have received much attention (rev. by Bach, 1975). While less studied, the sex sterioids including estrogens and androgens have been shown to suppress and sometimes enhance various immune functions (rev. by Ahlquist, 1976). DES is a recognized stimulant of the reticulo-endothelial system (RES) which causes increased hepatic (Kelly et al., 1962) and splenic (Steven and Snook, 1975) phagocytic activity of macrophages although the mechanisms for this response are unclear. Administration of DES to female mice in prenatal, postnatal or adult life induces thymic involution (Luster et al., 1979; Kalland et al., 1978; Greenman et al., 1977) and suppresses antibody responses to T-dependent (Sljivic et al., 1975) and T-independent antigens (Kalland, 1980a, Sljivic and Warr, 1974). However, the T-independent (LPS) antibody response in male mice exposed *in utero* (Luster et al., 1978) or *in vitro* (Kenny and Diamond 1975) is enhanced indicating that DES may directly affect immunocompetent B-cells. Suppression of cell-mediated immunity occurs in prenatal or postnatally exposed mice as evidenced by decreased lympho-proliferative responses to T-cell mitogens and delayed hypersensitivity responses (Luster et al., 1979; Kalland, et al., 1980; Kalland and Forsberg, 1978).

The purpose of these studies was to examine the effects of acute DES exposure in mice on various macrophage, immunological and bone marrow functions. Possible mechanisms of DES-induced immune dysfunction were also examined.

MATERIALS AND METHODS

Animals and Dosages

Female $B_6C_3F_1$ mice, 7 to 9 weeks of age, were obtained from NCI (Fort Detrick, MD). Animals were housed 10 per cage and allowed free access to food and water. DES (Sigma Chemical Company; St. Louis, MO) was dissolved in corn oil and so diluted that mice recived 0.01 ml per 2 g of body weight. Exposure was accomplished by subcutaneous (sc) injections into the back of the neck at dosages of 0.2, 2.0 and 8.0 mg/kg body weight for five successive days. Controls received corn oil alone. Various parameters were examined 3-5 days following the last exposure.

Hematology

Blood samples were obtained from CO_2–sacrificed animals by cardiac puncture. Hematological profiles included erythrocyte counts (RBC) leukocyte counts (WBC) and differential. Quantitation of splenic leuko-cytes with B- or T-lymphocyte markers was performed using fluorescien conjugated antisera to specific markers as decribed previously (Luster et al., 1979).

Macrophage Function Assays

Macrophages were obtained from noninduced (resident) peritoneal cells by aseptically flushing the peritonial cavity with 8.0 ml of Hank's balanced salt solution (HBSS) containing 1 unit per ml of heparin (pre-servative free; Fisher Sci.). Cells were centrifuged (800 g, 10 min, 4°C), resuspended and allowed to adhere to microexudate flasks according to the method of Mantovani et al. (1979). Cell counts were determined on a Model 2B Coulter Counter (Coulter Electronics, Hialeah, FL) and viability was performed by trypan blue exclusion (always > 95%). The adherent peritoneal mononuclear (PM) cells were evaluated for their ability to phagocytize SRBCs (Stuart et al., 1978), proliferate in response to colony stimulating factor (Hadden, 1979; Boorman and Luster sub-mitted) and inhibit the growth of MBL-2 leukemia target cells (Dean et al., 1979) as described previously.

Bone Marrow Assays

Bone marrow cells were aseptically collected from both femurs by cutting the ends at the epiphysis and flushing the shaft with MEM culture medium. The cells were dispersed and the number of nucleated cells determined with a Coulter Counter. Colony forming units in culture (CFU-C) and colony forming units in spleen (CFU-S) were determined in individual mice by the methods of Bradley and Metcalf (1966) and Till and Mculloch (1961), respectively, as modified in our laboratory (Luster et al., 1980).

Antibody Responses

Antibody responses were measured to a T-dependent antigen (SRBCs) and a T-independent antigen (lipopolysaccharide; LPS. E. coli 055:B5; Difco, Detroit, MI). Responses were determined four days following iv immunization with either 0.2ml or a 10% suspension of SFBCs or 5.0 μg of LPS in saline. SRBC antibody production was monitored by enumera-tion of direct splenic plaque forming cells (PFCs) by a modification of the Jerne plaque assay (Dresser and Greaves, 1973) and serum hemagglutina-tion titers using a microtiter technique (Cooke Engineering; Alexandria,

VA). LPS serum antibody titers were determined by passive hemagglutination (Veit and Michael, 1972).

Lymphoproliferative Responses

Splenic lymphoproliferative responses to the T-cell mitogens, phytohemagglutinin (PHA-P), conconavlin A (Con A) and *Staphylococcus* enterotoxin A (SEA), as well as to a B-cell mitogen (LPS), were performed in a microculture system as previously described (Luster et al., 1979), except 5% human AB serum was substituted for fetal calf. SEA was a gift from Dr. D. Archer (FDA, Cinn., OH). One–way mixed leukocyte cultures (MLC) were performed under similar condition except the media was also supplemented with 5×10^{-5} 2-mercaptoethanol employing 5×10^5 mitomycin-C (Sigma) treated splenic leukocytes per culture from DBA/2 mice. MLCs were harvested on day 5 of culture following an 18 hr pulse with ^{3}H-thymidine.

Examination for Suppressor Cell Activity

Suppressor cell activity was examined in DES treated mice (8 mg/kg dosage group) by coculturing MMC-blocked spleen cells from treated animals with cells from normal animals, followed by examination of LP responsiveness to mitogenic stimulation. Splenic cells to be assayed for suppressor activity or in MLC were incubated with MMC (50 μg/10^7 cells/ml) for 40 minutes at 37°C. Following three washes in RPMI-1640 media to remove excess MMC, these cells (2×10^5) and non-treated spleen cells from normal donors (2×10^5) were cocultured in wells of a microtiter plate and LP responsiveness examined. To determine whether suppressor activity resided in the macrophage population, adherent cells were selectively removed from spleen cells of normal mice using Sephadex G-10 columns (LY and Mishell, 1974). While this procedure has been reported to have little or no effect on the proportion of T- and B-lymphocytes (Berlinger et al., 1976), we obtained less than 0.2% macrophages remaining as determined by nonspecific esterase staining. Suppressor activity was then evaluated by examination of LP responses of normal macrophage-depleted spleen cells cocultured with adherent peritoneal macrophages from treated mice.

Delayed Hypersensitivity Response

Delayed hypersensitivity responses (DHRs) were measured to a T-dependent antigen, KLH (keyhole lymphet hemocyamin; Pacific Biomarine, Venice, CA) by a modification of a radiometric ear assay (Lefford, 1974). Briefly mice were injected sc with 0.1 mg equivalent of KLH emulsified in incomplete Freund's adjuvant (Difco, Detroit, MI) followed 9 days later with a second injection in a similar manner. Nine days following the booster injection, mice were injected intraperitoneally with 1.0 μCi/g body weight ^{3}H-thymidine (S.A. 20 Ci/mmole, New England Nuclear, Boston, MA). Twenty-four hours later, the left ear of each mouse was injected with 30 μg of purified KLH in a volume of 0.01 ml of saline while the right ear received saline alone. The following day 6 mm ear plugs were taken from both ears, solublized with tissue solublizer (NCS; Amersham Searle, Chicago, IL) and prepared for scintillation counting. The data were expressed as a DHR index:

$$\text{Index} = \frac{\text{CPM Sensitized ear}}{\text{CPM control ear}}$$

Statistical Analysis

The Mann-Whiteny U test was employed to assess the significance of treatment effects while the analysis of dose-response trends was determined by Jonckheere's test (1954).

RESULTS

Pathotoxicology

None of the mice died or revealed overt signs of toxicity during the study. The effects of DES on body weights and selected organ weights are depicted in Table I. Body weights were slightly affected by DES exposure as indicated by increased weight gains. Liver weights were increased in higher dosage groups and histologically revealed enhanced cytoplasmic vascuolization of hepatocytes. Thymus weights were severely decreased at all dosage levels and were histologically characterized by a progressive depletion of cortical lymphocytes. Splenomegaly with increased cellularity occurred in the highest dosage groups. Histological examination revealed smaller follicles, increased red pulp and marked hematopoiesis (both erythropoiesis and myelopoiesis) as a consequence of DES exposure.

Bone Marrow

The effects of DES on bone marrow cellularity and CFU assays are summarized in Table 2. A progressive decrease in cellularity occurred with increasing DES exposure although only the hypocellularity in the

Table 1. **Body Weights, Thymic Weights and Splenic Weights in Mice Exposed to DES.***

DOSAGE (MG/KG)	BODY WEIGHT (G)	LIVER WEIGHT (MG)	THYMIC WEIGHT (MG)	THYMUS/BODY WEIGHT RATIO ($\times 10^{-4}$)	SPLEEN WEIGHT (MG)	SPLEEN/BODY WEIGHT RATIO ($\times 10^{-4}$)
0	21.1 ± 0.2	1063 ± 59	49.2 ± 1.6	23.4 ± 0.9	137 ± 15	6.6 ± 0.7
0.2	21.4 ± 0.3	1294 ± 24 †	21.8 ± 1.1 ‡	10.2 ± 0.6 ‡	120 ± 12	5.5 ± 0.4
2.0	24.4 ± 0.3 ‡	1666 ± 66 ‡	14.5 ± 1.1 ‡	6.0 ± 0.5 ‡	187 ± 21	8.2 ± 0.9
8.0	26.0 ± 0.5 ‡	2070 ± 51 ‡	12.1 ± 0.7 ‡	4.7 ± 0.3 ‡	199 ± 20 *	9.0 ± 0.8 †
Dose Response (P)	< 0.01	< 0.01	< 0.01	< 0.01	< 0.01	< 0.05

* Mean value $\pm$ SE of 8 animals/group.
† p $<$ 0.05 vs controls.
‡ p $<$ 0.01 vs controls.

Table 2.   Mouse Bone Marrow Cellularity and CFU's Following DES Exposure *

| | | COLONY FORMING UNITS | |
DOSAGE (MG/KG)	NUCLEATED CELLS/ FEMUR ($\times 10^{-6}$)	IN CULTURE/ 5×10^5 CELLS	IN SPLEEN/ 5×10^4 CELLS
0	19.1 ± 1.6	54.4 ± 2.9	6.78 ± 0.67
0.2	15.7 ± 0.6	40.9 ± 4.1 †	6.56 ± 0.70
2.0	13.7 ± 0.9 †	34.6 ± 2.2 ‡	6.02 ± 0.64
8.0	12.9 ± 0.7 ‡	33.5 ± 4.6 ‡	4.00 ± 0.36 ‡
Dose Response (P)	< 0.01	< 0.01	< 0.01

* Mean ± SE of an average of 6 animals tested/group.
† p < 0.05 *vs* controls.
‡ p < 0.01 *vs* controls.

2.0 and 8.0 mg/kg dosage groups was statistically significant. The number of granulocyte-macrophage precursor colonies (CFU-GM) was depressed at all exposure levels while hematopoietic pleuripotent stem cell colonies (CFU-S's) were statiscally reduced only at the 8.0 mg/kg dosage group.

Hematology

Hematological examination revealed normal RBC counts but increased numbers of leukocytes at all dosage levels (Table 3). Leukocytosis was predominantly a result of increased lymphocytes although blood monocytes and to a lesser extent neutrophils were also elevated. Increased numbers of resident PM cells occurred as a consequence of DES treatment with a proportional increase in both monocytes and lymphocytes (Table 4). The percentage of adherent PM cells capable of phagocytizing SRBCs was increased at the 2.0 and 8.0 mg/kg dosage groups. The phagocytic activity was not affected at the 0.2 mg/kg dosage level.

Macrophage Function

PM cells from DES exposed mice showed a 2- to 3-fold increase in their ability to proliferate in the presence of macrophage growth factor (MGF) as determined *in vitro* by ³H-thymidine incorporation (Table 5). There were no changes in cell proliferation in treated mice without MGF present.
   The effect of DES exposure on activation of adherent PM cells was

Table 3.   Hematologic Profile in DES Treated Mice.*

PARAMETER	DOSAGE (MG/KG)				DOSE RESPONSE (P)
	0	0.2	2.0	8.0	
RBC $\times 10^6$/mm^3	5.5 ± 0.2	7.5 ± 0.2 ‡	5.1 ± 0.1	5.7 ± 0.1	> 0.05
Leukocytes $\times 10^3$/mm^3	3.8 ± 0.3	5.7 ± 0.6 †	8.4 ± 1.5 ‡	11.0 ± 1.0 ‡	< 0.01
Lymphocytes $\times 10^3$/mm^3	2.9 ± 0.2	4.4 ± 0.4 †	7.3 ± 1.3 ‡	9.1 ± 0.8 ‡	< 0.01
Lymphocytes (%)	77	78	86 †	84 †	< 0.01
Monocytes (mm^3)	90 ± 10	110 ± 20	220 ± 60 †	240 ± 30 ‡	< 0.01
Monocytes (%)	2.4	2.0	2.6	2.4	> 0.05
Neutrophils $\times 10^3$/mm^3	0.8 ± 0.1	1.1 ± 0.2	1.0 ± 0.1	1.6 ± 0.3 †	< 0.05
Neutrophils (%)	20	20	12 †	14 †	< 0.01

* Mean value $\pm$ SE of 8 mice/group.
† $p < 0.05$ vs control.
‡ $p < 0.01$ vs controls.

Table 4.   Effects of DES on Resident Peritoneal Exudate Cells.*

DOSAGE (MG/KG)	TOTAL NO. OF PE CELLS ± SE	DIFFERENTIAL (%)		SRBC PHAGOCYTIC INDEX
		MONOCYTES	LYMPHOCYTES	
0	2.76 ± 0.12	71.0 ± 2.5	25.6 ± 2.6	47.6 ± 7.9
0.2	3.50 ± 0.32 †	75.7 ± 3.7	21.3 ± 3.8	44.0 ± 7.2
2.0	4.40 ± 0.22 ‡	79.8 ± 2.5	17.4 ± 2.6	74.6 ± 2.8 †
8.0	5.62 ± 0.30 ‡	71.4 ± 6.5	26.0 ± 6.1	71.5 ± 4.7 †
Dose Response	< 0.01	> 0.05	> 0.05	< 0.01

* Mean Value ± SE of 8 animals/group.
† p < 0.05.
‡ p < 0.01.

assessed by their ability to inhibit the growth of MBL-2 leukemia target cells in a microculture growth inhibition assay (Table 6). A marked inhibition of target cell growth occurred at all exposure levels ranging from 28% in the 0.2 mg/kg dosage group to 90% inhibition in the 8.0 mg/kg dosage group compared to controls. Addition of macrophage activation factor (MAF) enhanced the inhibition of tumor growth in the control and 0.2 mg/kg groups but had no effect at high DES exposure levels.

Cell Mediated Immunity

The effects of DES exposure on delayed hypersensitivity responses (DHRs) to KLH are shown in Table 7. Similar responses were obtained

Table 5.   Effects of DES Exposure on ³H-Thymidine Uptake of PE Cells in the Presence of Varying Concentrations of Macrophage Growth Factor (MGF).*

DOSAGE GROUP	CPM ± SD OF ³H-TdR INCORPORATION		
	0% MGF	20% MGF	30% MGF
0	139 ± 60	389 ± 117	742 ± 313
0.2	158 ± 36	587 ± 124	1169 ± 374 †
2.0	136 ± 52	659 ± 295	1754 ± 444 ‡
Dose Response (P)	> 0.05	> 0.05	< 0.01

* Mean ± SD of 6 animals/group using 10⁴ PE cells.
† p < 0.06.
‡ p < 0.01.

Table 6.   Effects of DES on Macrophage Activation as Determined by Macrophage Cytostasis.*

DOSAGE GROUP (MG/KG)	MAE	^{3}H-TdR INCORPORATION CPM $\pm$ SE $\times$ 10^3	PERCENT INHIBITION
0	—	199.7 $\pm$ 7.9	—
	+	110.9 $\pm$ 5.5	—
0.2	—	99.3 $\pm$ 16.4 ‡	(50↓)
	+	79.6 $\pm$ 6.2 †	(28↓)
2.0	—	27.9 $\pm$ 5.7 ‡	(86↓)
	+	30.7 $\pm$ 8.8 ‡	(72↓)
8.0	—	19.4 $\pm$ 6.2 ‡	(90↓)
	+	20.5 $\pm$ 6.3 ‡	(82↓)
Dose Response (P)		< 0.01	< 0.01

* Mean of 4 pools per group.
† $p < 0.05$ vs controls.
‡ $p < 0.01$ vs controls.

Table 7.   Delayed Hypersensitivity Responses to KLH in DES Treated Mice.*

KLH SENSITIZATION *	DOSAGE (MG/KG)	^{3}H-TdR INCORPORATION (CPM + SE $\times$ 10^2) CONTROL EAR	CHALLENGED EAR	DHR INDEX $\pm$ SE
Post-DES Exposure	0	17.2 $\pm$ 1.6	41.2 $\pm$ 2.1	2.56 $\pm$ 0.34
	0.2	12.9 $\pm$ 1.0	35.8 $\pm$ 1.8	2.85 $\pm$ 0.24
	2.0	12.5 $\pm$ 1.2	40.2 $\pm$ 3.5	3.23 $\pm$ 0.28
	8.0	14.2 $\pm$ 1.2	40.0 $\pm$ 3.2	2.94 $\pm$ 0.33
	Dose Response (P)			> 0.05
Pre-DES Exposure	0	11.9 $\pm$ 1.0	26.7 $\pm$ 1.9	2.79 $\pm$ 0.17
	0.2	9.8 $\pm$ 0.8	25.4 $\pm$ 2.1	2.79 $\pm$ 0.22
	2.0	9.5 $\pm$ 0.9	19.3 $\pm$ 1.5	2.15 $\pm$ 0.20 †
	8.0	10.4 $\pm$ 0.9	13.3 $\pm$ 1.1	1.88 $\pm$ 0.15 ‡
	Dose Response (P)			< 0.01

*Mice were sensitized by injecting 100 μg KLH emulsified in ICFA SC followed by a subsequent immunization 9 days later. Animals were tested 10 days following the last injection. Mean $\pm$ SE of 8 animals per group.
† $p < 0.05$.
‡ $p < 0.01$.

in control and treated groups when mice were exposed to DES prior to antigen sensitization. However, when mice exposed to DES following sensitization, but prior to ear challenge, significant suppression of DHRs occurred in both 2.0 and 8.0 mg/kg dosage groups.

Table 8 summarizes the effects of DES administration on *in vitro* lymphoproliferative (LP) assays. LP responses to the T-lymphocyte mitogens, PHA, Con A and SEA, in treated mice were severely depressed from normal control values and ranged from approximately 30% depression in the 0.2 mg/kg dosage group to 70% in the 8.0 mg/kg dosage group. The B-cell LP response to LPS was not significantly affected at any dosage group although a 30% reduction in the highest dosage group occurred. The mixed leukocyte culture (MLC) responses were depressed at the 2.0 and 8.0 mg/kg dosage levels. Furthermore, a 25 percent decrease of splenic leukocytes stainable with FITC-conjugated antiserum to a T-cell marker (absorbed rabbit anti-C_3H mouse brain) was found at the highest dosage level when compared to controls. There was no difference in the percentage of B-cells at this dosage level as determined by enumeration of Ig-positive splenic leukocytes (data not shown).

A series of coculture experiments using several cell combinations and cell treatments followed by analysis of LP responses was used to determine whether DES exposure induced splenic suppressor cell activity (Table 9). Experiment I depicts the LP responses from spleens of a pool of normal or DES treated mice (8 mg/kg) showing depression of PHA, Con A and LPS LP responses. When normal spleen cells were cocultured with MMC-blocked spleen cells from treated mice, marked depression of normal LP response occurred (Expt. II) and was comparable to the suppression observed in experiment I. Depletion of adherent cells from spleen cells resulted in diminished Con A responses in control animals but in markedly enhanced responses in DES treated mice (Expt. III). Con A LP responses in cocultures containing macrophage depleted normal spleen cells and 10% adherent PM cells from treated mice revealed a 40% depression from appropriate controls, suggesting that the suppressed LP response in treated mice was due, at least in part, to suppressor cell activity that resided in the macrophage population (Expt. IV).

Humored Mediated Immunity

Direct antibody PFC responses to the thymus-dependent antigen (SRBC) was reduced approximately 25% in both the 2.0 and 8.0 mg/kg dosage groups compared to control mice when evaluated by PFC/10^6 leukocytes and 40% based upon PFC/total spleen cells, but not by hemagglutination

Table 8.   Effects of DES on the *In Vitro* Lymphoproliferative Response to Mitogens and Allogenic Cells As Well As the Number of Splenic Leukocytes Staining with a T-Cell Reagent.*

DOSAGE GROUP (MG/KG)	^{3}H-TdR INCORPORATION NCPM $\times 10^3$					% STAINED POSITIVE
	PHA	CON A	LPS	SEA	MLC	
0	27.5 ± 3.6	23.4 ± 2.8	8.2 ± 0.8	2.6 ± 0.2	4.0 ± 0.3	38.0 ± 0.8
0.2	17.3 ± 1.5 † (37.1↓)	16.1 ± 3.1 (31.2↓)	13.6 ± 1.0 (65.8↑)	2.9 ± 0.3 (11.5↑)	3.9 ± 0.4 (2.5↓)	ND
2.0	12.2 ± 1.5 ‡ (55.6↓)	12.1 ± 1.7 ‡ (48.3↓)	10.0 ± 0.9 (22.0↑)	1.6 ± 0.2 † (38.5↓)	2.8 ± 0.2 ‡ (30.0↓)	ND
8.0	4.8 ± 0.7 ‡ (82.5↓)	8.3 ± 0.8 ‡ (64.5↓)	5.8 ± 1.2 (29.3↓)	1.1 ± 0.1 ‡ (57.7↓)	3.0 ± 0.2 ‡ (25.0↓)	28.5 ± 2.3 ‡ (25↓)
Dose Response (P)	< 0.01	< 0.01	> 0.05	< 0.01	< 0.01	—

* Mean ± SE of 8 animals/group with % change from controls in parenthesis. The data is expressed as net CPM = counts per minute (CPM) in mitogen stimulated cultures—CPM in cultures without mitogen.
† p < 0.05 vs controls.
‡ p < 0.01 vs controls.
ND = Not Done.

Table 9.   Evidence for Suppressor Cell Activity in the Spleens of DES-Treated Mice.*

EXPERIMENT	DONOR	TREATMENT	^{3}H-TdR INCORPORATION (CPM $\times$ 10^3)		
			PHA	CON A	LPS
I	Normal	None	35.1	31.3	7.0
	DES	None	7.8	7.9	3.7
			(78%↓)	(75%↓)	(47%↓)
II	Normal	Co-Cultured with normal MMC-Treated cells	19.5	35.3	8.1
	Normal	Co-Cultured with DES MMC-Treated cells	3.9	11.3	3.3
			(80%↓)	(68%↓)	(59%↓)
III	Normal	Mø-Depleted	ND †	19.2	ND
	DES	Mø-Depleted		66.2	
				(227%↑)	
IV	Normal	Mø-Depleted and Co-Cultured with 10% normal PE cells	ND	67.2	ND
	Normal	Mø-Depleted and Co-Cultured with 10% DES PE cells		40.8	
				(39%↓)	

* DES-Treated mice received 5 daily injections of 8.0 MG/KG of DES. Values represent mean net CPM of triplicated microcultures from pools of at least 4 mice with % change from appropriate control in parenthesis.
† ND = Not done.

(Table 10). Antibody response to the T-independent antigen (LPS) was also reduced at the two highest dosage groups, but particularly at the 8.0 mg dosage level, as measured by passive hemagglutination. Antibody responses to both SRBC and LPS in the 0.2 mg/kg exposure level were similar to controls.

DISCUSSION

In the present studies we demonstrate a marked alteration of immunocompetence in female mice as a consequence of acute adult exposure to pharmacologically relevant doses of DES. These studies provide further insight into earlier reports demonstrating suppression of various immune functions following prenatal or postnatal exposure to DES and helps explain the increased RES activity observed following acute adult exposure. While the lower dosage employed in the present studies can be considered pharmacologically equivalent to current theraputic dosages,

Table 10.*   The Effects of DES Treatment on the Antibody Response to SRBC and LPS.

DOSAGE GROUP (MG/KG)	SRBC PFC/ 10^6 SPLEEN CELLS	SRBC PFC/ SPLEEN	SRBC HA TITER (LOG 2)	LPS P-HA TITER (LOG 2)
0	1003 ± 34	1.6×10^5	5.88 ± 0.12	6.67 ± 0.21
0.2	1039 ± 55	1.3×10^5	6.00 ± 0.19	6.00 ± 0.26
2.0	742 ± 65 ‡	8.7×10^4 ‡	5.50 ± 0.19	5.67 ± 0.21 †
8.0	775 ± 88 §	9.1×10^4 §	5.62 ± 0.18	3.67 ± 0.49 ‡
Dose Response (P)	< 0.01	< 0.01	> 0.05	< 0.01

* Mean ± SE of 8 animals/group. All mice received iv injection of 0.2 ml of a 10% suspension of SRBC or 5 μg LPS 4 days prior to sacrifice.
† p < 0.05.
‡ p < 0.01.
§ p < 0.1.

the higher dosages examined are not currently administered. These higher dosages, however, are comparable to those previously used for treatment of threatened abortions in pregnant women. Dosages in this earlier theraputic application of DES ranged from 175 mg to 47 g during pregnancy with an average daily dose estimated to be ~100 mg (Heinonen, 1973). It has been estimated that anywhere between one-half to two million women received DES during its period of greatest use (rev. by McLachlin and Dixon, 1976).

Hematological profiles indicated marked leukocytosis that was not a consequence of bone marrow stimulation, since decreases in bone marrow celluarity, macrophage-granulocyte progenitor cells and pleuripotent stem cell proliferation occurred following DES exposure. Examination of the spleen revealed splenomegaly, hypercelludarity and histological evidence of increased hematopoiesis in treated mice. This may indicate that the spleen serves as the primary hematopoietic organ following DES exposure and is similar to a number of other agents (e.g., cycloposphamide) which induces bone marrow depression with the spleen compensating as the primary hematopoietic organ (Pannacciulli et al., 1977). The leukocytosis may not entirely be due to increased splenic hematopoiesis, however, since adherent PM cells from DES treated animals revealed enhanced proliferation in the presence of MGF indicating a possible direct effect by DES on the mature macrophage population.

A dichotomous effect on the immune response was evident from these studies with B- and T-lymphocyte mediated functions markedly depressed and the mononuclear phagocytic system stimulated as a consequence of DES exposure. In many respects natural estrogens show similar effects but to a much lesser degree (reviewed by Ahlquist, 1976). Suppression of immunity was evidenced by depressed antibody responses, DHRs and LP responses to T-cell mitogens, B-cell mitogens and allogeneic cells. Since suppressed DHRs were only obtained when antigen sensitization preceded DES treatment these data can be construed to indicate that the immuno-suppressive effects are not particularly persistent. On the other hand, a direct effect on memory cell function cannot be readily dismissed. In this respect earlier studies have suggested that DES administered during prenatal (Luster et al., 1979) or early postnatal development (Kalland et al., 1978) induces relatively long lasting effects on immune responses while suppression of LP responses following adult exposure may be temporary (Kalland et al., 1980).

While peripheral lymphocytosis and splenomegaly occurred following DES treatment, there was a decreased percentage of splenic T-cells as determined by staining with an anti-T cell antiserum. Since the percentage of Ig-positive splenic leukocytes was not altered, an absolute increase in lymphocytes without detectable T- or B-lymphocyte markers resulted from DES exposure. These cells may represent null cells or immature T-cells not possessing this T-cell marker and occurring as a result of thymo-cyte mobilization of immature T-cells, since histological evidence in-dicated severe depletion of cortical thymcytes without evidence of cell necrosis. Alternatively, this may result from the inhibition of normal T-cell maturation resulting from loss of the normal thymic environment since severe thymic atrophy occurs follow DES treatment. It has been well established that T-cell precursors enter the thymus and mature under the influence of the thymic epithelium leading to expression of T-cell markers (reviewed Stutman 1978). Recent evidence has indicated that mice exposed neonatally to DES also reveal decreased percentages of splenic T-cells (Kalland, 1980a). Furthermore, an increase in the number of cells possessing the Ly 1, 2, 3 marker (precommitted T-cells) and decreased number of Ly 1 cells (T-helper) were found indicating a selective effect on T-cell immunity.

The role of suppressor cells and their products has achieved wide-spread recognition in the regulation of the immune response. Spleen cell populations in laboratory animals capable of suppressing a variety of *in vitro* lymphocyte responses have been characterized in different systems as belonging to the monocyte/macrophage series, having properties of B-cells or immature T-cells. The inhibitory effects of these suppressor cells appear to be exerted at the level of lymphocyte DNA synthesis (Kirchner et al., 1975) suggesting that *in vitro* coculture experiments followed by examination of LP responses represents a simple means to assay for suppressor cells. The present studies demonstrate that suppressor activity resides within adherent PM cells of DES treated mice which is capable of suppressing LP responses from spleen cells of normal mice. This was evidenced by marked suppression of LP responses of spleen cells when cocultured with MMC-blocked spleen cells from DES exposed mice since MMC treatment blocks DNA synthesis, but has no immediate effect on elaboration of supernatant factors. The enhanced LP response that occurs in DES treated mice following removal of adherent cells is consistent with LP suppressed tumor bearing mice which demonstrates enhanced LP responsiveness following removal of adherent cells (Rudcz-ynski and Mortensen, 1978). The observation that suppressor cell activity resided in the adherent population is not particularly surprising consider-ing the activated nature of the macrophage population following DES exposure. The nature of macrophage suppressor activity is currently un-certain although it has been postulated to occur through synthesis of prostaglandins (Webb and Nowowiejski, 1978). These studies do not exclude the possibility that suppressor activity residing in the lymphocyte population also exists and preliminary evidence has suggested this to be the case.

Macrophage functions were potentiated by DES treatment as evidenced by increased phagocytosis, proliferation and tumor growth inhibition by adherent PM cells. The ability of natural and synthetic estrogens to stimulate phagocytic activity has been well documented (Heller, et al., 1957; Nicol et al., 1963). DES, itself, causes increased hepatic phagocytic activity of macrophages (Kelly et al., 1962; Loose and Diluzio, 1976). Whether the RES stimulation is due to increased macrophage prolifera-tion, hyperphagocytosis or enlargement of RES organs is uncertain, al-though indirect evidence suggests that it is due to liver or spleen enlarge-ment (Loose and DiLuzio, 1976). Evidence from the present studies would indicate that increased RES activity at least in part, was due to increased macrophage activation, although an additive contribution by increased RES organ weights cannot be excluded since livers and spleens were enlarged at the highest dosage levels.

A panel of host susceptibility assays indicated that DES treatment resulted in decreased resistance to endotoxin, bacterial, parasitic and tumor cell challenges (see Dean et al. this book). Although endotoxin detoxification is probably a macrophage dependent process (Braude et al., 1955), animals treated with various RES stimulants such as BCG

(Sater, 1964), zymosan (Benacerraff et al., 1959) or glucan (Crafton and Diluzio, 1979) are more susceptible to endotoxin. This has been taken as evidence that host susceptibility to endotoxin is related to the "endotoxin-detoxifying" ability of the liver and spleen rather than phagocytic activity. Since sulfhydryl containing enzymes (e.g., glutathione-S-transferase) are important for endotoxin detoxification, it would be relevant to examine the activity of several of these enzymes in mononuclear cells from DES treated animals.

Unlike endotoxin, defense against facultatiave intracellular bacteria as well as *Trichnella spiralis* is dependent upon a collaborative effort between antigen sensitized T-lymphocytes and cells from the mononuclear phagocytic system although recent studies have suggested resistance to *Listeria monocytogenes* may well be a bone marrow dependent function (Bennet et al., 1976). Thus, the decreased resistance observed following DES exposure can be interpreted as indicating: 1) a T-cell mediated defect; 2) depression of bone marrow function; 3) and/or a nonphagocytic related defect of macrophage function such as alterations in lysozomal enzymes and subsequent loss of macrophage-dependent bacterial killing. While similar reasoning can be applied to the increased susceptibility to tumor cell challenge, the increased ability of adherent PM cells to inhibit tumor cell growth *in vitro* would suggest that macrophage-mediated cytostasis does not correlate to tumor resistance, at least, as a consequence of DES exposure. A further consideration is that natural killer (NK) cell activity is depressed following DES treatment. In this respect, recent studies by Kalland (1980b) have demonstrated depressed NK activity in neonatally DES exposed mice.

The role of DES-induced immunological alterations in the development of malignant alterations in genital tracts of mice treated *in utero* with DES (rev. by McLachlin and Dixon, 1976) and in carcinogenicity in mice exposed as adults (rev. by McMartin et al., 1970) remains to be determined. Immunological studies in women who have developed vaginal clear-cell adenocarcinoma following exposure to DES *in utero* (Herbst, 1971) would be of interest to examine.

SUMMARY

Diethylstilbestrol (DES), a nonsteroidal compound possessing estrogenic activity, is a potent stimulant of the RES. The compound has been used extensively as a therapeutic agent in humans as estrogen replacement and treatment of certain cancers and as a growth-promoting agent in sheep and cattle. In the present studies, female $B_6C_3F_1$ adult mice were administered subcutaneous injections of DES in corn oil at dosages of 0, 0.2, 2.0 and 8.0 mg/kg body weight for 5 days. While increased numbers of peripheral lymphocytes and monocytes occurred, severe depression of various immune parameters resulted. These included depressed antibody responses (PFCs) to SRBCs and lipopolysaccharide (LPS), delayed hypersensitivity responses, and lymphoproliferative response to both mitogens and allogeneic cells. Bone marrow examination revealed hypocellularity and decreased proliferation (colony formation) of both hemopoietic stem cells and granulocyte-macrophage precursors. In contrast, various macrophage functions were enhanced including phagocytosis, proliferation in response to macrophage growth factor and activation as determined by cytostasis. Coculture experiments revealed the presence of suppressor activity residing in the macrophage population which was capable of suppressing lymphoproliferative responses from normal animals. These results indicate that DES, while an RES stimulant, severely depresses specific immunity and that suppression, at least in part, is due to macrophage suppressor cell activity.

REFERENCES

Ahlquist, J. Endocrine influences on lymphatic organs, immune responses, inflammation and autoimmunity. Acta endocrinologica *83*:1 (1976).

Bach, J. F. 1975. Corticosteroids. In *Modes of Action of Immunosuppressive Agents* (A. Neuberger, and L. A. Tatum, eds.), pp. 21–70. North-Holland Publishing Co., Amsterdam, Netherlands.

Bailer, J. C. and Byar, D. P. Estrogen treatment for cancer of the prostrate: Early results with 3 doses of diethylstilbestrol and placebo. Cancer *26*:257 (1976).

Benacerraf, B., Thorbecke, G. J. and Jacoby, D. Effect of zymosan on endotoxin toxicity in mice. Proc. Soc. Evp. Biol. Med., *100*:796 (1959).

Bennet, M., Baker, E. E., Eastcott, J. W., Kumar, V. and Yonkosky, D. Selective elimination of bone marrow precursors with the bone-seeking isotope, 89, Sr. J. Retic. Soc., *20*:71 (1976).

Berlinger, N. T., Lopez, C. and Good, R. A. Facilitation or attenuation of mixed leucocyte culture responsiveness by adherent cells. Nature *260*:145 (1976).

Boorman, G. A. and Luster, M. I. Macrophage proliferation in liquid cultures as measured by tritiated thymidine uptake. J. Ret. Endo. Soc. (1980) in press.

Bradley, T. R. and Metcalf, D. The growth of mouse bone marrow cells *in vitro*. Aust. J. Exp. Biol. Med. Sci., *44*:287, (1966).

Braude, A. I., Carey, F. J. and Zalesky, M. Studies with radioactive endotoxin. J. Clin. Invest. *34*:858, (1955).

Crafton, C. G. and DiLuzio, N. R. Relationship of reticuloendothelial functional activity to endotoxin lethality. Amer. J. Physiol., *217*:736 (1969).

Cutler, B. S., Forbes, A. P., Ingersoll, F. M. and Scully, R. E. Endomentrial carcinoma after stilbestrol therapy in gonadal dysgenesis. N. Engl. J. Med., *287*:628 (1972).

Dean, J. H. Padarathsingh, M. L. Response of murine leukemia to combined BCNU-MUE therapy and correlation with macrophage activation by MUE in the *in vitro* growth inhibition assay. Cancer Treat., *62*:1807 (1978).

Dodds, E. C. The significance of synthetic oestrogenic agents. Acta. Med. Scand. (Suppl.) *90*:141 (1939).

Dresser, D. W. and Greaves, M. F. *Handbook of Experimental Immunology* (D. M. Weir, Ed.) Oxford: Blackwell Scientific Inc. (1978).

Greenman, D. L., Dooley, K. and Breeden, C. R. Strain differences in the response of the mouse to diethylstilbestrol. J. Toxicol. and Environm. Hlth., *3*:589, (1977).

Hadden, J. W., Sadlik, J. R. and Hadden, E. M. 1978. The induction of macrophage proliferation *in vitro* by a lymphocyte produced factor. J. Immunol., *121*:231 (1978).

Heinonen, O. P. The Boston collaborative drug surveillance program: Diethylstilbestrol in pregnancy. Cancer *31*:573 (1973).

Heller, J. H., Meier, R. M. Zucker, R. and Mast, G. W. The effect of natural and synthetic estrogens on reticuloendothelial system function. Endocrinol., *61*:235 (1957).

Herbst, A. L., Ulfelder, H., and Poskanzer, D. C. Adenocarcinoma of the vagina. Association of maternal stilboestrol therapy with tumor appearance in young women. N. Engl. J. Med., *284*:878 (1971).

IARC Monographs Evaluation of carcinogenic risk. V. G. Lyon: IARC (1974).

Jonckheere, A. R. A distribution-free K-sample test against ordered alternatives. Biometrika, *41*:133 (1954).

Kalland, T. Alterations of antibody response in female mice after neonatal exposure to diethylstilbestrol. J. Immunol. (1980a) In press.

Kalland, T. 1980b. Reduced natural killer activity in female mice after neonatal exposure to diethylstilbestrol J. Immunol. (1980b) In press.

Kalland, T. and Forsberg, J. Delayed hypersensitivity response to oxazolone in neonatally estrogenized mice. Cancer Letters 4:141, (1978).

Kalland, T. Forsberg, T. M. and Forsberg, J. G. 1978. Effect of estrogen and corticosterone on the lymphoid system in neonatal mice. Explt. Molec. Path., *28*:76, (1978).

Kalland, T., Strand, O. and Forsberg, J. Long term effects of neonatal estrogen treatment on mitogen responsiveness of mouse spleen lymphocytes. JNCI (1980c) In press.

Kelly, L. S., Brown, B. A., and Dobson, E. L. Cell division and phagocytic activity in liver reticulo-endothelial cells. Proc. Soc. Exp. Biol. Med.,*110*:555 (1962).

Kenny, J. F. and Diamond, M. Immunological responsiveness to Escherichia coli during pregnancy. Infec. Immun., *16*:174 (1977).

Kirchner, H., Muchmore, A. V. and Chused, T. M. Inhibition of proliferation of lymphoma cells and T-lymphocytes by suppressor cells from spleens of tumor-bearing mice. J. Immunol., *114*:206 (1975).

Lefford, M. J. The measurement of tuberculin hypersensitivity in rats. Int. Arch. Allergy Appl. Immunol. *47*:570 (1974).

Loose, L. D. and DiLuzio, N. R. 76 Dose related reticuloendothelial system stimulation by diethylstilbestrol. J. Reticuloendothelial Soc., *20*:457 (1976).

Luster, M. I., Boorman, G. A., Harris, M. W., and Moore, J. A. Laboratory studies on polybrominated biphenyl-induced immune alterations following low-level chronic or pre/postnatal exposure. Int. J. Immunopharmacol. (1980) In press.

Luster, M. I., Faith, R. E., and McLachlan, J. A. Modulation of the antibody response following in utero exposure to diethylstilbestrol. Bull. Environ. Contam. Toxicol., *20*:433 (1978).

Luster, M. I., Faith, R. E., McLachlin, J. A. and Clark, G. C. Effect of *in utero* exposure to diethylstilbestrol on the immune response in mice. Toxicol. Applied Pharmacol., *47*:279 (1979).

Ly, I. A. and Mishell, R. I. Separation of mouse spleen cells by passage through columns of Sephadex G-10. J. Immunol. Meth., *5*:239 (1973).

Mantovani, A., Jerrells, T. R., Dean, J. H. and Herberman, R. B. Cytolytic and cytostatic activity on tumor cells of circulating human monocytes. Int. J. Cancer, *23*:18 (1979).

McLachlan, J. A. and Dixon, R. L. Advances in Modern Toxicology. Hemisphere. New York (1976).

McMartin, K. E., Kennedy, K. A., Greenspan, P., Alam, S. N., Greiner, P. and Yam J. Diethylstilbestrol: A review of its toxicity and use as a growth promotant in food-producing animals. J. Environm. Path. and Toxicol., *1*:297 (1978).

Nicol, T., Cordingley, J., Charles, L., McKelvie, P. and Bailey, D. Effect of reticulo-endothelial stimulation on experimental infection. In *Role du System Reticulo-endothial dans L'Immunite. Antibacterienne et Antitumorole.* Paris Colloques Internationaux du C. N. R.s Nolls, p. 165 (1963).

Pannacciulli, I. M., Massa, G., Saviane, A. G., Bianchi, G., Bagliolo, G. V. and Ghio, R. The effects of chronic administration of cyclophosphamide on haemo-poietic stem cells. Scand. J. Haematol., *19*:217 (1977).

Rudczynski, A. B. and Mortensen, R. F. Suppressor cells in mice with murine mammary tumor virus-induced mammary tumors. I. Inhibition of mitogen-induced lymphocyte stimulation. J. Natl. Cancer Inst., *60*:205 (1978).

Sater, E. Hyperreactivity to endotoxin in infection. In *Bacterial Endotoxins* (M. Landy and W. Braun, eds.) Rutgers, State Univ. Press, New Brunswick, N.J. (1976).

Sljivic, V. S., Clark, D. W. and Warr, G. W. Effects of oestrogens and pregnancy on the distribution of sheep erythrocytes and the antibody response in mice. Clin. Exp. Immunol., *20*:179 (1975).

Sljivic, V. S. and Warr, G. W. Activity of the RES and the antibody response III. The fate of type III pneumococcol polysaccharide and the antibody response. Immunology., *27*:1009 (1974).

Steven, W. M. and Snook, T. The stimulatory effects of diethylstilbestrol and diethylstilbestrol diphosphate on the reticuloendoendothelial cells of the rat spleen. Am. J. Anat., *144*:339 (1975).

Stuart, A. E., Habeshaw, J. A. and Davidson, A. E. In *Handbook of Experimental Immunology.* (D. M. Weir Ed.) Blackwell Scientific, Oxford England 1978.

Stutman, O. Intrathymic and extrathymic T-cell maturation Immunological Rev., *42*:138 (1978).

Till, J. E. and McCulloch, E. A. A direct measurment of the radiation sensitivity of normal mouse bone marrow cells. Radiation Research, *14*:213 (1961).

Veit, B. C., and Michael, J. G. The lack of thymic influence in regulating the immune response to Escherichia coli 0127 endotoxin. J. Immunol. *109*:547 (1972).

Webb, D. R. and Nowowiejski, I. Mitogen induced changes in lymphocyte prostaglandin levels: A signal for the induction of suppressor cell activity. Cell Immunol., *41*:72 (1978).

DISCUSSION

SPREAFICO: One comment and one question, Dr. Luster: I'm glad to hear your data, because we have published studies on a series of contraceptive agents, using the three estrogen-progesterone combinations which are more frequently employed in Europe. We find that all of them are immunodepressant when employed in chronic treatment at the lowest dosage giving 100 percent antifertility effect. Our data differ somewhat from yours in that, in our conditions, the T-cells seem to be the most compromised, but there is one question that I would like to ask you. Have you checked on the effect of DES in other species? In our hands the mouse was far more susceptible to the effects of contraceptive steroids than was the rat, for instance. Do you have any information on this?

LUSTER: We haven't looked at other species but what I have seen with receptors for DES is quite a lot of species variation in organ distribution; also one sees differences in the toxicological effects and metabolites of DES.

One statement: I'm not suggesting that there are more severe effects on B-cells than T-cells. I don't think we can make that statement.

KALLAND: I would also like to emphasize that DES may have profound effects on the immune system in humans as well. DES-phosphate is widely used for treatment of prostatic cancer, as mentioned by Dr. Luster. We have performed studies on the natural killer activity in patients before and during treatment, and have found a profound effect on the natural killer activity. It is clearly reduced. We can see the effect after about one week of treatment but we have no indications as to how long the effects will last after the treatment is stopped. These studies are done in collaboration with Dr. Haukos.

If we treat the neonatal mouse with DES, as already mentioned by Dr. Luster, there are profound effects on the immune system.

We have also studied the effects on natural killer activity in these mice. Table 1 shows results. It shows the effect of neonatal treatment with DES on the natural killer activity in adult animals, using the standard assay for natural killer activity, measuring killing of YAC-1 or MPC-11 cells. As indicated, both in inbred BALB/c and C57 strains and also in outbred NMRI mice, the activity on natural killing is dramatically reduced.

The relevance of these findings is further underlined by the development of tumors in these animals. Tumors of the classical estrogen-target organs

Table 1.   Effect of Neonatal DES-Treatment on NK Activity

ANIMAL	NEONATAL TREATMENT	% CYTOTOXICITY [a]	
		YAC-1	MPC-11
BALB/c	Olive Oil	40.2 ± 3.7	25.0 ± 3.2
BALB/c	DES	18.7 ± 2.7***	10.2 ± 2.3***
C57BL/6	Olive Oil	49.5 ± 4.8	35.7 ± 3.0
C57BL/6	DES	12.6 ± 3.2***	8.1 ± 1.8***
NMRI	Olive Oil	34.3 ± 3.5	22.5 ± 2.9
NMRI	DES	24.7 ± 4.5*	15.4 ± 2.6[n.s.]

[a] Mean % cytotoxicity $\pm$ SE of 10 female mice assayed individually at an effector to target cell ratio of 50:1. Asterices indicate statistical significance of reduction by neonatal DES treatment.

are well known following neonatal DES treatment but, recently, we have also performed studies on general tumor incidence in these animals; neonatally DES-treated animals also have shown an increased incidence of methyl-cholanthrene-induced sarcomas.

LaVIA: I have two comments on your somewhat contradictory results with the T-independent antigen and activated T-suppressor cells. We have a similar phenomenon in an entirely different system, but there is one possible explanation for this, and I wonder whether you have looked into it. There is a series of papers in Cellular Immunology in 1978 and 1979 by Masuda and Miyama suggesting that there may be some suppressor factors secreted by Fc receptor negative B lymphocytes. Have you had any indication of anything like this?

LUSTER: No. We're thinking of looking at that, as a matter of fact.

I would like to comment on Dr. Kalland's studies. I think what both of us would like to emphasize is the fact that in utero exposure, or early post-natal exposure, appears to have a persistent effect on the immunological system. We feel adult exposure is not persistent. It may change, last only a month or two. One of the questions that should be addressed is why no one has looked at human females exposed in utero to DES for immuno-logical responses.

SIGEL: I think it ought to be clarified that the LPS is not strictly a thymus-independent response. That part of the LPS response is thymus dependent.

LUSTER: I was aware of that.

THURMAN: I would like to ask if you analyzed the cells that were removed on the G-10 column, since we know that certain T-cells are adherent to macrophages? I wondered if you might have moved a population of suppressor T-cells with the adherent cells.

LUSTER: No. All we did was to enumerate the total T-cells and total B-cells and saw no variation in the percentage of T- and B-cells isolated. It's always a possibility that one can be selecting for a specific LY marker but, from earlier studies that I have seen, no type of T-cell was selectively decreased or selectively increased following G-10 passage.

12
Effects of Alkylating Agents on the Immune Response

**Martin L. Padarathsingh, Jack H. Dean
and Lenwood Keys**

*Department of Immunology, Litton Bionetics, Inc., Kensington, MD
Environmental Biology Branch and Environmental Chemistry
Laboratory, National Institute of Environmental Health Sciences
Research Triangle Park, N.C.*

INTRODUCTION

Suppressed general and cell-mediated immune (CMI) responses have been
reported in studies conducted in mice treated with low doses of heavy
metals (Koller, 1973; Koller et al., 1976). General impaired immunocompetence has likewise been observed in animals with 2,3,7,8-tetrachlorodi-
benzop-dioxin (TCDD) (Vos and Moore, 1974; Faith and Moore, 1977);
polybrominated biphenyls (PBB) (Luster et al., 1978). In addition, immune dysfunction has been reported by Bekesi and co-workers (1978)
among Michigan dairy farmers exposed to polybrominated biphenyls.
Studies from our laboratory (Dean et al., 1979) as well as others
(Winkelstein, 1973; Milton et al., 1976) with cyclophosphamide (CY), a
well known alkylating agent, have shown depressed CMI responses following CY exposure. Likewise, studies with the flame retardant Tris (2-3-
dibromopropyl phosphate) have shown this compound to be mutagenic
in bacterial systems (Blum and Ames, 1977; Prival et al., 1977). Other
studies have shown Tris to be carcinogenic in mice (Consumer Product
Safety Commission, 1977) and to induce both benign and malignant
tumors in mice (Van Duuren et al., 1978).

Recently, our laboratory has focused on the application of general and
cell-mediated immune competence assays for measuring immune dysfunction. We have attempted to correlate *in vivo* parameters including tumor
susceptibility; the isotopic footpad assay (IFP) for measuring cutaneous

176

delayed type hypersensitivity to recall antigens; Cunningham's modification of the Jerne Plaque Assay (PFC) which examines the number of antibody producing cells; and the lymphocyte proliferative (LP) response to general mitogens for assessing lymphocytes (T- and B-cell) function.

The purpose of the present study was to examine the general immune competence of cells within the spleens of BALB/c mice treated with Tris or CY relative to the PFC response against sheep red blood cells (SRBC), LP responses to T- and B-cell mitogens and the IFP responses to tumor-associated antigens (TAA) of sarcoma mKSA. We also measured susceptibility of treated animals to transplantable tumors.

MATERIALS AND METHODS

Mice

Female inbred BALB/c mice weighing 20 to 24 gm were obtained from the production colonies of the National Institutes of Health (NIH) and used throughout these studies.

Drugs

CY was obtained from Mead Johnson and Company (Evansville, IN) and was dissolved in sterile saline immediately prior to use. Animals were injected IP in doses of 180 mg/kg to 1.08 mg/kg. Commerical Tris was obtained from K and K Laboratories (Plainview, NY). The drug was dissolved in commercially available corn oil (Mazola, Best Foods, Englewood Cliffs, NJ) and administered IP at 500 to 0.5 mg/kg of body weight.

Tumors

The mKSA tumor-cell line was developed by Kit et al., (1969) by the transformation of primary BALB/c kidney cell cultures with SV40. The tumor line has been maintained in our laboratory for several years by *in vivo* serial passage.

Tumor Susceptibility Assay

A sensitive assessment of general immunocompetence is reflected in the ability of a mouse to resist challenge with a syngeneic transplantable tumor given at a low tumor cell dose (TD) which produces tumors in 10-20% (TD_{10}-TD_{20}) of injected animals. The ability to resist a low tumor cell dose is thought to reflect general immune surveillance indicative of normal lymphocyte function.

Tumor susceptibility testing was performed in BALB/c mice exposed to graded doses of CY and Tris two days prior to subcutaneous (SC) challenge with 5×10^2 mKSA tumor cells. Animals were weighed and palpated twice weekly for changes in body weights and tumor development through day 90. Data were expressed as: (1) the number of tumor takes/number of mice challenged; and (2) the mean latency (in days) to tumor detection.

Isotopic (^{125}I) Footpad Assay (IFP)

BALB/c mice were immunized with mKSA-TU5 tissue culture adapted cells by four weekly SC injections of 1×10^6 tumor cells. Two to six weeks following the last immunization, control, Tris and CY treated animals were challenged with viable mKSA ascites tumor cells to measure the delayed cutaneous hypersensitivity (DHS) response in the footpad using the IFP assay previously described in detail (Dean et al., 1977). Results were expressed as the footcount ratio (FCR) $=$ $\dfrac{\text{CPM test foot}}{\text{CPM contralateral control foot}}$. Significance between positive IFP responses to test antigen in immune and normal mice was determined by Student's t-test.

Plaque-Forming Cell (PFC) Assay

The plaque-forming cell (PFC) response to sheep red blood cells (SRBC) was performed as described in Cunningham (1965). Mice were injected IV with 0.1 ml of a 10% SRBC suspension 4 days before PFC's were determined. The data were expressed as: PFC/10^6 spleen cells; PFC/spleen and percent change relative to response of normal (non-drug-treated) BALB/c donors.

Lymphocyte Proliferation (LP) Assay

The microculture LP assay previously described by Dean et al. (1975) utilizing the mitogens [Phytohemagglutinin (PHA), Concanavalin A (Con A) and *E. coli* lipopolysaccharide (LPS)] was employed to assay the proliferative potential of immunocompetent spleen cells. These data were expressed as: the mean CPM ($\bar{x}$CPM) of the four replicate experimental cultures (E) which usually had standard errors (SE) of $\pm 5\%$; and percent change, which is the net CPM of the drug-treated mice divided by the net CPM of the normal mice minus one × 100.

$$\text{Percent Change} = 1 - \frac{\text{nCPM of Drug-Treated Mice}}{\text{nCPM of Normal Mice}} \times 100.$$

RESULTS

Experiments were performed to determine the effects of CY on normal resistance to a titrated dose of mKSA sarcoma cells that would produce tumors in approximately 10% of non-treated animals. The level of tumor cells used for challenge was selected to determine the minimal level of cells which would measure chemical induced alterations of normal host resistance. In these experiments, normal BALB/c mice were treated with CY at 180 mg/kg two days prior to challenge with mKSA ascites tumor cells at concentrations between 5×10^4 to 5×10^1. The number of tumors and the mean latency to tumor detection were recorded (Table 1). Challenge of CY treated mice with mKSA at 5×10^3 to 5×10^2 enhanced the development of tumors (80–90% takes) when compared to untreated animals which had only 20 and 10 percent tumor takes, respectively. In addition, the mean latency to tumor detection ranged between 10.5 and 19 days among drug-treated, tumor-challenged mice, compared with a

Table 1.   The Effect of Cyclophosphamide in Promoting the Growth of mKSA Sarcoma in BALB/c Mice When Administered Before Tumor Inoculation.

CY (MG/KG) GIVEN ON DAY −2	CONCENTRATION OF mKSA CHALLENGE [1]	NUMBER OF TUMORS / NUMBER OF MICE INOCULATED	PERCENT TUMORS	MEAN TIME TO TUMOR DETECTION (DAYS)
0	5×10^4	8/10	80	10
0	5×10^3	2/10	20	21
0	5×10^2	1/10	10	30
0	5×10^1	0/10	—	—
180	5×10^4	10/10	100	8.5
180	5×10^3	10/10	90	10.5
180	5×10^2	8/10	80	19
180	5×10^1	0/10	—	—

[1] Mice were challenged SC with tumor cells on day 0 and then palpated three times weekly for tumor formation. Last day of observation was on day 60.

Table 2.   Effects of Graded Doses of Tris or CY Administered to BALB/c Mice Prior to Inoculation with mKSA Sarcoma.

TREATMENT SCHEDULE	DOSE (MG/KG) ON DAY −2	TUMOR TAKES [1] NUMBER OF ANIMALS INOCULATED	PERCENT TUMOR TAKES
None	—	2/20	10
Tris	500	4/10	40
Tris	50	2/10	20
Tris	5	1/10	10
Tris	0.5	0/10	—
CY	108	6/10	60
CY	23	3/10	30
CY	9	2/10	20
CY	3	1/10	10
CY	1.08	0/10	—

[1] Mice were challenged with 5×10^2 mKSA ascites cells SC on day 0 and palpated three times weekly for tumor formation. Last day of observation was on day 60.

latency of 21 to 30 days among the untreated animals challenged at the same tumor cell level. These data indicate that CY administered at 180 mg/kg depressed the immune response and enhanced susceptibility to sarcoma mKSA.

Mice were treated with graded doses of CY (180 to 1.08 mg/kg) or with Tris (500 to 0.5 mg/kg) and then challenged with 5×10^2 mKSA ascites tumor cells (Table 2). Treatment of normal mice with Tris enhanced tumor susceptibility to between 20–40%. Increased tumor susceptibility (20–60%) was observed in BALB/c mice treated with CY at 9-180 mg/kg. These data demonstrate that low levels of CY and Tris enhanced tumor susceptibility to mKSA sarcoma.

Studies were then undertaken to examine the effects of chemical exposure on the delayed-type hypersensitivity responses to tumor-associated antigens (TAA) of mKSA-TU5 utilizing the isotopic footpad (IFP) assay. The effects of CY and Tris on the CMI responses to syngeneic mKSA tumor cells as measured by ^{125}I footpad incorporation are demonstrated in Table 3. BALB/c mice immunized to mKSA and treated with CY or Tris were challenged ID in the right hind footpad (RHFP) with 10^6 mKSA-TU5 cells followed by ^{125}I human serum albumin given IP. The mean footcount ratio for the non-treated immune mice were approximately three times

Table 3.   Effect of Tris or CY on Delayed Hypersensitivity Response to mKSA-TU5 TAA in Immune Mice Using the IFP Assay.

TEST GROUP	TREATMENT SCHEDULE	I^{125} CONTROL FOOT CPM	TUMOR CELL I^{125} CHALLENGED FOOT CPM	FOOTCOUNT RATIO [1] ($\pm$SE)
Non-Immune	None	3,669	4,130	1.13 (0.02)
mKSA-TU5 Immune [2]	None	3,221	6,919	2.84 (0.08)*
mKSA-TU5 Immune	CY 180 mg/kg	3,153	4,457	1.41 (0.12)
mKSA-TU5 Immune	Tris 500 mg/kg	2,953	4,002	1.36 (0.15)

[1] Values represent the mean footcount ratio of six mice/group.
[2] BALB/c mice were immunized by 4 to 6 weekly SC injections of 1×10^6 mKSA-TU5 tissue cultured grown cells.
* Significantly different than in control feet at $p < 0.01$ by Student's t-test.

greater than the footcount ratio of the non-immune controls. Moreover, when mice with established DHS to mKSA were treated with CY or Tris and tested two days later, the DHS response to mKSA became non-reactive. A single injection of CY at 180 mg/kg or Tris at 500 mg/kg abrogated the DHS responses of these immune animals to the syngeneic mKSA tumor. These data indicate that CY or Tris abrogated the anti-tumor DHS response.

Attention was next focused on the measurement of non-specific parameters in normal mice treated with CY or Tris. The antibody plaque-forming cell (PFC) responses to the T-cell dependent antigen sheep red blood cells (SRBC) were measured in normal and drug-treated animals given 4×10^8 SRBC IV four days prior to the PFC assay (Table 4). A single dose of CY at 180 mg/kg severely suppressed (77%) the PFC response of BALB/c mice. Likewise, a single dose of Tris at 50 or 500 mg/kg suppressed the PFC response (30 and 50% respectively).

Spleen cells from BALB/c mice treated with CY or Tris were evaluated for proliferative responses to T- and B-cell mitogens. Table 5 demonstrated mitogen data (PHA, Con A and LPS) from non-treated mice and mice treated with CY or Tris. Seven days following a single treatment of CY at 180 mg/kg, the proliferative response to PHA was reduced by 61% and to Con A by 67%. The lymphoproliferative response to LPS was reduced by 70%. Reduced LP responses were also observed in mice treated with Tris. These results indicate that both the T- and B-cell mitogen responses of mice treated with CY or Tris were suppressed.

Table 4. **The Effect of Tris or Cyclophosphamide on the Antibody PFC Response of BALB/c Mice to SRBC.**

TREATMENT [1]	DOSE MG/KG	MONONUCLEAR CELLS PER SPLEEN	MEAN PFC PER 10^6 SPLEEN CELLS	PERCENT CHANGE [2]
None	—	2.2×10^8	1,438	—
Tris	500	1.43×10^8	719	50*↓
Tris	50	1.57×10^8	1,006	30*↓
Tris	5	1.97×10^8	1,581	10↑
CY	180	9.75×10^7	340	77*↓

[1] Six normal or treated BALB/c mice/group were injected IV with 4×10^8 SRBC four days prior to PFC assay.
[2] Percent change relative to response of normal BALB/c donors.
* Significantly different from control values at $p < 0.05$ by Student's t-test.

**_Table 5._ Lymphoproliferative Responses to Mitogens in Spleen
Cells from Normal BALB/c Mice Treated
with Tris or Cyclophosphamide.[1]**

| | | NET CPM OF ^{3}H-TdR INCORPORATION [2] | | |
| | | PHA
($\pm$SE) | CON A
($\pm$SE) | LPS
($\pm$SE) |
TREATMENT	DOSE MG/KG	% CHANGE	% CHANGE	% CHANGE
None	—	226,058 (6,227)	244,450 (4,873)	11,626 (235)
Tris	500	130,030 (7,025) 42*↓	69,772 (2,462) 71*↓	3,992 (155) 66*↓
Tris	50	106,827 (20,231) 52*↓	106,637 (9,315) 56*↓	8,631 (828) 26*↓
Tris	5	197,790 (5,358) 13 ↓	268,988 (2,003) 10 ↑	12,174 (141) 5 ↑
CY	180	88,594 (6,956) 61*↓	80,141 (4,322) 67*↓	3,486 (327) 70*↓

[1] Six normal drug-treated BALB/c mice were sacrificed and their spleen cells pooled in each group and assayed on the same day.
[2] Values from optimum blastogenic concentration of mitogens were used: PHA (0.25µg/ well), Con A (0.5µg/well) and LPS (5µg/well).
* Significantly different from control at $p < 0.05$

DISCUSSION

The indications of immunologic impairment following exposure of experimental animals or man to certain chemicals are of great concern relative to the selection of methodology for routine assessment of immunobiological effects induced by chemicals. Methodology selected should encompass a high degree of reproducibility, be relatively easy to perform, economical and above all should be relevant to the human experience. With these considerations, a series of immunobiological assays were utilized to more specifically define the effect of alkylating agents on the immune responses of normal BALB/c mice. Evaluation of these chemicals was also made in mice bearing progressively growing tumors which often produce some degree of immunological suppression (Howell et al., 1975).

A series of immunocompetence assays were validated in BALB/c mice following treatment with CY or Tris to measure immune dysfunction. In addition, we studied the effects of these compounds on susceptibility to transplantable syngeneic tumors to examine the ability of these agents to alter host resistance to a graded dose of tumor cells which produced tumors in only ten percent of non-treated mice. This tumor cell challenge level was selected since previous studies had shown that tumor cell challenge was a sensitive endpoint to measure immune dysfunction in the drug-treated host (Dean et al., 1979).

The battery of general and CMI assays utilized in these studies demonstrated severe immune suppression in BALB/c mice following treatment with CY or Tris. The tumor susceptibility assay appeared to be quite sensitive in detecting immune depression following administration of low levels of CY (9 mg/kg). This level of CY results in enhanced growth of sarcoma mKSA and confirmed our previous studies (Dean et al., 1979). Recently Van Duuren and his co-workers (1978) have shown commercial grade Tris to be carcinogenic in mice given 10 mg skin application. One should be extremely careful in analyzing these data since commerical Tris contains impurities which have been shown to be mutagenic in bacterial systems (Blum and Ames, 1977) and caused a high incidence of squamous carcinoma of the stomach in mice and rats by gastric intubation (Olson et al., 1973).

The delayed-type hypersensitivity response to mKSA ascites tumor cells was easily quantitated by the IFP assay with approximately a three-fold response in the mKSA immunized animals when compared to the non-immune control mice. However, when these immunized mice were treated with a single dose of Tris or CY, the IFP responses were reduced to the level of the normal, non-immune, non-treated mice. It appears that CY or Tris depleted the memory responses to TAA in these immunized animals. Studies by Moore and Faith (1976) have shown that the chemical TCDD can deplete the DHR.

The PFC response to SRBC which represents a T-cell dependent antigen response, appeared to be sensitive for detecting B-cell suppression in animals exposed to test compounds prior to immunization with SRBC. Our data demonstrated strong immunosuppressive action of CY and Tris on the PFC responses in mice treated seven days following drug treatment. Similar results have been shown in studies with a variety of environmental chemicals including: TCDD (Vos et al., 1973); PCB (Vos and Van Driel-Grootenhuis, 1972); and heavy metals (Koller et al., 1976).

The measurement of LP responses in drug-treated mice appear efficacious for detecting immune suppression using selective T- and B-cell mitogens. Results of our study demonstrated that LP responses in Tris or CY treated mice were strongly suppressed in both the T- and B-cell compartments of the CMI response. Studies from our laboratory (Dean et al., 1979) and those of others (Stockman et al., 1973) have shown CY to depress mitogenic reactivity. LP suppression following exposure to environmental chemicals such as TCDD (Vos and Moore, 1974); PBB (Bekesi et al., 1978) and organometals (Seinen et al., 1977) have been observed similar to that produced by CY or Tris.

In summary, the general and cell-mediated immunity assays as described and performed in these studies provided evidence of immune dysfunction induced by CY and Tris. This panel of tests measured effects to both humoral and cell-mediated immunity as well as susceptibility to transplantable tumors. The tumor susceptibility and DHR assays appeared to be good *in vivo* correlates of altered immunocompetence as measured by *in vitro* assays such as the PFC and LP responses.

CONCLUSION

General and cell-mediated immune parameters were investigated utilizing a series of *in vivo* and *in vitro* assays to measure immunological effects of the chemicals Tris or cyclophosphamide. BALB/c mice treated with these chemicals prior to tumor inoculation demonstrated a higher frequency of tumors and a shorter mean time to tumor detection as compared with the non-treated and tumor inoculated mice. Moreover, these agents abrogated specific delayed-hypersensitivity responses to recall antigens as demonstrated by the isotopic footpad assay in immunized mice. The results of the antibody plaque-forming cell and lymphocyte proliferation assays in treated mice correlated well with *in vivo* responses; in that, antibody plaque numbers following sheep erythrocytes challenge and lymphoproliferative responses to general mitogens were markedly suppressed in BALB/c mice treated with these chemicals.

ACKNOWLEDGMENTS

We greatly appreciate the help and cooperation of Ms. Carolyn Fox for her assistance in the preparation of this manuscript.

REFERENCES

Bekesi, J. G., Holland, J. F., Anderson, H. A., Fischbein, A. S., Rom, W., Wolff, M. S. and Selikoff, I. J.: Lymphocyte function of Michigan dairy farmers exposed tto polybrominated biphenyls. Science, *199*:1207 (1978).

Blum, A. and Ames, B. N.: Flame-retardant additives as possible hazards. Science, *195*:17-23 (1977).

Consumer Product Safety Commission: Tris and fabric yarn or fiber containing Tris. Additional interpretations as banned hazardous substances. Federal Register, *42*:60-64 (1977).

Cunningham, A. J.: A method of increased sensitivity for detecting single antibody-forming cells. Nature, *207*:1106-1107 (1965).

Dean, J. H., McCoy, J. L., Lewis, D. D., Appella, E. and Law, L. W.: Studies of lymphocyte stimulation by intact tumor cell and solubilized tumor antigens. Int.

Dean, J. H., Lewis, D. D. Padarathsingh, M. L., McCoy, J. L., Northing, J. W., J. Cancer, *16*:465-475 (1975).

Natori, T. and Law, L. W.: Cellular immunity to SV40-induced tumor cells and solubilized tumor-associated antigens in immune mice using an isotopic footpad assay. Int. J. Cancer, *20*:951-959 (1977).

Dean, J. H., Padarathsingh, M. L., Jerrells, T. R., Keys, J. and Northing, J. W.: Assessment of immunobiological effects induced by chemicals,, drugs or food additives. II. Studies with cyclophosphamide. Drug and Chemical Toxicology, *2*:133-153 (1979).

Faith, R. E. and Moore, J. A.: Impairment of thymus-dependent immune function by exposure of the developing immune system to 2,3,7,8-tetrachlorodibenzo-p-dioxin (TCDD). J. Toxicol. Environ. Health, *3*:451-464 (1977).

Howell, S. B., Dean, J. H. and Law, L. W.: Defects in cell-mediated immunity during growth of a syngeneic Simian virus-induced. Int. J. Cancer, *15*:152-169 (1975).

Kit, S., Kurimura, T. and Dubbs, D. R.: Transplantable mouse tumor line induced by inection of SV40 transformed mouse kidney cells. Int. J. Cancer, *4*:384-392 (1969).

Koller, L. D.: Immunosuppression produced by lead, cadmium and mercury. Am. J. Vet. Res., *34*:1457-1458 (1973).

Koller, L. D., Exon, J. H. and Roadn, J. G.: Humoral antibody response in mice after single dose exposure to lead cadmium. Proc. Soc. Exp. Biol. Med., *151*:339 (1976).

Luster, M. I., Faith, R. E. and Moore, J. A.: Effects of polybrominated biphenyls (PBB) on immune response in rodents. Environ. Health. Perspec., In press (1980).

Milton, J. D., Carpenter, C. B. and Addison, I. E.: Depressed T–cell reactivity and suppressor activity of lymphoid cells from cyclophosphamide treated mice. Cellular Immunol., *24*:308 (1976).

Moore, J. A. and Faith, R. E.: Immunologic response and factors affecting its assessment. J. Natl. Cancer Inst., *81*:125 (1976).

Olson, W. A., Haberman, R. T., Weinburger, E. K., Ward, J. M. and Weisbruger, J. H.: Induction of stomach cancer in rats and mice by halogenated aliphatic fumigants. J. Natl. Cancer Inst., *51*:1993-1995 (1973).

Prival, M. H., McCoy, E. C., Gutter, B. Rosenkranz, H. S.: Tris (2,3-dibromo-propyl) phosphate: Mutagenicity of a widely used flame retardant. Science, *195*:76-78 (1977).

Seinen, W., Vos, J. G., Van Krieken, R., Penninks, A., Brands, R. and Hooykas, H.: Toxicity of organotin compounds. III. Suppression of thymus-dependent immunity in rats by di-n-butyltindichloride and di-n-octyltindichloride. Toxicol. Appl. Pharmacol., *42*:213 (1977).

Stockman, G. D., Heim, L. R., South, M. A. and Trentin, J. J.: Differential effects of cyclophosphamide on the B- and T-cell compartments of adult mice. J. Immunol., *110*:282 (1973).

Van Duuren, B. L., Loweengart, G., Seidman, I., Smith, A. C. and Melchionne, S.: Mouse skin carcinogenicity tests of the flame retardants Tris (2,3-dibromopropyl) phosphate, Tetrakis (hydroxymethyl) phosphonium chloride and polyvinyl bromide. Cancer Res.,*38*:3236 (1978).

Vos, J. G. and Van Driel-Grootenhuis, L.: PCB-induced suppression of the humoral and cell-mediated immunity in guinea pigs. Sci. Total Environ., *1*:289 (1972).

Vos, J. G., Moore, J. A. and Zinkl, J. G.: Effect of 2,3,7,8-tetrachlorodibenzo-p-dioxin on the immune system of laboratory animals. Environ. Health Perspec., *5*:149 (1973).

Vos, J. G. and Moore, J. A.: Suppression of cellular immunity in rats and mice by maternal treatment with 2,3,7,8-tetrachlorodibenzo-p-dioxin. Int. Arch. Allergy Appl. Immunol., *47*:777-794 (1974).

Winkelstein, A.: Mechanisms of immunosuppression: Effects of cyclophosphamide on cellular immunity. Blood, *41(2)*:273-283 (1973).

DISCUSSION

LaVIA: Dr. Padarathsingh, you indicated that the PFC responses occurred after 7 days in one instance and after 14 days in the other?

PADARATHSINGH: That is correct.

LaVIA: In the second one you had a decrease in suppression at the low Tris dosage and an increase in suppression at the higher Tris dosage, as I recall. Have you looked at both the IgM and IgG PFC's?

PADARATHSINGH: Just one, the IgM.

LaVIA: I wonder what would have happened if you had looked at both. There may be some interesting differences.

PADARATHSINGH: I agree. You know—I did not point it out—but in some of the low doses with Tris, we found that there was enhancement of the PFC response. What that means, I'm not sure. I know that Drs. Dean and Luster have obtained similar results with low doses of Tris.

GHAFFAR: Where treatment of tumor-bearing mice with aniline mustard resulted in unresponsiveness to PHA, was there resistance to a second tumor challenge?

PADARATHESINGH: Not at day 14, but if you would allow about two additional weeks or so, then tumor challenge (on day 28), the animals which received aniline mustard alone will be immune competent and as such will resist the second tumor challenge with the syngeneic ADJ-PC5 plasmacytoma.

GHAFFAR: They will resist a secondary challenge?

PADARATHSINGH: Yes, they will resist, not on day 14, but by day 28.

HINSDILL: I've always been in favor of doing challenge type experiments to conclude research trying to show immunosuppressive effects, but I'm trying to get a feel for how tumor challenge compares with some of the more classic challenge-type of experiments, e.g., with Listeria, *Strep. pneumoniae,* or endotoxin challenge. Maybe Dr. Luster would want to speak to this also. What advantage do you feel it has over some of the microbial challenges that are perhaps easier and quicker to do?

PADARATHSINGH: I think at this point in time it's not an all-or-none phenomenon. I certainly agree with what you are saying, in that it would be interesting to look at the other factors of host resistance assays, the bacterial, fungal or viral susceptibilities. The debate continues concerning health risks associated with industrial chemicals and much of the discussion is focused on cancer. As such our reason for selection of the tumor susceptibility assay, even though we fully recognize the other health effects, needs to be considered as well.

HINSDILL: Has either of you ever noticed a major discrepancy where, for example, challenge with Listeria would show one thing and challenge with tumors would show a completely different picture?

PADARATHSINGH: As far as bacteria, let me give way to Dr. Luster because I have no experience with the bacterial system.

LUSTER: No, we haven't seen any large discrepancies. We are attempting to correlate the two assays to see how well they really do correlate. I don't believe one is going to be able to select one bacteria over another. I think the bottom line is going to be that you should be doing both host susceptible as well as immunological assays.

We assume that these are immunologically mediated events. I think we are going to do some correlations to prove to toxicologists that they are immunologically oriented, by performing correlative studies. I think what's needed with host-susceptibility assays is a validation time and eventual development of a panel of different tumors and bacteria, that will arouse everyone's interest in immunotoxicology.

ZWILLING: Could you give us an idea of how the levels that you obtained by injection correlate with the levels obtained through the natural exposure to Tris, which I understand is through absorption through the skin?

PADARATHSINGH: Would you mind repeating the question.

ZWILLING: Yes. As I understand natural exposure to Tris, it's by absorption through the skin, and I'm curious as to how the levels you used by the injection of Tris compare to levels obtained by absorption.

PADARATHSINGH: I think that the levels Van Duuren used in these studies was 10 mg per skin application. In our case we demonstrated tumor susceptibility with doses of 500 mg/kg which is equivalent to the 10 mg per skin application of Van Duuren.

ZWILLING: Well, the point I'm trying to make is that, if you paint 10 mg on the skin, it does not ensure that 10 mg will be absorbed and, if you are seeing effects at dosages of 500 mg or perhaps 50 mg, it may not be relevant to what the individual or animal is actually being exposed.

PADARATHSINGH: On a milligram per kilogram basis, the actual amount that the animal receives is approximately one fiftieth of the scheduled regimen and as such is consistent with the dose range of Tris reported to be carcinogenic in the literature.

SIGEL: Actually my comments concern this last question. I was going to speak to the very same point and also to the previous question on the difference in delayed type hypersensitivity evoked with microbial or cellular antigens. With regard to this point I was going to ask the same question: The only convincing suppression with Tris was at 50 mg/kg. At 50 were you getting fewer tumor takes?

PADARATHSINGH: Yes, at 50 mg/kg, the tumor susceptibility was 20 percent as compared with 40 percent at 500 mg/kg.

SIGEL: You were getting more or less borderline results; even 50 mg is far above what one would expect to get through skin absorption. If this program is to have acceptance in the real world of toxicology and exposure, we should be looking at the scale of dosage. I'm sure one can induce tumors and suppression with anything in this room if we use it in a high enough dose. We have to be more circumspect as to what dosages we are applying in our measuring schemes. I think it's a very important point.

Regarding the two types of measurement of delayed-type hypersensitivity, the work by Hahn and Kaufmann in Germany clearly shows that the cells involved in DTH evoked by microbial agents are different from those involved in cell-induced hypersensitivity, thus you may be measuring entirely different phenomena.

Moreover, since delayed hypersensitivity has two phases, the inductive and the effector phases, one has to reckon with inflammatory infiltration of macrophages in the latter phase. Therefore one should use non-specific skin reactivity such as that induced by turpentine as a control to see what is being compromised, the effector or inducer phase of the reaction.

DEAN: I don't agree with Dr. Zwilling's concern that the acute exposure dosage of Tris used by Dr. Padarathsingh might be too high and not mimic the real-life situation. The LD_{50} of Tris in mice is greater than 2.5 grams/kg; therefore I don't believe the dose was too high for an acute exposure. Secondly, the amount or form of a chemical applied to a garment may not reflect the amount or form which comes from the garment. Estimates of real-life exposure are practically impossible. In addition, the real-life exposure is chronic with possible bioaccumulation. Chronic low-level or topical exposure would be in order if acute studies demonstrated an immunologic alteration.

13
Modulation of the Immune Response in Laboratory Animals by Lead and Cadmium

Loren D. Koller

Department of Veterinary Medicine,
University of Idaho, Moscow, Idaho

INTRODUCTION

Lead and cadmium are environmental contaminants that affect both man and animals. Exposure to lead in the environment can occur from many sources. Some of these are: lead based paints, dust and dirt, ambient air (burning of coal and leaded gasoline), industrial (lead ore smelters, data reproduction, ceramics, printing (plastics) and moonshine (Haley, 1968; Ziegfield, 1964; Morgan et al., 1966). Recent studies have shown levels of lead to be elevated in soils, vegetation, and humans in close proximity to major urban highways with heavy traffic density (Hemphill et al., 1974; Caprio et al., 1974). Another important consideration is that a larger percentage of lead is absorbed from the gastrointestinal tract of children than adults. Approximately 53% of ingested lead is absorbed in children, while 10% is absorbed in adults. The biological half-life of lead is relatively short, approximately 20 to 30 days.

Cadmium is found in water, meats, grains, dairy products, pigments, plastics, stabilizers, alloys, batteries, cigarette smoke and industrial processes such as electroplating (Christensen and Olson, 1957; Fleischer et al., 1974; Flick et al., 1971; Morgan, 1971; Menden et al., 1972; Nadi et al., 1969). Forty percent of inhaled cadmium is absorbed while only

190

5% of that injected is absorbed (Morgan, 1971). The biological half-life of cadmium is extremely long and considered to be somewhere between 10 to 25 years.

Exposure of humans to lead is often constant due to release of lead from automobile exhausts after combustion of gasoline. However, in adults the most serious exposures come from mining and smelters while paints are responsible for major poisonings in children. Cadmium, on the other hand, is not a major problem to the majority of the population. Cadmium accumulates over the years with large concentrations found in older people. Cigarette smoke is a common source of cadmium.

Both lead and cadmium compromise the immune system of experimental animals. This report will describe modulation of the immune responses in laboratory animals resulting from exposure to lead or cadmium and compare the responses produced by these two metals.

RESULTS AND DISCUSSION

Immunotoxicology of Lead

There is considerable evidence that lead exerts adverse effects on the resistance of the body to disease. The ability of lead salts to induce a profound sensitization to endotoxicosis in rats, mice (Selye et al., 1966; Schumer and Erve, 1973; Rippe and Berry, 1973) and chickens (Truscott, 1970) has been well documented. Lead has also been shown to increase the susceptibility of rats to bacterial (*E. Coli*) challenge (Cook et al., 1975), and of mice to *Salmonella typhimurium* (Hemphill et al., 1971), encephalomyocarditis virus (Gainer, 1977; Exon et al., in press), Langet virus (Thind et al., 1977), or *Hexamita muris* (Exon et al., 1975).

Although the exact mechanism by which lead alters the host response has not been fully clarified, alteration of reticuloendothelial system and hepatic function has been predicted (Trejo et al., 1972). In addition, more recent evidence suggests that the enhanced mortality in metal-exposed animals may be due to an immunosuppressive effect of metals.

Lead treated animals subsequently subjected to procedures of active immunization developed lesser quantities of serum globulin, complement levels underwent progressive diminution, and anti-typhoid antibody titers were reduced (DeBruin, 1971). Interference with the phagocytic activity of polymorphonuclear leukocytes (Ward et al., 1975) and a reduction of lysozyme activity (DeBruin, 1971) were also reported following lead exposure.

In our laboratory, lead has consistently suppressed the immune system of experimental animals. Lead has resulted in increased susceptibility to encephalomyocarditis virus in mice (Exon et al., in press), reduced antibody titers in rabbits to pseudorabies virus (Koller, 1973), impaired antibody synthesis (Koller and Kovacic, 1974), interfered with complement receptors on B lymphocytes (Koller and Brauner, 1977), inhibited the memory response (Koller and Roan, 1979a) and enhanced tumor growth (Kerkvliet, 1979a). However, lead did not significantly alter lymphocyte transformation to mitogens Con A and LPS (Koller et al., 1979) or responsiveness in mixed lymphocyte cultures (Koller and Roan, 1979b). Nevertheless, others have shown lead to inhibit proliferation of lymphocytes to mitogens PHA and PWM (Garworski and Sharma, 1978) as well as impair delayed hypersensitivity (Faith et al., 1179). Further, specific CMI investigations must be conducted by the use of a variety of techniques to determine if other segments of the cellular immune system are compromised.

Immunotoxicology of Cadmium

The immunosuppressive properties of cadmium are rather ambiguous compared to those of lead. Cadmium has produced a profound increase in susceptibility of rats to challenge inoculation of bacterial endotoxins (Cook et al., 1974; Cook et al., 1975) and encephalomyocarditis virus (EMCV) (Gainer, 1977). However, in two other studies (Exon et al., in press; Exon et al., 1979), mice which were exposed to cadmium acetate in drinking water and subsequently inoculated with EMCV had reduced mortality compared to non-cadmium inoculated mice. These conflicting reports could partially be accounted for by differences in species, dosages, length of exposure, virulence of virus, etc.

The effects of cadmium on the immune system of laboratory animals have been controversial. Cadmium injected into rats seven days after an antigen suppressed serum antibody, but when injected 14 days prior to antigen, enhanced the antibody titer (Jones et al., 1971). In our laboratory we have shown that chronic exposure of mice to cadmium produces a significant decrease in antibody titer (Koller, 1973) and antibody synthesis (Koller et al., 1975) and that this suppression persists for several weeks after discontinuance of exposure. The IgG response was most markedly suppressed an indication that the memory cell or T helper cell may be involved. This impaired antibody production by cadmium has been confirmed by others (Bozelka et al., 1978; Graham et al., 1978). Recently, however, the memory response was reported (Koller and Roan, 1979a) to be actually augmented, rather than impeded, in cadmium exposed animals. Cadmium also has inhibited EAC rosette formation of B cells, an assessment of the complement receptor activity (Koller and Brauner, 1977).

Cadmium also affects macrophages. Cadmium exposure promoted intravascular clearance of particles (Cook et al., 1974) and stimulated phagocytosis by macrophages (Koller and Roan, 1977). Conversely, cadmium impaired EA rosette formation of alveolar macrophages, a measure of the Fc receptor activity (Hadley et al., 1977). Further, cadmium has been demonstrated to be directly cytoxic to phagocytic cells (Loose et al., 1978).

Cell-mediated responses induced by cadmium exposure have varied considerably. Cadmium inhibited lymphocyte transformation by mitogens PHA and PWM (Garworski and Sharma, 1978) while Con A had no effect and LPS, a B cell mitogen, actually stimulated blastogenesis (Koller et al., 1979). To further confuse the issue, when lymphocytes obtained from cadmium exposed animals were tested in mixed lymphocyte cultures, there was no appreciable effect (Koller and Roan, 1979b). Finally, cadmium has impaired the growth of transplant tumors as well as promoted repression of those tumors which did develop (Kerkvliet et al., 1979b). Correlating with decreased tumor growth *in vivo,* cell-mediated cytotoxicity of tumor cells *in vitro* was enhanced by exposure of the animals to cadmium. These data, as viewed in the context of current formation, indicate that cadmium can deter certain segments of the immune system but augment others. The mechanisms by which cadmium compromises the immune system need to be further elucidated.

CONCLUSION

Lead appears to consistently suppress most all segments of the immune system of experimental animals. This environmental contaminant has contributed to increased susceptibility to infectious agents and toxins, reduced humoral antibody responses such as titers, synthesis, memory and receptor activity, inhibited phagocytosis of macrophages, suppressed cell mediated immunity and promoted growth of neoplasms.

Cadmium, on the other hand, has produced mixed reactions. This chemical has resulted in enhanced mortality to infectious agents in some instances and reduced mortality in others. Generally, cadmium impedes antibody production but in certain cases has augmented immune responses as well as memory. Mitogen responses after cadmium exposure have ranged from stimulatory to unresponsive to diminished. Phagocytosis by macrophages has generally been potentiated. Cadmium also appears to protect a host against tumor growth by amplifying the cytotoxic ability of lymphocytes.

Therefore, lead essentially affects all immune systems tested to date adversely while cadmium seems to stimulate some and inhibit other immune responses and, thus, appears to be selective in its site of action. Many of these changes occur at levels well below those which produce overt clinical signs or symptoms of toxicity in the host. Whether similar conditions occur in humans exposed to these metals has yet to be determined. However, it is apparent that these two environmental contaminants as well as others can affect regulatory systems in the body at very low dosages emphasizing that caution should be taken to minimize exposure to these chemicals whenever possible.

REFERENCES

Bozelka, B. E., Burkholder, P. M. and Chang, L. W.: Cadmium, a metallic inhibitor of antibody-mediated immunity in mice. Environ. Res., *17*:390 (1978).

Caprio, R. J., Margulis, H. L. and Joselow, M. M.: Lead absorption in children and its relationship to urban traffic densities. Arch. Environ. Health, *28*:195 (1974).

Christensen, F. C. and Olson, E. C.: Cadmium poisoning. Arch. Ind. Health, *16*:8-15 (1957).

Cook, J. A., Marconi, E. A. and DiLuzio, N. R.: Lead, cadmium, endotoxin interaction: Effect on mortality and hepatic function. Toxicol. Appl. Pharmacol., *28*:292 (1974).

Cook, J. A., Hoffman, E. O. and DiLuzio, N. R.: Influence of lead and cadmium on the susceptibility of rats to bacterial challenge. Proc. Soc. Exptl. Biol. Med., *150*:741 (1975).

DeBruin, A.: Certain biological effects of lead upon the animal organism. Arch. Environ. Health, *23*:249 (1971).

Exon, J. H., Patton, N. M. and Koller, L. D.: Hexamatiasis in cadmium exposed mice. Arch. Environ. Health, *31*:463 (1975).

Exon, J. H., Koller, L. D. and Kerkvliet, N. I.: Lead-cadmium interaction: Effects on viral-induced mortality and tissue residues in mice. Arch. Environ. Health (in press).

Exon, J. H., Koller, L. D. and Kerkvliet, N. I.: Tissue residues, pathology and viral-induced mortality in mice chronically exposed to different cadmium salts. J. Environ. Path. Toxicol., in press (1979).

Faith, R. E., Luster, M. I. and Kimmel, C. A.: Effect of chronic developmental lead exposure on cell-mediated immune function. Clin. Exp. Immunol., *35*:413 (1979).

Fleischer, M., Sarofim, A. F., Fasset, D. W., et al.: Environmental impact of cadmium. A review by the panel on hazardous trace substances. Environ. Health Perspec., *7*:253-323 (1974).

Flick, D. F., Kraybill, H. F. and Dimitroff, J. M.: Toxic effects of cadmium: A review. Environ. Res., *4*:71-85 (1971).

Gainer, J. H.: Effects of heavy metals and of deficiency of zinc on mortality rates in mice infected with encephalomyocarditis virus. Am. J. Vet. Res., *38*:869 (1977).

Garworski, C. L. and Sharma, R. P.: The effects of heavy metals on ^{3}H-thymidine uptake in lymphocytes. Toxicol. Appl. Pharmacol., *46*:305 (1978).

Graham, J. A., Miller, F. J., Daniels, M. J., Payne, E. A. and Gardner, D. E.: Influence of cadmium, nickel, and chromium on primary immunity in mice. Environ. Res., *16*:77 (1978).

Hadley, J. G., Gardner, D. E., Coffin, D. L. and Menzel, D. B.: Inhibition of antibody-mediated rosette formation by alveolar macrophages: A sensitive assay for metal toxicity. J. Reticuloendothel. Soc., *22*:417 (1977).

Haley, T. J.: A review of the toxicology of lead. *Air Quality Monograph 69-7,* American Petroleum Institute, New York, p. 53 (1968).

Hemphill, R. E., Kaeberle, M. L. and Buck, W. B.: Lead suppression of mouse resistance to *Salmonella typhimurium.* Science, *173*:1031 (1971).

Hemphill, D. D., Marienfeld, C. J., Reddy, R. S., et al.: Roadside lead contamination in the Missouri lead belt. Arch. Environ. Health, *28*:190 (1974).

Jones, R. H.,Williams, R. L. and Jones, A. M.: Effects of heavy metals on the immune response. Preliminary findings for cadmium in rats. Proc. Soc. Expl. Biol. Med. *137*:1231 (1971).

Kerkvliet, N. I., Koller, L. D., Beacher, L. G. and Brauner, J. A.: Effect of cadmium exposure on primary tumor growth and cell-mediated cytotoxicity in mice bearing MSB-6 sarcomas. J. Natl. Cancer Inst., *63*:479 (1979a).

Kerkvliet, N. I.: Personal communication (1979b).

Koller, L. D.: Immunosuppression produced by lead, cadmium and mercury. Am. J. Vet. Res., *34*:1457 (1973).

Koller, L. D. and Kovacic, S.: Decreased antibody formation in mice exposed to lead. Nature, *250*:148 (1974).

Koller, L. D., Exon, J. H. and Roan, J. G.: Antibody suppression by cadmium. Arch. Environ. Health, *30*:598 (1975).

Koller, L. D. and Brauner, J. A.: Decreased B cell response after exposure to lead and cadmium. Toxicol. Appl. Pharmacol., *42*:621 (1977).

Koller, L. D. and Roan, J. G.: Effects of lead and cadmium on mouse peritoneal macrophages. J. Reticuloendothel. Soc., *21*:7 (1977).

Koller, L. D. and Roan, J. G.: Effects of lead, cadmium and methymercury on immunological memory. J. Environ. Path. Toxicol., in press (1979a).

Koller, L. D. and Roan, J. G.: Response of lymphocytes from lead, cadmium, and methylmercury exposed mice in the mixed lymphocyte culture. J. Environ. Path. Toxicol., in press (1979b).

Koller, L. D., Roan, J. G. and Kerkvliet, N. I.: Mitogen stimulation of lymphocytes in CBA mice exposed to lead and cadmium. Environ. Res., *19*:177 (1979).

Loose, L. D., Silkworth, J. B. and Warrington, D.: Cadmium-induced phagocyte cytotoxicity. Bull. Environ. Contam. Toxicol., *20*:582 (1978).

Menden, E. E., Elia, V. J., Michael, L. W., et al.: Distribution of cadmium and nickel of tobacco during a cigarette smoking. Environ. Sci. Technol., *6*:830-832 (1972).

Morgan, J. M., Hartley, N. W. and Miller. R. E.: Neuropathy in chronic lead poisoning. Arch. Int. Med., *118*:17 (1966).

Morgan, J. M.: Tissue cadmium and zinc content in emphysema and bronchogenic carcinoma. Chron. Dis., *24*:107-110 (1971).

Nadi, M., Sloan, D., Jick, H., et al.: Cadmium content of cigarettes. Lancet, *2*:1329-1332 (1969).

Rippe, D. F. and Berry, L. J.: Metabolic manifestations of lead acetate sensitization to endotoxin in mice. J. Reticuloendothel. Soc., *13*:527 (1973).

Schumer, W. and Erve, P. R.: Endotoxin sensitivity of adrenalectomized rats treated with lead acetate. J. Reticuloendothel. Soc., *13*:122 (1973).

Selye, H., Tuchweber, B. and Bertok, L.: Effect of lead acetate on the susceptibility of rats to bacterial endotoxins. J. Bacteriol., *91*:884 (1966).

Thind, I. S., Thind, G. S. and Louria, D. B.: Potentiation of viral infections due to trace metal intoxication. Internatl. Symp. on Clin. Chem. and Chemical Toxicol. of Metals, Monte Carlo (1977).
Trejo, R. A., Diluzio, N. R., Loose, L. D. and Hoffman, E.: Reticuloendothelial and hepatic functional alterations following lead acetate administration. Exptl. Mol. Path., *17*:145 (1972).
Truscott, R. B.: Endotoxin studies in chicks: Effects of lead acetate Can. J. Comp. Med., *34*:134 (1970).
Ward, P. A., Goldschmidt, P. and Greene, N. D.: Suppressive effects of metal salts of leukocyte and fibroblastic function. J. Reticuloendothel. Soc., *18*:313 (1975).
Ziegfield, R. L.: Important uses of lead. Arch. Environ. Health, *8*:202 (1964).

DISCUSSION

GRAY: We have conducted experiments using Cd^{2+} and $P6^{2+}$, as well as Cr^{3+}, but I'll keep my remarks to cadmium and lead. Although our experiments are somewhat different from Dr. Koller's, in a number of ways they are analogous. We have used a concentration of the chlorides of each of the ions, from .01 ppm to 5 ppm in drinking water. Our animals, which are Balb/c mice, are tested after four weeks on the drinking water under test.

One group was challenged with MOPC-104E in its soluble form after the four-week experiment. Unfortunately in our first experiments, we used too many cells, and all animals died. However, the rate of death was significantly decreased by as much as 40 percent, both for lead and cadmium, at these levels.

Using the Cunningham modification of the plaque technique, we found a peak for plaque formation at about 0.1 ppm, in drinking water, for Cd^{2+}, and somewhat higher, about 0.5 ppm, for the Pb^{2+}.

Using MOPC-104E tumor cells as targets cells and the metal-treated lymphocytes as effector cells, a chromium-release assay also showed a peak at the same concentration of ions in drinking water. When the splenocytes were tested for this immunoproliferative response, we found that cell stimulation was enhanced in the metal-treated animals. When tested in the presence of either PHA or LPS, the stimulating effects of both mitogens were also enhanced.

An interesting recent finding was the result of binding studies carried out, using labeled 109 Cd^{2+}. These were *in vitro* studies, with the cadmium concentration ranging from $10^{-3} - 10^{-7}M$. In the absence of the mitogen LPS, we found a logarithmic relationship between ion concentration and amount bound indicated essentially one type of binding. In the presence of LPS we found a break in the curve indicating an increased binding or association of the ions with the lymphocytes. This break occurred at about $10^{-5}M$.

Using the calculated regression lines, we can extrapolate each line to an intersection point which we've termed the "critical concentration" below which cadmium does not appear to get into the cell. While above that concentration per lymphocyte, there is an influx into the cell and some of the toxic effects of cadmium may be seen.

These results are supported by those of Dr. Koller except at a much lower concentration.

It is interesting to note that, at the concentration of lead that we used, there was an immediate influx into the cell and the criterical concentration was far below that which we had been using.

KALLAND: I just would like to mention some experiments done in collaboration with Dr. Wesenberg on natural killing cell after cadmium exposure. When rats were exposed to 30 ppm cadmium between four and eight weeks of age, we could find either no effect or a slight enhancement of natural killer activity.

In this connection I would like to ask if you have any data on the tumor incidence in these animals in long-term follow-up studies? Further, what do these animals die of when they finally die? You said you could expose them to 300 ppm without clinical signs of toxicity. What do you mean by clinical signs of toxicity? When we expose rats to 300 ppm cadmium we get proteinuria. I think that's a very significant sign of toxocity.

KOLLER: No. That has not been separated out. I have looked at it clinically, e.g., weight loss, serum enzyme changes, or any overt clinical symptom where you might see a change in that animal. One of the diagnostic features of lead toxicity is the occurrence of acid-fast inclusion bodies in cells of the renal tubules, renal cells, of animals exposed to lead. We often cannot identify these bodies in rats or mice. They are visible under the microscope as eosinophilic inclusion bodies with H&E stain, but not visible with acid-fast staining as in humans, cattle, or some other animals. Therefore, one sees different responses and different changes.

The other part is that we usually, by the end of 18 months, kill these animals to determine some immunological parameters. We have not carried them on for longer than 18 months.

The same is true with cadmium. We have not determined the effect cadmium would have on spontaneous or long-term tumors. Our studies have all been short-term.

LaVIA: I have a question. You showed a compilation of data indicating enhancement or no effect or depression. Has anyone looked at this in terms of strain of mice and dosage?

KOLLER: No. That has not been separated out. I have looked at it generally and it is difficult to compare the data, which is one of the current problems in immunotoxicology. Everyone uses his own assay, his own animals, his own dosages. Thus, a comparison becomes very difficult and is something we need to improve on in the future. However, it appears, from looking at it generally, that most of this work is done in different dosages.

14
Direct and Induced Suppression of *in Vitro* Antibody Production by Selected Phenols: A Comparison to Virus-Type Interferon

**Douglas L. Archer, Bennett G. Smith
and Howard M. Johnson**

*Department of Health, Education and Welfare,
Public Health Service, Food and Drug Administration,
Division of Microbiology, Cincinnati, Ohio
Department of Microbiology, University of Texas Medical Branch,
Galveston, Texas*

INTRODUCTION

We previously reported that BHA, PG and GA could suppress the *in vivo* primary anti-SRBC PFC response of mouse spleen cells (Archer et al., 1978) with immunosuppression kinetics similar to those reported for VIF (Archer et al., 1977a; Johnson et al., 1979). Also, the suppression caused by adding GA directly to cultures was reversed by adding 2-mercaptoethanol (2ME) to the GA-treated cultures even when the addition of 2ME was delayed for 48 hr (Archer et al., 1977a); 2ME is also capable of reversing suppression of the anti-SRBC PFC response caused by the direct addition of VIF (Johnson, 1978) to cultures. Recent studies showed that VIF is capable of inducing both lymphoid and non-lymphoid cells to produce a substance capable of suppressing the anti-SRBC PFC response (Johnson and Ohtsuki, 1979), which is not related to the antiviral activity of VIF (Johnson and Ohtsuki, 1979) but may be related to its antitumor properties (Johnson and Blalock, in press). Because of the observed similarities between VIF and certain phenolic compounds, a study was designed to determine if BHA and GA, in particular, might also induce cells to become suppressive.

METHODS

Mice

Six- to 8-week old BDF_1 (C57B1/6 × DBA/2)F_1 female mice were obtained from Laboratory Supply Co., Indianapolis, IN.

Chemicals

The source and purity of BHA, GA, and PG are stated elsewhere (Archer et al., 1978; Archer and Wess, 1979). The VIF used in these studies was mouse fibroblast interferon (50,000 U/ml stock), as previously described (Johnson and Ohtsuki, 1979).

Antigen, Biological Reagents and Cell Cultures

SRBC, fetal bovine serum and general cell culture methods for the anti-SRBC response have been described elsewhere (Archer and Wess, 1979; Mishell and Dutton, 1967).

Experimental Design

Cultures exposed to chemicals consisted of 10×10^6 BDF_1 spleen cells/ml. Culture medium consisted of RPMI-1640, with 10% fetal bovine serum, and penicillin, streptomycin and gentamicin added to the final concentrations of 100 U/ml, 100 and 10 μg/ml, respectively. BHA, PG and GA were solubilized in absolute ethanol and administered to cultures by applying the ethanol in a 10 μl spot to 35-mm plastic cell culture dishes and permitting the ethanol to evaporate before the addition of the cells. Final concentrations of BHA, PG and GA in each culture were 100, 25 and 25 μg/ml, respectively. Control culture dishes were spotted with absolute ethanol. VIF was added to a final concentration of 400 U/ml in culture medium. Cultures were incubated on rocker platforms for 24 hr. Nonadherent cells were then removed from dishes, pooled by chemical group and washed three times with the culture medium by centrifugation. Pooled cells were enumerated in a hemacytometer, and culture viability was determined by trypan blue dye exclusion. Viabilities at 24 hr of culture generally were $> 95\%$. Viable cell numbers were adjusted to twice the desired concentration in culture medium, and 500 μl was added to culture dishes containing 500 μl of fresh BDF_1 spleen cells at 3×10^7/ml. Cultures were then immunized with 3×10^6 SRBC and 2ME was added to a final concentration of 5×10^{-5} M where indicated. Cultures were fed daily with nutritional cocktail (Mishell and Dutton, 1967) and the PFC response was determined on day 5 of culture, according to the method of Cunningham and Szenberg (1968). Data are presented as the mean of triplicate cultures; the standard error of the mean did not exceed 10%. Background PFC/culture did not exceed 5% of the SRBC-induced PFC response.

RESULTS

Similarities of Biological Activities of VIF, GA, and BHA

Table 1 summarizes some of the previously observed similarities (No. 1 through 6, Table 1) in the immunologic and biological activities of VIF, GA and BHA, which led to this investigation (Nos. 7 and 8, Table 1). Names in paraentheses (Table 1) cite references to the original observation of each characteristic.

Induced Suppressive Activity of Cells Treated with BHA, PG, GA and VIF

Data presented in Figure 1 show the results obtained when 1-, 5- and 10×10^5 BDF_1 spleen cells, pretreated with PG, GA BHA, VIF or nothing (C) and washed 3X, were co-cultivated with 15×10^6 fresh BDF_1 spleen cells immunized with SRBC concomitant with the addition of chemical-treated cells. The results indicate that the three phenolic compounds tested, all of which may function as antioxidants, can induce cells to become suppressive to fresh spleen cell cultures. PG- and GA-treated cells (5×10^5) were, in fact, more effective suppressors in the co-culture than an equal number of VIF-treated (400 U/ml) cells. When greater numbers of treated cells (10×10^5) were used, percents of suppression relative to the control for PG-, GA- and VIF-treated cells were similar. BHA-treated cells appeared somewhat less capable of suppression at corresponding cell numbers. The increase in PFC observed in control cultures

Table 1. **A Comparison of Some Biological Characteristics of Virus-Type Interferon, Gallic Acid (GA) and Butylated Hydroxyanisole (BHA).**

CHARACTERISTIC	VIRUS-TYPE INTERFERON	GA	BHA
1. Antiviral activity	+ (Isaacs and Lindenmann, 1957)	− (Archer and Johnson, 1978)	?
2. Antitumor activity	+ (Strander, 1977)	?	+ (Emanuel and Lipchina, 1958)
3. Suppresses anti-SRBC PFC response	+ (Johnson et al., 1975)	+ (Archer et al., 1977a)	+ (Archer et al., 1977b)
a. added at 24 hr of culture	+ (Johnson et al., 1975)	+ (Archer et al., 1977a)	+ (Archer et al., 1977b)
b. added at 48 hr of culture	− (Johnson et al., 1975)	+ (Archer et al., 1977a)	− (Archer et al., 1977b)
4. Primary anti-SRBC response suppression reversed by 2ME	+ (Johnson, 1978)	+ (Archer et al., 1977a)	− (Archer and Wess, 1979)
5. Secondary anti-SRBC response suppression reversed by 2ME	?	+ (Archer and Wess, 1979)	+ (Archer and Wess, 1979)
6. Suppresses thymus-independent antibody response of Nu/Nu	+ (Johnson et al., 1975)	− (Archer et al., 1977a)	+ (Johnson, 1978)
7. "Induces" suppressor of PFC response	+ (Johnson and Ohtusuki, 1979)	+	+
8. "Induced" suppression *not* reversed by 2ME	+	+	+

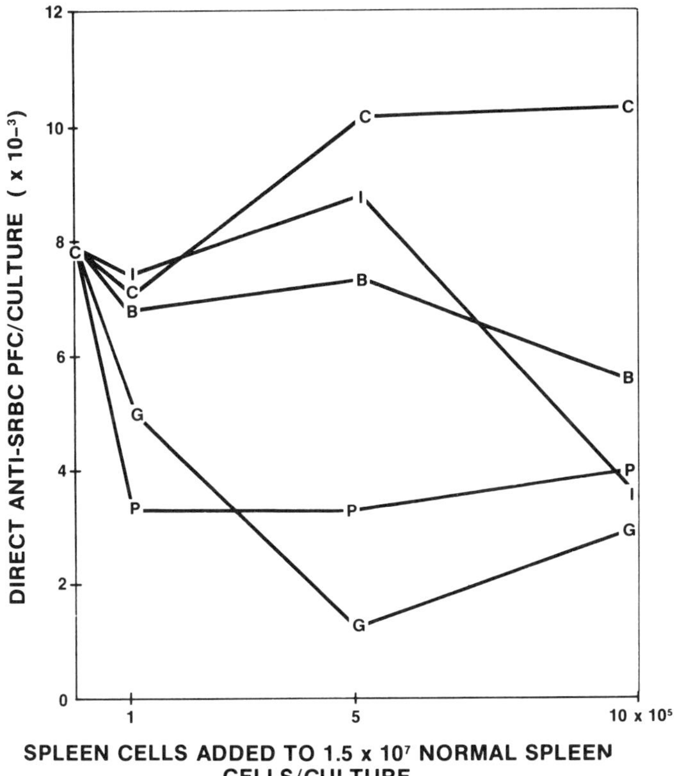

**SPLEEN CELLS ADDED TO 1.5 x 10⁷ NORMAL SPLEEN
CELLS/CULTURE**

Figure 1. The effect of adding varying numbers of spleen cells treated with VIF (I), BHA (B), PG (P), GA (G) or nothing (C) on the primary anti-SRBC PFC response of mouse spleen cells not exposed to chemical.

was probably due to an increase in the number of antigen-responsive cells in cultures.

BHA-Induced PFC Suppression—Effect of 2ME and Increasing Number of Cells Co-Cultivated

Figure 2 shows the effect of co-cultivating increasing numbers of BHA-treated cells with fresh SRBC-immunized BDF_1 spleen cells. The data indicate that the greater the number of untreated control cells added to fresh spleen cells, the greater the resulting day 5 PFC response. In contrast, BHA-pretreated cells co-cultivated with fresh spleen cells resulted in

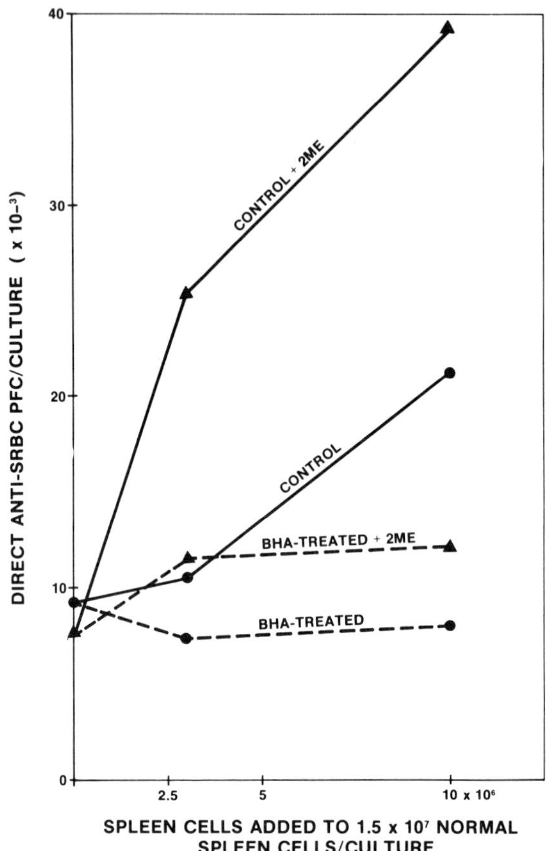

Figure 2. The effect of adding greater numbers of BHA-treated spleen cells on the anti-SRBC PFC response of normal spleen cells in the presence or absence of 2ME.

a suppressed PFC response. The suppression resulting from the addition of 10×10^6 BHA-treated cells ($\approx 64\%$) was greater than that observed when 3×10^6 BHA-treated cells ($\approx 29\%$) were added. The addition of 2ME to cultures co-cultivated with control cells enhanced the resulting PFC response. Cultures which were co-cultivated with 3×10^6 and 10×10^6 BHA-treated cells and to which 2ME were added demonstrated percents of suppression (54 and 70%, respectively) of the PFC response greater than those observed in cultures not treated with 2ME. That 2ME can enhance the anti-SRBC PFC response is well documented (Click et al.,

1972), but 2ME can also function as a reducing agent and, thus, can protect the integrity of protein sulfhydryl groups.

VIF- and GA-induced PFC suppression—Effect of 2ME

As previously stated, GA and VIF, added directly to concomitantly immunized spleen cell cultures, produce suppression that is reversible when 2ME is added to culture (Archer et al., 1977a; Johnson et al., 1975) In contrast, results presented in Figure 3 show that the presence of 2ME in cultures enhances GA- and VIF-induced suppressor cell activity. It should be noted that the VIF-induced suppressive factor isolated by Johnson and Ohtsuki (1979) required the presence of dithiothreitol (a reducing agent and sulfydryl group stabilizer) to retain its suppressive activity.

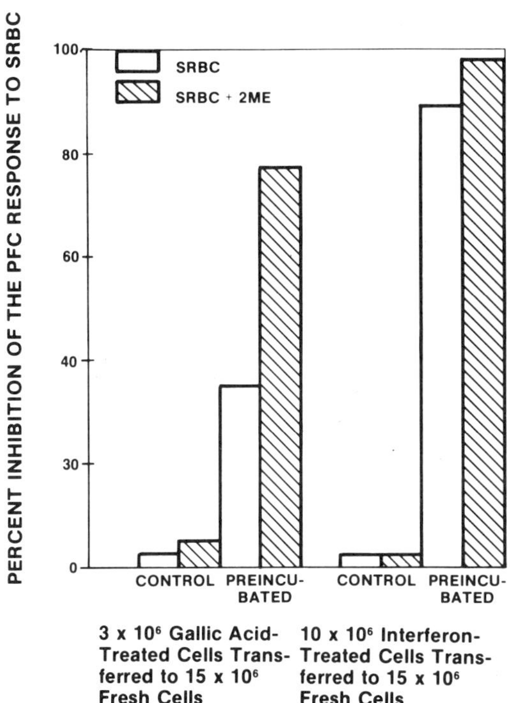

Figure 3. The suppressive effects of GA- and BHA-treated cells on the anti-SRBC PFC response of normal spleen cells in the presence or absence of 2ME.

DISCUSSION

The data presented in Figures 1 and 2 demonstrate that the phenols examined in this study are capable of inducing cells to become suppressive to fresh SRBC-immunized spleen cells in co-culture. GA, BHA and PG do not activate suppressor T-lymphocytes; in fact, they abrogate T-lymphocyte function (Archer and Johnson, 1978). Macrophages are also unlikely to become activated to a suppressive state by these compounds because a) GA abrogates macrophage support functions for T-lymphocytes (Archer et al., 1977a), and b) only nonadherent cells were collected and washed thoroughly before co-culture.

The ability of VIF to induce a suppressive effect has been previously established by Johnson and Ohtsuki (1979). Once the suppressive state has been induced, thiols such as 2ME fail to reverse suppression [as they can reverse the initial direct effect (Johnson, 1978)] and, in fact, potentiate the suppression (Figure 3). GA follows exactly the same pattern as VIF in that once the suppressive state was induced, 2ME failed to reverse the suppression and, in fact, enhanced suppression (Figure 3). Previous studies showed that the suppression of the primary anti-SRBC PFC response caused by directly adding BHA to cultures was not reversed by 2ME (Archer and Wess, 1979), therefore, it was not surprising that 2ME also failed to reverse the BHA-induced suppression of the primary PFC response (Figure 2).

There is no evidence to date that BHA or GA enters lymphoid cells. GA, in particular, would be highly charged in aqueous medium and would likely be excluded at the cell membrane surface. The ability of several sulfhydryl reagents to inhibit mitogen-induced lymphocyte activation was recently reported (Chaplin and Wedner, 1978). A surface sulfhydryl reagent p-hydroxymercuriphenylsulfonic acid, was found to inhibit lymphocyte activation when added to lymphocyte cultures, together with lectin mitogens, or at any time up to 48 hr after the addition of mitogen; this effect is similar to the PFC and blast transformation inactivation kinetics that were observed with GA (Archer et al., 1977a). Chemical interference with surface sulfhydryl groups has been shown to block concanavalin A- and endotoxin-induced activation of the hexose monophosphate pathway in human polymorphonuclear leukocytes (Tsan et al., 1976a), and this pathway plays a primary role in NADPH production (Tsan et al., 1976b). Direct interaction between GA and surface sulfhydryl groups remains unproven, but evidence, such as the reversibility of GA's immunosuppressive activity by 2ME (Archer et al., 1977a) and L-cysteine (unpublished data), suggests this as a possible mechanism. In contrast to GA, BHA is hydrophobic and is likely to enter cells. This does not preclude the possibility that BHA interacts with sulfhydryl groups since N-ethylmalmeimide, a sulfhydyl reagent known to enter cells, has also been shown to inhibit lymphocyte activation (Chaplin and Wedner, 1978). Investigations are under way to determine the possible interaction of GA and BHA with sulfhydryl groups.

Johnson and Ohtsuki (1979) recently showed that the PFC response-suppressor factor induced by VIF is a protein capable of blocking translational events. Although the suppressor factor inhibited the anti-SRBC PFC response, it failed to demonstrate antiviral activity (Johnson and Ohtsuki, 1979). Furthermore, the inhibitory factor preparation was shown to contain seven times greater levels of protein kinase activity than non-VIF-induced cells (Johnson and Ohtsuki, 1979). Protein kinases can be activated when the internal reduction-oxidation potential of the cell is unbalanced; thus activated, they are capable of inhibiting translational events by phosphorylating eukaryotic initiation factor-2 (Ernst et al., 1979).

The existing similarities in biological activity of VIF and the phenolic antioxidants suggest that similar mechanisms may play a role in the immunosuppressive activity of these compounds. Johnson and Blalock (in press) recently presented evidence that the VIF-induced suppressor factor may play a role in normal and tumor cell growth regulation. Since BHA has been reported to have antitumor activity (Emanuel and Lipchina, 1958), further work with PG, GA and BHA seems warranted and may result in a better understanding of tumor cell growth regulation.

REFERENCES

Archer, D. L., Bukovic-Wess, J. A. and Smith, B. G.: Suppression of macrophage-dependent T-lymphocyte function(s) by gallic acid, a food additive metabolite. Proc. Soc. Exp. Biol. Med., *156*:465-469 (1977a).

Archer, D. L., Bukovic-Wess, J. A. and Smith, B. G.: Inhibitory effect of an antioxidant, butylated hydroxyanisole, on the primary *in vitro* immune response. Proc. Soc. Exp. Biol. Med., *154*:289-294 (1977b).

Archer, D. L., Smith, B. G. and Bukovic-Wess, A. J.: Use of an *in vitro* antibody producing system for recognizing potentially immunosuppressive compounds. Int. Arch. Allergy Appl. Immunol., *56*:90-93 (1978).

Archer, D. L. and Johnson, H. M.: Blockade of mitogen induction of the interferon lymphokine by a phenolic food additive metabolite. Proc. Soc. Exp. Biol. Med., *157*:684-687 (1978).

Archer, D. L. and Wess, J. A.: Chemical dissection of the primary and secondary *in vitro* antibody response with butylated hydroxyanisole and gallic acid. Drug Chem. Toxicol., *2*:155-166 (1979).

Chaplin, D. D. and Wedner, H. J.: Inhibition of lectin-induced lymphocyte activation by diamide and other sulfydryl reagents. Cell Immunol., *36*:303-311 (1978).

Click, R. E., Benck, L. and Alter, B. J.: Enhancement of antibody synthesis *in vitro* by mercaptoethanol. Cell. Immunol., *3*:155-160 (1972).

Cunningham, A. J. and Szenberg, A.: Further improvements in the plaque technique for detecting single antibody-forming cells. Immunology, *14*:599 (1968).

Emanuel, N. M. and Lipchina, L. P.: Leukosis in mice and its development during interaction with inhibitors of chain oxidative processes. Dokl. Akad. Nauk S.S.S.R., *121*:141-144 (1958).

Ernst, V., Lerin, D. H. and London, I. M.: Inhibition of protein synthesis initiation by oxidized glutathione: Activation of a protein kinase that phosphorylates the α subunit of eukaryotic initiation factor-2. Proc. Natl. Acad. Sci., USA, *75*:4110-4114 (1979).

Isaacs, A. and Lindenmann, J.: Virus interference. I. The interferon. Proc. R. Soc. London Ser. B., *147*:258-267 (1957).

Johnson, H. M., Smith, B. G. and Baron, S.: Inhibition of the primary *in vitro* antibody response by intreferon preparations. J. Immunol., *114*:403-409 (1975).

Johnson, H. M.: Differentiation of the immunosuppressive and antiviral effects of interferon. Cell. Immunol., *36*:220-230 (1978).

Johnson, H. M. and Ohtsuki, K.: Suppression of *in vitro* antibody response by ribosome-associated factor(s) from interferon-treated cells. Cell. Immunol., *44*:215-230 (1979).

Johnson, H. M. and Blalock, J. E.: Interferon induced suppressor factor: Possible regulator of normal and tumor cells. J. Clin. Hematol. Oncol., (in press).

Mishell, R. I. and Dutton, R. W.: Inmmunization of mouse spleen cell cultures from normal mice. J. Exp. Med., *126*:423-442 (1967).

Strander, H.: Anti-tumor effects of interferon and its possible use as an antineoplastic agent in man. Tex. Rep. Biol. Med., *35*:429-435 (1977).

Tsan, M-F., Newman, B., Chusid, M., Wolff, S. M. and McIntyre, P. A.: Surface sulphydryl groups and hexose monophosphate pathway activity in resting human polymorphonuclear leucocytes. Br. J. Haematol., *33*:205-211 (1976a).

Tsan, M-F., Newman, B. and McIntyre, P. A.: Surface sulphydryl groups and phagocytosis-associated oxidative metabolic changes in human polymorphonuclear leucoytes. Br. J. Haematol., *33*:189-204 (1976b).

DISCUSSION

HADDEN: I have two questions. One, it wasn't clear to me what concentrations of gallic acid and the phenols you were using and how this might relate to levels that you would see with natural exposure.

Two, I wonder about the mechanism involved in the suppression. Interferon has been reported by Yaron to be an inducer of prostaglandin metabolism and it's apparent that this action does not relate to its antiviral activity. This action may account for certain aspects of its antiproliferative activity, and it seems to me what you are describing in the Mishell-Dutton system could very well be an action on the macrophage to induce prostaglandin. Have you tried treating your cultures with aspirin or indomethacin?

ARCHER: Yes. In response to the second part of your question, we were unable to reverse the suppression of the PFC response caused by virus-type or immune interferon with indomethacin, but we could reverse LPS-induced suppression. These were crude interferons, however, so the involvement of prostaglandins cannot be entirely excluded.

As to the question of dose, the direct addition of as little as 1 ppm gallic acid to *in vitro* cultures completely abrogates the antibody response to sheep erythrocytes. In terms of a human dose, the question is more difficult. We have studied one gallic-acid-containing food, tea. On a dry weight basis, tea was as suppressive to *in vitro* antibody production as was pure gallic acid, and the suppression caused by tea was likewise reversed by 2-mercaptoethanol. An average teaspoon of dry tea contains approximately 235 mg of material, or 235,00 times the amount of material required to suppress the Mishell-Dutton system. Gallic acid does affect DNA synthesis of human peripheral lymphocytes at doses similar to those which suppress mouse lymphocyte DNA synthesis. We have no data on gallic acid's effect on human *in vitro* antibody production.

On a weight basis, gallic acid is the most potent suppressant. Propyl gallate is also quite potent. Methyl paraben and BHA are less potent by three-to-five fold. One interesting thing we consistently noted was the lack of correlation of structure with function; that is, small modifcations of the phenol structure caused large variations in biological activity.

LA VIA: Did you try to take a supernatant and add it to your cells instead of co-culturing?

ARCHER: Yes. Our efforts were unsuccessful. We currently favor the idea of cell-to-cell contact as being either required or more efficient. This is in agreement with what's known about the interferon system.

GHAFFAR: I think you mentioned that both these agents inhibit oxidation. Did you look at the oxidative part with macrophages? What effects do these agents have?

ARCHER: I'm glad you brought that up. It should be stressed that these compounds are antioxidants. There is no evidence that these compounds enter cells, in fact, it is unlikely that gallic acid does, owing to its charge distribution. The immunologic phenomena we see could all involve binding of these substances to surface sulfhydryl groups, at which stage thiol compounds can effect reversal. The second step is the internal induction of a suppressive substance which may be a natural response to an upset in the reduction-oxidation potential of a cell. This mechanism has been demonstrated *in vitro* for the regulation of heme production and proposed for virus-type interferon.

15
Selective Action of Alkylating Agents on Helper and Suppressor Functions

A. Ghaffar and R. D. Paul, W. Lichter, L. L. Wellham, and M. M. Sigel

Department of Microbiology and Immunology,
University of South Carolina School of Medicine,
Columbia, South Carolina
Department of Microbiology and Immunology,
University of Miami School of Medicine, Miami, Florida

Environmental chemicals and therapeutic agents can cause effects ranging from total irreversible ablation of all immune responses through moderate selective, often subtle, changes to imperceptible effects. In large measure, the gradation of effects depends on the agent, its concentration and duration of action. Since cells of the lymphoreticular system which constitute the immune mechanism are derived from common precursors in bone marrow, it follows that any agent which severely affects stem cells would interfere with the generation of all cell types and result in total failure of the immune system. On the other hand, if an environmental or chemotherapeutic agent should damage only a terminally differentiated cellular set, the result would be abrogation of a single function. When life was simple, the immunologist was concerned only with the PMN's, macrophages, lymphocytes and antibodies. Based on the state of knowledge in the 40's and 50's, one expected that the elimination of macrophages and PMN's would result in debilitation of the primitive, nonspecific defense mechanism defined by phagocytosis. Likewise, if an agent caused lymphopenia, it was expected to compromise the antibody-forming capacity of the host. There was little inkling in those days that the macrophages played much more sophisticated roles in presentation of antigen to subsets of lymphocytes and in the initiation of humoral immune responses. Nor was it appreciated that lymphocytes could be subdivided into a variety of classes and subclasses with specialized functions performed in humoral and cell-mediated responses as well as in their regulation.

The Diversity of Targets for Action by Chemical Agents

In order to understand how chemical agents affect immune responses, it is first necessary to restate the current principal dogma of immunology: all immunologic responses are complex processes involving multiple sets of interacting cells. Even if we limit the analysis to a single major function of the immune mechanism, antibody production, the process involves a large number of steps including antigen presentation and recognition, membrane perturbation, activation of DNA synthetic processes, cellular proliferation and differentiation, activation of protein synthetic processes, which lead to the production of immunoglobulins and other immunologically relevant molecles, and secretion of these proteinaceous products. It was once thought that with the so-called thymus-independent antigens, the cells involved in these various steps were mainly of the B lineage and that T cells played little or no role. This oversimplified view of the thymus-independent (TI) humoral response has given way to newer concepts which include a diversity of types of B cells with preferential responses to different kinds of TI antigens (Mosier et al., 1976; Mosier et al., 1977; Zitron et al., 1977; Tittle and Rittenberg, 1980). The antigens have now been subdivided into at least two subclasses, with TNP-LPS representing TI-1 antigens and TNP-Ficoll and pneumococcal polysaccharide (SIII) representing TI-2 antigens (Mosier et al., 1977). Moreover, there are observations which indicate that B cells may also serve as helper cells to other B cells (Schott and Merchant, 1979) and possibly T cells (Ho et al., 1980). Although TI antigens do not require an obligatory participation of TH cells to initiate an immune response, their activity may be magnified or curtailed by T cells (Baker and Prescott, 1979).

Thymus-dependent (TD) responses are even more complex in their induction and regulation. The B cells involved in TD responses appear to be different from at least one subset of B cells responsive to TI antigens (Playfair and Purves, 1971; Tittle and Rittenberg, 1980). Macrophages appear to play a central role in coordinating presentation of antigen to T and B cells, thus providing the signal(s) which triggers proliferative and differential responses culminating in antibody production (Rosenthal and Schevach, 1973; Benacerraf, 1978; Cowing et al.,1978; Schwartz et al., 1979). The T cells which interact with B cells have been subdivided into several subsets, namely, T helper (TH), T amplifier (TA) and T suppressor (TS) cells (Katz and Benacerraf, 1972; Gershon, 1974; Markham et al., 1977; Muirhead and Cudkowicz, 1978). Positive control by T cells entails more than facilitation of antibody production as T cell cooperation with B cells also determines antibody class (Kishimoto and Ishizaka, 1973) and cell type (Herzenberg et al., 1976). Although one is wont to speak of *a* T helper cell, the fact of the matter is that the term denotes a multitude of cells of T lineage capable of providing a positive input to the immune response. The heterogeneity of TH cells has recently been emphasized by the discovery that, in addition to T cells which provide help after priming by a carrier linked to the hapten (in Tada's terminology, cognate interaction), there exists another kind of T cell which helps after priming by an unlinked irrelevant carrier (Tada et al., 1978). A similar dichotomy in TH cells has been described by Lubet and Kettman (1979), and their findings are especially relevant to the subject at hand because the cell providing nonspecific help is more resistant to at least one immunosuppressive agent, radiation, than is the specific TH cell. Another type of heterogeneity was described by Janeway (1979) who demonstrated the participation of two helper cells, one recongnizing Ig on B cells and the other recognizing the carrier. Since these observations were based on experiments utilizing primed T cells, it is conceivable that one of these cell populations may represent memory TH cells. Another type of heterogeneity derives from the fact that a given population of T cells contains TH precursors along-side functional TH cells. All of these considerations are relevant to the analysis of the effects of immunodulatory agents and certain aspects of this will be brought out in connection with our findings on the action of alkylating agents.

A negative regulatory signal is produced by T suppressor cells which carry the membrane phenotype of Ly23. According to the observations of several investigators, the Ly1 and Ly23 cells are differentiated from the Ly123 precursors (Huber et al., 1976; Cantor et al., 1978a; Cantor et al., 1978b; McDougal et al., 1979). The suppression by T cells has been the subject of very extensive investigations leading to the establishment of several experimental models (Feldmann et al., 1977; Benacerraf and Germain, 1979; Cantor and Gershon, 1979). One of these is depicted in Figure 1. Two Ly1 cells are shown, one bearing the additional phenotypic marker $Qa1^+$ and the other $Qa1^-$. The two cells appear to be required for activation of B cells toward differentiation to plasma cells and the pro-

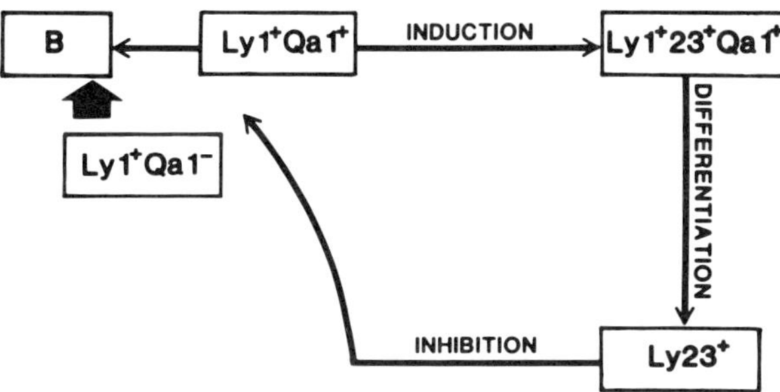

Fig. 1. Experimental model for mechanism of suppression by T cells.

duction of antibodies. What is more important to negative regulation is that the LY1Qa1⁺ cell is believed to serve as the inducer of suppressor cells. It acts on the Ly123Qa1⁺ precursors, causing them to differentiate to the Ly23 suppressor cell which performs a dual function. It exerts a suppressive effect on antibody production and also provides a feedback inhibition to the Ly1Qa1⁺ cell suppressing its inductive function and thereby preventing further generation of suppressor cells. More recently, information has been gathered to indicate that a short-circut may exist between the Ly1 and Ly 23 cells whereby a precursor or non-active Ly23 cell becomes activated to full suppressive activity by the Ly1Qa1⁺ cells (Eardley et al., personal communication).

The communication between the various subsets of T cells may be accomplished through molecules on the cell surfaces or secreted into the microenvironment (Mozes, 1978; Taussing et al., 1979; Pierce et al., 1979; Feldmann et al., 1979). These often contain products of the immunoregulatory region of the major histocompatibility complex (Ia antigens). Furthermore, it is now believed that the communication between cells including delivery of molecules or signals is performed by macrophage-type cells (Benacerraf, 1978; Cowing et al., 1978; Unaue, 1978; Ptak et al., 1977; Schwartz et al., 1979). Macrophages have also been implicated as the ultimate cell in exerting suppression under the influence of TS cells which simply provide the proper molecules for arming macrophages toward immunosuppressive activity (Pierce et al., 1979).

The intensity of the immune response (the quantitative level), as well as the quality of the response, are determined to a large extent by T cells. The other determinants are products of the I region and the antigen itself. Depending on the physicochemical nature of the antigen and its concentration, as well as the route of injection, the target cell activated by the antigen may be the one associated with the positive or negative regulation (Adorini et al., 1979; Baskin et al., 1980). The existence of so many variables which collectively and individually affect immune response in a positive or negative manner is at once a bane and a boon for the immunotoxicologist. It is a bane because it creates the complexity which leads to ambiguities and difficulties in interpreting results of experiments measuring the effects of various toxic agents. It is a boon because it provides an opportunity to study these effects on specific cell subsets, their functions and their interactions, thus providing an approach toward dissection of the immune mechanism.

Experiments Demonstrating Differential Effects of Alkylating Agents

We have been studying the effect of several anticancer chemo- and immunotherapeutic agents on various facets of the immune function (Ghaffar et al., 1978; Ghaffar and Sigel, 1978; Sigel et al 1979; Sigel et al., 1980; Ghaffar et al., 1980). In this chapter we will summarize previous and new observations on the effects of alkylating agents, cyclophosphamide (Cy), melphalan (Mel), 1, 3-bis (2-chloroethyl)-1-nitrosourea (BCNU), 1-(2-chloroethyl)-3-cyclohexyl-1-nitrosourea (CCNU) and 1-(2-chloroethyl 3-methyl-cyclohexyl)-1-nitrosourea (MeCCNU) on: (1) primary and secondary antibody responses to sheep erythrocytes (SRBC); (2) primary antibody responses to pneumococcal polysaccharide (SIII); and (3) induction of specific suppressor cells with high dose antigen (SRBC).

Effects on Primary and Secondary Responses

The effects of alkylating agents on TD response was determined in young adult male BDF_1 or Balb/C mice injected with the drug 2 days before or 2 days after immunization with 1×10^9 SRBC i.p. SRBC were also used as the antigen when the effects of drugs on secondary antibody responses were measured. In this instance, mice were injected i.p. with 1×10^8 SRBC 16 days apart and the drug was administered 2 days before or after the priming or 2 days before or after the secondary challenge with SRBC. Both primary and secondary responses to SRBC were measured 4 days after the final immunization by a modification of Jerne's technique for detecting antibody plaque-forming cells (PFC) (Cunningham and Szenberg, 1968). SIII antigen kindly provided by Dr. P. J. Baker of the NIAID, NIH, was used as the TI antigen and the drugs were injected 2

Table 1. Effect of Alkylating Agents on Immune Response to Thymus-Dependent and Thymus-Independent Antigens.

| | | PERCENT SUPPRESSION [2] | | | |
| | | SRBC | | SIII | |
DRUG [1] TREATMENT	DOSE MG/KG	PRE	POST	PRE	POST
Cy	100	99	99	26	98
Mel	8	99	98	variable	99
BCNU	30	98	97	98	98
McCCNU	30	14	−57	97	73
CCNU	30	84	96	n.t.	n.t.

[1] Drugs injected i.p. 2 days before (Pre) or 2 days after (Post) i.p. immunization with 1×10^9 SRBC or 0.5 μg SIII.

$$^2\ 1 - \left(\frac{\text{PFC per spleen in drug-treated mice}}{\text{PFC per spleen in control mice}} \right) 100.$$

Negative values represent higher responses in drug-treated mice than in controls.
n.t. = not tested.

days before or after i.p. immunization with 0.5 μg of this antigen. PFC responses were measured 5 days after immunization (Baker et al., 1969).

In Table 1 are summarized data on the effects of various alkylating agents employed in doses of approximately one LD $_{10}$ on primary and secondary anti-SRBC responses. It is apparent that Cy (100 mg/kg), Mel (8 mg/kg), BCNU and CCNU (30 mg/kg), severely suppressed primary anti-SRBC responses whether injected before or after the antigen. By contrast, MeCCNU (30 mg/kg), failed to be suppressive under either schedule. Although all agents except MeCCNU, were profoundly suppressive of the primary anti-SRBC PFC response when injected before antigen, they all failed to affect the secondary response when administered 2 days before priming (Table 2). The slight suppression caused by Mel was not significant. All agents caused suppression when injected 2 days after priming. The magnitude of this suppression varied from agent to agent. Cy and Mel were the most potent suppressors and CCNU and MeCCNU were only moderately suppressive; BCNU fell in the middle of the range. All agents were relatively more effective in suppressing PFC responses when injected 2 days before the secondary challenge and, with the exception of MeCCNU, were equally or more suppressive when injected 2 days after the secondary challenge.

Antibody response to SIII was not affected by either Cy or Mel when injected before the antigen (Table 1). The 26% suppression by Cy in-

Table 2.   Effect of Alkylating Agents on Secondary Immune Response to SRBC.

DRUG [1] TREATMENT	DOSE MG/KG	PERCENT SUPPRESSION [2]			
		PRIMING		SECONDARY	
		PRE	POST	PRE	POST
Mel	8	19	68	82	86
Cy	100	− 3	85	86	99
BCNU	30	3	59	88	76
MeCCNU	30	−20	37	74	−16
CCNU	30	− 1	34	66	99

[1] Drug injected i.p. 2 days before (Pre) or 2 days after (Post) priming or secondary challenge with 1×10^8 SRBC.

[2] $1 - \left(\dfrac{\text{PFC per spleen in drug-treated mice}}{\text{PFC per spleen in control mice}} \right) 100$.

Negative values indicate higher responses in drug-treated mice than in control animals. None of the negative values is statistically significant.

jected prior to the antigen was statistically not significant, and Mel caused a slight to modest suppression in some experiments and a slight enhancement in other experiments. By contrast, both BCNU and MeCCNU injected before antigen caused a consistent suppression of the anti-SIII response. Four of the agents tested suppressed anti-SIII responses when injected after antigen (CCNU was not tested).

Effects on Generation and Function of T Suppressor Cells

Suppressor cells were induced by the supraoptimal immunization (SOI) of BDF_1 mice with 4×10^9 SRBC and the expression of suppressor cell activity was measured by the i.v. transplantation of SOI splenocytes into syngeneic normal mice which were simultaneously immunized with 1×10^8 SRBC (Whisler and Stobo, 1976). PFC responses of recipients were measured 4 days later.

The genesis of suppressor activity (which is mediated by T cells and can be abrogated by anti-Thy-1 plus complement) is a slow process. Two days after SOI there is minimal activity measured by adoptive transfer. This progressively increases to a maximum suppressor activity by day 10 and persists at about the same level for at least 28 days. We shall refer to cells transferred after day 14 as T suppression effectors (TSe), to cells in the 2-12 day interval as activated T suppression inducers (TSi) (probably intermixed with increasing numbers of TSe), and to cells prior to SOI as non-activated precursors of TSi and TSe.

Donors of suppressor cells immunized with 4×10^9 SRBC were treated with an alkylating agent at different times in relation to SOI. The choice of times of treatment was dictated by several considerations. There are reports in the literature which indicate that resting precursors of suppressor cells are susceptible to Cy (Zembala and Asherson, 1976; Sy et al., 1977; Schwartz et al., 1978; Cantor et al., 1978a). On the other hand, there are also reports that Cy may actually induce suppressor cells (Milton et al., 1976; L'Age-Stehr and Diamantstein, 1978). Since we have shown that, under some circumstances Cy can exert differential effects on cells in different stages of differentiation (e.g., in the secondary response with drugs given at different times in relation to priming and secondary challenge), we asked the question whether Cy and the other alkylating agents would exert differential effects on the induction of T suppressor cells. Animals were therefore treated at 2 days before and at intervals after SOI. The data summarized in Table 3 indicate that none of the alkylating agents injected 2 days before SOI prevented the induction of TSe capable of exerting suppression in the adoptive host. When injected 2 days following SOI, both Cy and BCNU caused a dramatic reduction in

Table 3. **Effects of Alkylating Agents on Induction of Suppressor Cells by Supraoptimal Immunization.**

| | | PERCENT SUPPRESSION [2] | |
| | DOSE | | |
TREATMENT [1]	MG/KG	2D PRE SOI	2D POST SOI
Saline		86	88
Cy	100	92	2 [3]
BCNU	30	82	1 [3]
CCNU	30	84	92
MeCCNU	30	65	89
Mel	8	91	81

[1] Mice were injected i.p. with drugs either 2 days before or 2 days after immunization with 4×10^9 SRBC; 14 days later splenocytes from these mice were injected i.v. into syngeneic recipients which were simultaneously immunized with 1×10^8 SRBC. PFC in recipients' spleens were examined 4 days post cell transfer.

$$[2]\; 1 - \left(\frac{\text{PFC per spleen in mice receiving SOI splenocytes}}{\text{PFC per spleen in mice receiving non-immune splenocytes}} \right) \times 100.$$

[3] Significantly different from non-drug treated groups (line 1 above). All other differences were statistically not significant.

Table 4.   Differential Sensitivity of Suppressor Cells to Cy and BCNU with Maturation.

TREATMENT [1]	DRUG MG/KG	PERCENT SUPPRESSION WHEN TREATED ON DAY [2] POST SOI		
		+2	+12	+26
Saline	—	88	89	83
Cy	50	2 [3]	23 [3]	53 [3]
BCNU	30	1 [3]	77	n.t.

[1] Mice were injected i.p. with 4×10^9 SRBC or saline and treated with drugs 2, 12 or 26 days later. Ten days following drug treatment on day +2 or 2 days following drug treatment on days +12 or +26, splenocytes from SOI and control mice were transferred to syngeneic recipients which were simultaneously immunized with 1×10^8 SRBC. PFC in recipients' spleens were examined 4 days post cell transfer.

[2] $1 - \left(\dfrac{\text{PFC per spleen in mice receiving splenocytes}}{\text{PFC per spleen in mice receiving non-immune splenocytes}} \right) 100.$

[3] Significantly different from non-drug treated groups (line 1 above). All other differences were statistically not significant.

the capability of donor splenocytes to induce suppression in the secondary host. Mel, MeCCNU and CCNU were ineffective. There was further disparity between BCNU and Cy in their effects on suppressor cell function which was detectable in experiments where the drug was injected 12 days after SOI. It is apparent from Table 4 that on day 12 post SOI Cy still caused significant reduction in the suppressor effect while BCNU had no such effect. It is also evident from data summarized in Table 4 that, with the passing of time after SOI, as the suppressor cells matured, their sensitivity to Cy gradually diminished. Thus, while on day 2, 50 mg/kg of Cy could totally alleviate suppressor activity, the same dose of Cy alleviated only 77% and 47% of this activity on days 12 and 26, respectively.

We interpret our data in the light of the previously described kinetics of induction of transferable suppressor activity and the assumption that TSe dominated after 14 days of induction, whereas prior to this time there were variable ratios of TSi and TSe (the latter increasing with the passage of time after SOI). The fact that none of the drugs diminished the induction of suppressor cells signifies that resting precursors are resistant to alkylating agents. At first glance these findings contradict the findings of others who have demonstarted that Cy eliminates precursors of TSe (Zembala and Asherson, 1976; Sy et al., 1977; Schwartz et al., 1978; Cantor et al., 1978a). In the terminology of the feedback inhibition model (Figure 1) the precursor is the Ly123 cell which, according to Cantor et al. (1978a) is sensitive to Cy. In fact our findings do not argue against the sensitivity of such precursors because our experimental approach is based on an adoptive transfer to normal syngeneic recipients whose precursors have not been disturbed by drugs. Thus, if such cells are required for the generation of TSe they would be provided by the recipient. What the recipients are lacking are the activated TS inducer cells (TSi) which may correspond to the Ly1Qa1$^+$ cell in Figure 1. Our findings suggest that it is the precursors of TSi or resting TSi that are resistant to all alkylating agents. After activation, the proliferating TSi becomes susceptible to CY and BCNU but not to the other alkylating agents. The ultimate suppressor cell, TSe, is still susceptible to Cy (albeit to a lesser degree) but is resistant to BCNU.

DISCUSSION

Alkylating agents such as Cy, Mel, BCNU and CCNU can inhibit the development of a primary response when injected before or after a thymus-dependent antigen. By contrast, the secondary response is affected only when the drug is injected after exposure to the antigen. This implies that precursors of memory cells are relatively resistant to these alkylating agents and they become sensitive only after exposure to the antigen.

The fact that precursors of memory cells are resistant to alkylating agents sets them apart from precursors of cells involved in the primary response which are susceptible to most of the alkylating agents studied. We have observed other differential aspects in the sensitivity of primary and memory responses to suppression using T suppressor cells. For example, TS cells which can interrupt the generation of the primary response cannot prevent the activation of the secondary response (unpublished observations).

Results obtained with the TI antigen indicated that B cells which respond to SIII are resistant to Cy and Mel while in the resting state but become sensitive when stimulated with antigen. By contrast, the resting B cells are susceptible to BCNU and MeCCNU just as they are sensitive after exposure to the antigen. This produces a paradox: if resting B cells are susceptible to MeCCNU this agent should not spare the primary anti-SRBC response. The apparent discrepancy may represent a differential susceptibility of B cells involved in TD and TI responses. As cited in the introduction, there is ample evidence for heterogeneity among B cells with respect to their participation in TI and TD responses (Playfair and Purves, 1971; Tittle and Rittenberg, 1980) and even in relation to their recognition and responsiveness to different types of TI antigens (Mosier et al., 1976; Mosier et al., 1977; Zitron et al., 1977; Tittle and Rittenberg, 1980). The selective action of Cy and Mel demonstrated against anti-SIII and anti-SRBC responses when the drugs were given prior to immunization should also be considered in this light. The two agents inhibited the anti-SRBC responses but not the anti-SIII response, indicating that resting B cells specific for this antigen are relatively resistant to Cy and Mel whereas resting cells participating in the primary SRBC response are susceptible. At this time it is not possible to state whether in our system it is the resting TH cell or the resting SRBC-reactive B cell that is sensitive to Cy and Mel. Using a different approach Shand (1978) demonstrated that both non-activated B and T cells are susceptible. Even though resting B cells specific to SIII were found to be resistant to Cy, a recent publication by Berenbaum (1979) shows that resting B cells responsive to LPS can be eliminated by Cy. It is interesting that SIII is a TI-2 antigen which triggers a different subset of B cells from that triggered by LPS, a TI-1 antigent. Thus, alkylating agents seem to differentiate between different subsets of B cells and with respect to a TI-2 response, the nitrosoureas are inhibitory for resting B cells while Cy and Mel are not.

There is considerable precedent for selective action of Cy. It eliminates resting T cells which react to mitogens (Winkelstein et al., 1972; Sigel et al., 1980), depletes precursors of GVH cells (Owens and Santos, 1971) and destroys precursors of DTH suppressor cells (Zembala and Asherson, 1976; Sy et al., 1977; Schwartz et al., 1978), but not the precursors of T cells affecting DTH (Sy et al., 1977). Activated DTH T cells are apparently susceptible (Sy et al., 1977). Our results indicate that at least one type of T cell involved in suppressor activity, presumably the resting TSi (or its precursor) is resistant to all alkylating agents prior to activation by antigen. This cell becomes susceptible to Cy and BCNU but not to Mel, MeCCNU or CCNU immediately after activation. Mature TSe were found to be susceptible only to CY and with the passage of time their susceptibility seemed to decrease.

It is clear from these studies that chemotherapeutic agents can cause differential effects on different components of the immune system. Thus, all alkylating agents can discriminate between primary and secondary TD responses; some can distinguish between cells responding to TD and TI antigens and some can differentiate between positive and negative regulation.

In the context of the theme of this conference we would like to conclude by making three observation:

(1) Immunologic methods are highly useful for detecting *differential*

effects of chemical agents which may go undetected or not be recognized as subtly differential by other methods.

(2) No single immunologic method is sufficient to demonstrate selective or unique effects and it is therefore obligatory that a battery or immunologic techniques be brought into a study of various effects, especially subtly modulatory effects. It is no longer sufficient to compare overall humoral and cell-mediated responses. The new battery of tests must address immunologic interactions comprised of inductive and regulatory networks and pathways within the humoral and cell-mediated responses. This requires the acquisition of more knowledge about the cellular and molecular components of these networks and circuits.

(3) The fact that immunosuppressive agents exert selective activity should make them suitable as probes for future studies on induction and regulation of immune responses.

ACKNOWLEDGMENTS

A portion of this work was supported by USPHS Contract No. NO1–CM–57041 from the National Cancer Institute. Technical assistance by Sheila Long and Sharon Robinson is appreciated.

REFERENCES

Adorini, L., Harvey, M. A., Miller, A. and Sercarz, E. E. Fine specificity of regulatory T cells. II. Suppressor and helper T cells are induced by different regions of hen egg-white lysozyme in a genetically nonresponder mouse strain. J. Exp. Med., *150*:2931306 (1979).

Baker, P. J., Stashak, P. W. and Prescott, B. Use of erythrocytes sensitized with purified pneumococcal polysaccharides for the assay of antibody and antibody-producing cells. Appl. Micro-biol., *17*:442-426 (1969).

Baker, P. J. and Prescott, B. Regulation of the antibody response to pneumococcal polysaccharide by thymus-derived (T) cells. Mode of action of suppressor and amplifier T cells. In: *Immunology of Bacterial Polysaccharides* (J . A. Rudback and P. J. Baker, eds.), p. 67. Elsevier-North Holland, New York (1979).

Baskin, B. L., Blake, J. T. and Rosenthal, A. S. Determinant specific suppression of antigen-induced T cell proliferation in the guinea pig. II. Determinant specific suppression of *in vitro* T cell responsiveness parallels a seleceive suppression of anti-hapten but not anti-carrier antibody responses. J. Immunol., *124*:189-193 (1980).

Benacerraf, B. A hypothesis to relate the specificity of T lymphocytes and the activity of I region-specific Ir genes in macrophages and B lymphocytes. J. Immunol., *120*:1809-1812 (1978).

Benacerraf, B. and Germain, R. N. The immune response genes of the major histocompatibility complex. Immunol. Rev., *38*:72-119 (1978).

Benacerraf, B. and Germain, R. N. Specific suppressor responses to antigen under I region control. Fed. Proc., *38*:2053-2057 (1979).

Berenbaum, M. C. Time-dependence and selectivity of immunosuppressive agents. Immunol., *36*:355-365 (1979).

Cantor, H., McVay-Boudreau, L., Hugenberger, J., Naidorf, K., Shen, F. W. and Gershon, R. K. Immunoregulatory circuits among T cell sets. II. Physiologic role of feedback inhibition *in vivo:* Absence in NZB mice. J. Exp. Med., *147*:1116-1124 (1978a).

Cantor, H., Hugenberger, J., McVay-Boudreau, L, Eardley, D. D., Kemp, J., Shen, F. W. and Gershon, R. K. Immunoregulatory circuits among T-cell sets. Identification of a subpopulation of T-helper cells that induces feedback inhibition. J. Exp. Med., *148*:871-877 (1978b).

Cantor, H. and Gershon, R. K. Immunological circuits: Cellular composition. Fed. Proc., *38*:2058-2064 (1979).

Cowing, C., Pincus, S. H., Sachs, D. H. and Dickler, H. B. A subpopulation of adherent accessory cells bearing both I-A and I-E or C subregion antigens is required for antigen-specific murine T lymphocyte proliferation. J. Immunol., *121*:1680-1686 (1978).

Cunningham, A. J. and Szenberg, A. Further improvements in the plaque technique for detecting single antibody-forming cells. Immunol., *14*:599-600 (1968).

Feldmann, M, Beverley, P. C. L., Woody, J. and McKenzie, I. F. C. T-T interactions in the induction of suppressor and helper T cells: Analysis of membrane phenotype of precursor and amplifier cells. J. Exp. Med., *145*:793-801 (1977).

Feldmann, M., Erb, P., Kontiainen, S., Todd, I. and Woody, J. N. Comparison of antigen-specific I-region-associated cell interaction factors. In: *Subcellular factors in Immunity* (H. Friedman, ed.). Ann. N. Y. Acad. Sci.,*332*:591-604 (1979).

Ghaffar, A., Lichter, W., Wellham, L. L. and Sigel, M. M. Effect of anticancer chemothreapeutic agents on immune reactions of mice. I. Comparison of two nitrosoureas: 1,3-bis(2-chloroethyl)-1-nitrosourea and 1-(2-chloroethyl)-3-(4-methylcyclohexyl)-1-nitrosourea. J. Nat. Cancer Inst., *60*:1483-1487 (1978).

Ghaffar, A. and Sigel, M. M. Immunomodulation by *Corynebacterium parvum.* I. Variable effects on anti-sheep erythrocyte antibody responses. Immunol., *35*:1-9 (1978).

Ghaffar, A., Paul, R. D., Sigel, M. M., Lichter, W. and Wellham, L. L. Immunomodulation by *Corynebacterium parvum.* In: *Proceedings of the Conference on Immunmodulation by Bacteria and Their Products.* In press (1980).

Gershon, R. K. T cell control of antibody production. In: *Contemporary Topics in Immunobiology* (M. D. Cooper and N. L. Warner, eds.). Plenum Publishing Corp., New York. *3*:1-40 (1974).

Herzenberg, L. A., Okumura, K., Cantor, H., Sato, V. L., Shen, F. W., Boyse, E. A. and Herzenberg, L. A. T-cell regulation of antibody responses: Demonstration of allotype-specific helper T cells and their specific removal by suppressor T cells. J. Exp. Med., *144*:330-344 (1976).

Ho, M.-K., Kong, A.-S. and Morse, S. I. The *in vitro* effects of *Bordetella pertussis* lymphocytosis-promoting factor on murine lymphocytes. V. Modulation of T cell proliferation by helper and suppressor lymphocytes. J. Immunol., *124*:362–369 1980).

Huber, B., Cantor, H., Shen, F. W. and Boyse, E. A. Independent differentiative pathways of Ly1 and Ly23 subclasses of T cells: Experimental production of mice deprived of selected T cell subclasses: J. Exp. Med., *144*:1128-1133 (1976).

Janeway, C. A. Jr. Helper T cell interactions. Fed. Proc., *38*:2071–2074 (1979).

Katz, D. H. and Benacerraf, B. The regulatory influence of activated T cells on B cell responses to antigen. Adv. Immunol., *15*:1–94 (1972).

Kishimoto, T. and Ishizaka, K. Regulation of antibody response *in vitro*. VI. Carrier-specific helper cells for IgG and IgE antibody response. J. Immunol., *111*:720 (1973).

L'Age-Stehr, J. and Diamantstein, T. Induction of autoreactive T lymphocytes and their suppressor cells by cyclophosphamide. Nature, *271*:663–665 (1978).

Lubet, M. T. and Kettman, J. R. Regulation of the primary immune response to ovalbumin in mice: Activation of T cells mediating delayed-type hypersensitivity, nonspecific help, and specific help, and their sensitivity to radiation. J. Immunol., *123*:426–433 (1979).

McDougal, J. S., Shen, F. W. and Elster, P. Generation of T helper cells *in vitro*. V. Antigen-specific Ly1$^+$ T cells mediate the helper effect and induce feedback suppression. J. Immunol., *122*:437–442 (1979).

Markham, R. B., Reed, N. D., Stashak, P. W., Prescott, B., Amsbaugh, D. F. and Baker, P. J. Effect of Concanavalin A on lymphocyte interactions involved in the antibody response to type III pneumococcal polysaccharide. II. Ability of suppressor T cells to act on both B cells and amplifier T cells to limit the magnitude of the antibody response. J. Immunol., *119*:1163–1168 (1977).

Milton, J. D., Carpenter, C. B. and Addison, I. E. Depressed T-cell reactivity and suppressor activity of lymphoid cells from cyclophosphamide-treated mice. Cell. Immunol., *24*:308–317 (1976).

Mosier, D. E., Scher, I. and Paul, W. E. *In vitro* responses of CBA/N mice: Spleen cells of mice with an x-linked defect that precludes immune responses to several thymus-independent antigens can respond to TNP-lipopolysaccharide. J. Immunol., *117*:1363-1369 (1976).

Mosier, D. E., Mond, J. J., Zitron, I., Scher, I. and Paul, W. E. Functional correlates of surface Ig expression for T-independent antigen triggeriing of B cells. In: *Immune System: Genetics and Regulation* (E. E. Sercarz, L. A. Herzenberg and C. F. Fox, eds.), pp 699–706. Academic Press, New York, 1977.

Mozes, E. Some properties and functions of antigen specific T cell factors. In: *Ir Genes and Ia Antigens* (H. O. McDevitt, ed.), pp 475-485. Academic Press, New York, 1978.

Muirhead, D. Y. and Cudkowicz, G. Subpopulations of splenic T cells regulating an anti-hapten antibody response. II. Distinct functions of, and sequential requirement for, helper and amplifier cells. J. Immunol., *121*:130-137 (1978).

Owens, A. H. and Santos, G. W. The effect of cytotoxic drugs on the graft-*vs*-host disease in mice. Transplant., *11*:378-382 (1971).

Pierce, C. W., Tadakuma, T. and Kapp, J. A. Role of nonspecific and specific suppressor factors in immunity. In: *Subcellular Factors in Immunity* (H. Friedman, ed.). Ann. N. Y. Acad. Sci., *332*:336-344 (1979).

Playfair, J. H. L. and Purves, E. C. Anitbody formation by bone marrow cells in irradiated mice. I. Thymus-dependent and thymus-independent responses to sheep erythrocytes. Immunol., *21*:113-121 (1971).

Ptak, W., Zembala, M. and Gershon, R. K. Intermediary role of macrophages in the passage of suppressor signals between T-cell subsets. J. Exp. Med., *146*:424-434 (1977).

Rosenthal, A. S. and Schevach, E. M. Function of macrophages in antigen recognition by guinea pig T lymphocytes. I. Requirement for histocompatible macrophages and lymphocytes. J. Exp. Med., *138*:1194-1212 (1973).

Schott, C. F. and Merchant, B. Carrier-specific immune memory to a thymus-independent antigen in congenitally athymic mice. J. Immunol., *122*:1710–1718 (1979).

Schwartz, A., Askenase, P. W. and Gershon, R. K. Regulation of delayed-type hypersensitivity reactions by cyclophosphamide-sensitive T cells. J. Immunol., *121*:1573-1576 (1978).

Schwartz, R. H., Yano, A., Stimpfling, J. H. and Paul, W. E. Gene complementation in the T-lymphocyte proliferative response to poly $(Glu^{55}Lys^{36}Phe^9)n$. A demonstration that both immune response gene products must be expressed in the same antigen-presenting cell. J. Exp. Med., *149*:40-57 (1979).

Shand, F. L. The capacity of microsomally activated cyclophosphamide to induce immunosuppression *in vitro*. Immunol., *35*:1017-1025 (1978).

Sigel, M. M., Paul, R. D. and Ghaffar, A Adult thymectomy and cyclophosphamide have selective effects on immunoregulatory T cells and their precursors. In: *The Molecular Basis of Immune Cell Function* (J. G. Kaplan, ed.), pp 671-675. Elsevier-North Holland, Amsterdam, 1979.

Sigel, M. M., Lopez, D. M., Epstein, R. S., Paul, R. D., Lichter, W., Wellham, L. L. and Ghaffar, A. T and B lymphocytes under stress—tumor growth or chemotherapy. In: *Immunology of Parasitic infections*. In press (1980).

Sy, M.-S., Miller, S. D. and Claman, H. N. Immune suppression with supraoptimal doses of antigen in contact sensitivity. I. Demonstration of suppressor cells and their sensitivity to cyclophosphamide. J. Immunol., *119*:240-244 (1977).

Tada, T., Takemori, T., Okumura, K., Nonaka, M. and Tokuhisa, T. Two distinct types of helper T cells involved in the secondary antibody response: independent and synergistic effects of Ia^- and Ia^+ helper T cells. J. Exp. Med., *147*:446-458 (1978).

Taussig, M. J., Corvalán, J. R. F. and Holliman, A. Characterization of an antigen-specific factor from a hybrid T-cell line. In: *Subcellular Factors in Immunity* (H. Friedman, ed.). Ann. N. Y. Acad. Sci., *332*:316-335 (1979).

Tittle, T. V. and Rittenberg. M. B. IgG B memory cell subpopulations: Differences in susceptibility to stimulation by TI-1 and TI-2 antigens. J. Immunol., *124*:202-206 (1980).

Unanue, E. R. The regulation of lymphocyte functions by the macrophage. Immunol. Rev., *40*:227-255 (1978).

Whisler, R. L. and Stobo, J. D. Heterogeneity of murine regulatory T cells. I. Subpopulations of amplifier and suppressor T cells. J. Exp. Med., *144*:398-413 (1976).

Winkelstein, A., Mikulla, J. M., Nankin, H. R., Pollock, B. H. and Stolzer, B. L. Mechanisms of immunosuppression: Effects of cyclophosphamide on lymphocytes. J. Lab. Clin. Med. *80*:506-513 (1972).

Zembala, M. and Asherson, G. L. The effect of cyclophosphamide and irradiation on cells which suppress contact sensitivity in the mouse. Clin. Exp. Immunol., *23*:554-561 (1976).

Zitron, I. M., Mosier, D. E. and Paul, W. E. The role of surface IgD in the response to thymic-independent antigens. J. Exp. Med., *146*:1707-1718 (1977).

DISCUSSION

SPREAFICO: At variance with some of your data on MeCCNU, we find that it's much more a depressant than BCNU in the systems that you employed. So it well might be strain differences in these kinds of things.

GHAFFAR: I accept that fact but, unfortunately, we can't go on to all different strains and test each one for every parameter.

HINSDILL: I thought your system was a fascinating one, and it's too bad that Dr. Robert Speirs can't be here because, as you may or may not know, he has worked with cyclophosphamide as a prototype for some time. One of the interesting findings that he made was that cyclophosphamide can induce a very high IgE level at a time when it's knocking out IgM and IgG response. I think the theory was always that it was knocking out T-suppressor cells for IgE response, and it would seem that this would be a marvelous opportunity to check that out and perhaps learn the mechanism for turning on IgE.

GHAFFAR: Thank you. I presume it was a comment rather than a question. I would agree that this agent should be examined in that situation.

BRUSICK: I would like to make a couple of general comments, rather than to ask any questions. The subject of testing problems came up earlier this morning in discussions concerning concentrations needed to elicit responses in these types of tests, and I'd like to address this topic. The primary thrust of this particular session dealt with environmental agents, and I believe that one or two real environmental agents, other than chemotherapeutic agents, were actually discussed.

The problems of test concentration and the significance of toxicity one gets at only high levels are important. Most of the chemicals mentioned such as the alkylating agents, cytoxin, Tris, DES, BCNU and so on, all produced immunotoxic responses at high concentrations. If one looks at the total toxicology of these chemicals, such endpoints as mutagenesis, carcinogenesis, and teratogenesis occur at lower concentrations. If one focuses only on immunological responses, a considerable amount of these materials must be used. For example, it is somewhat disturbing to me that one would have to look at 500 mg/kg of Tris to detect a biological response since other endpoints as mutation and carcinogensis occur at only low concentration, or, in the case of cytoxin, 180 mg/kg. These are relatively lethal dose levels.

My point is that if all types of toxicity measurements are made as Dr. McCoy mentioned last night in his discussion of batteries of tests that data from immunotoxicity describe only one of several parameters. Cancer, for example, may be the product of several cellular intrusions, e.g., genetic, promoting, and immunosuppressive. Only in the context of this combined approach would a weak immunosuppressive effect be meaningful. On another point, it would be very helpful to know in the immunological systems, what kind of dose-response curves you get down at very low dose levels; e.g., are they linear; do you see a threshold effect? You will have to use, I believe, at least in the "Tumor Take" type assay, for example, more than ten animals. You are going to have to use many more animals to define the shape of the dose-response curves.

If the test compound is not only an immunosuppressive but also an initiating compound (e.g., Tris initiates transformation of cells at very low concentrations), or is a tumor promoting agent (perhaps a very small concentration of Tris, DES, or one of these other agents) acting as an immunosuppressive agent, the test compound might have a tremendously enhancing effect on the total process of carcinogenesis that one would not normally notice if one were looking at immunosuppression as the primary mechanism.

GHAFFAR: I agree with the dose response. I can only talk about the deviation of the immune responses. There has to be a stepping stone. One cannot introduce all parameters and all tests at once. It has to be staged in such a way that the basic observations should be made in a limited protocol using a limited dosage, preferably a high dosage so that one cannot miss the effect. From there on, the next step should be to extend studies to other parameters. If we overload the system, by including all parameters and all variables, we are never even going to start doing any of the tests.

BRUSICK: Absolutely right. I didn't want to discourage anyone. I think, initially, qualitative assessment is important, but the next critical step is quantitative assessment, because before one can apply this to toxicological safety evaluation, quantitation is an absolute necessity.

HADDEN: I wanted to reinforce the relevance of mouse strains in relation to the question by Dr. Spreafico. In the immunostimulation area we find that strains vary considerably, for example, the C57/black mouse is relatively resistant to the action of several immunopotentiators. Dr. Faanes has found this strain relatively more susceptible to suppressive effects of cytotoxic agents. Thus, in order to have a meaningful picture of the action of both potentiators and inhibitors on immune response, it's relevant to take into account these differences in strain, particularly the difference of the C57-black-related animals from other strains, such as Balb/c or C_3H. What strain do you use?

GHAFFAR: In these experiments they were BDF_1's. In some studies, we used BALB/c, but both parameters compared in both strains are similar. I agree with your comment on strain variation; unfortunately, until we come across a model where we can perform cell transfers in humans from one individual to the other, we have to stick to inbred strains of laboratory animals.

SIGEL: I couldn't agree more with the previous speaker's observation of addressing various parameters in various disciplines that may bear on the question of impact of various environmental and therapeutic agents. I think this was the purpose of delineating the action of various drugs, not on the immune system as a whole, but components of the system, because these may behave differently, as Dr. Ghaffar has indicated. What was not done today, because there was no time, was to show that some of the same agents which suppress antibody formation will actually enhance macrophage function or other cell-mediated responses. Unless we fully recognize the precise target and modes of action and define the active principle in the agents, we will always be at a loss to explain discrepancies and the multiplicity of effects that one observes in the complex of carcinogenesis and environmental effects. I would like to cite an example of a single drug which, when tested by one procedure, will be found to be suppressive and, when tested by another, will be shown to be ineffective. When mice are treated with cyclophosphamide their splenocytes lose their blastogenic responsiveness to PHA. Yet, these splenocytes respond to PHA with the production of a cytotoxic lymphokine (experiments by Ronald Paul and Diana Lopez). Thus, while this agent causes what appears to be death of the replicative potential, it does not appear to impair biosynthesis of protein. This supports the contention of Drs. Dean and McCoy, that we should be looking at multiple parameters of action by various agents.

McCOY: Actually, Dr. Sigel just answered, or attempted to answer, most of the questions I was going to pose to the audience: Are we ready today to introduce the idea of testing with a battery of tests? Again, in attempting to drive the point home that Dr. Brusick was getting at, I think that looking strictly at immunologic phenomena is only one small part of the total picture, and I would be very strong in advocating the idea of using a battery of immunological and non-immunological tests to evaluate toxological effects of chemicals.

GHAFFAR: I'd like to make one comment. I agree with Dr. McCoy's suggestion that we have to test these things in different parameters—in different systems and at different levels. But where we have to be careful is that we cannot introduce an agent at the level where some of the basics are unknown. Let's face it. Cyclophosphamide has been around for decades. All the work on immunosuppression has been done. So why bother with it? Because there are models now becoming available where we can test it at a different level. We cannot do this with agents where there is no background and where there is no information on the basic effects. For example, in immunology itself, if the agent is totally innocuous, it seems futile to me to go over and test for suppressor-cell function, for effect on suppressor cells. Therefore, we should have these stages and levels in the screening program and some agents should come into the program at a higher level than the others.

SECTION IV
HOST SUSCEPTIBILITY AND LUNG DEFENSE MECHANISMS: INTRODUCTION

INTRODUCTION

Chairman: Jack H. Dean

The purpose of the concluding session of this conference is to review two major aspects of immunotoxicology including host susceptibility models for examining chemical-induced immune alterations and methods to study inhalation exposure and the resultant effects on immunological responses of the lymphoid elements of the lungs. The lungs have a major interactive role with man's environment because of the vast amount of airborne pollutants and microorganisms they encounter daily. Host susceptibility models represent an important parameter to study since the "bottom-line" following chemical exposure (inhalation, oral or injection) would appear to be whether host resistance to neoplasia or infectious agents has been altered.

The observations of altered host resistance and immunologic dysfunction following low level exposure of rodents as well as man to certain chemical pollutants have prompted the methodical evaluation of immunologic methods for application to routine assessment of alterations in immunocompetence following chemical exposure. The panel of assays selected for immunotoxicologic evaluation should include procedures to study impaired immune responsiveness, hypersensitization and altered host resistance. The assay panel should be selected with certain practical considerations such as simplicity, reproducibility, cost and application to routine toxicology studies. Approaches for evaluating host susceptibility following challenge with small numbers of bacteria or transplantable tumor cells (LD_{10} or TD_{10}) will be described in this session. Information provided by this test panel should provide a reasonable and sensitive data base from which judgements can be made regarding the safety of the test drug or chemical. Immunologic assays may represent more sensitive endpoints then currently employed methods in general toxicity assessment since functional as well as cell-cell cooperation responses are examined using bone marrow and lymphoid cells.

The literature has become replete with clinical observations suggesting a relationship between spontaneous neoplasia or increased susceptibility to certain bacterial, viral, fungal or parasitic agents and immunologic alterations. For example, individuals born with severe immunologic dysfunction or receiving chemotherapeutic drugs to maintain an immunosuppressive state, to sustain an organ or bone marrow transplant, have significantly higher frequency of cancer and infectious diseases. More recently, altered host resistance to infectious agents has been observed following experimental exposure in rodents to certain chemicals of environmental concern such as 2,3,7,8-tetrachlorodibenzo-p-dioxin, polychlorinated biphenyls, hexachlorobenzene, arsenicals and diethylstilbestrol. Depressed host resistance following exposure to some of the above chemicals will be described during this session.

However, minimal effort has been directed during the past few years to correlate tests of immunologic function with assays of host resistance to define which immunologic parameters might predict altered host resistance. In addition, marginal progress has been achieved at developing or refining host resistance endpoints as sensitive and reproducible assays. These would appear to be the major immediate challenges of immunologists wishing to study chemical-induced immunotoxicity. The papers presented in this session represent the first step in addressing the challenge of developing and applying host resistance assays to measure immunologic alteration following chemical exposure.

Drs. Gardner and Bice will describe methods under development in their respective laboratories to study altered host resistance and immunologic function in the deep lung following inhalation exposure. Dr. Loose and I will describe changes in immunologic parameters and host susceptibility following systemic exposure by injection or ingestion.

16
Host Resistance Models as Endpoints for Assessing Immune Alterations Following Chemical Exposure: Studies with Diethylstilbestrol, Cyclophosphamide and 2,3,7,8-Tetrachlorodibenzo-p-dioxin

Jack H. Dean, Michael I. Luster,[1] Gary A. Boorman,
Martin L. Padarathsingh,[2] Robert W. Luebke and Mary E. Clements

*Environmental Biology Branch and Environmental Chemistry
Laboratory[1], National Institute of Environmental Health
Sciences, Research Triangle Park, North Carolina
and Department of Immunology[2], Litton Bionetics, Inc.,
Kensington, Maryland*

INTRODUCTION

The application and refinement of host resistance assays to study animals exposed to chemicals of real or potential environmental concern is now a major developmental emphasis in immunotoxicity assessment. This interest has been generated by the evidence that exposure to certain chemicals can result in immune alterations in experimental animals (reviewed by Vos, 1977; Faith et al., 1978; Dean et al., 1979a; Koller et al., 1979; Luster et al., 1979) which often leads to altered host resistance to bacterial

(Thigpen et al., 1975; Hemphill et al., 1971), viral (Friend and Trainer, 1970; Gainer and Pry, 1972; Fairchild et al., 1972), protozoan (Loose et al., 1978), or transplantable tumor cell challenge (Dean et al., 1979a) as well as spontaneous tumor development (Shimkin and Grady; 1940; Theiss et al., 1979). Studies have also shown that low-level exposure of humans to certain chemicals may induce immunologic alterations similar to that which occurs in experimental animals (Bekesi, et al., 1978). Burnet proposed (1970) that the immune system, principally the thymus-dependent lymphocytes and accessory macrophages provided primary resistance to neoplastic or tranformed cells, transplanted foreign tissue and intracellular parasites (i.e., immune surveillance). This concept has been substantiated by studies such as Law et al. (1972) who demonstrated that neonatal thymectomy increased the susceptibility of mice to polyoma virus transformation and tumor development. In addition, exposure to certain chemicals has been shown for some time to increase tumor frequency (Shimkin and Brady, 1940) and to reduce host resistance to transplantable syngeneic tumor cells in experimental animals (Dean et al., 1979b). Humans exposed to immunosuppressive drugs to sustain organ transplants have also been shown to have an unusually high frequency of spontaneous tumors (Penn, 1978) and increased frequency of bacterial and viral infections (Allen, 1976). Thus, it is well established that altered immune function results in decreased host resistance.

Cyclophosphamide (CY) is an efficient and widely used alkylating agent with potent immunosuppressive and cancer chemotherapeutic properties (Goodman and Gilman, 1975). It has been widely used in the therapy of acute and chronic lymphocytic leukemia, multiple myeloma and lymphomas and as an immunosuppressive agent to sustain organ transplants. CY requires metabolic activation to the phosphoramide mustard by hepatic microsomal enzymes (Brock and Hohorst, 1967) which is particularly efficient in inhibiting DNA synthesis in rapidly dividing cells by dimer formation among guanine bases (Goodman and Gilman, 1975). Cells of the lymphoid series are particularly sensitive to CY with up to 70% lymphoid cell depletion in the mouse within 1 day following CY treatment and 95% depletion within 3 days (Willer and Sluis, 1977). Earlier reports (Turk and Poulter, 1972) suggested CY selectively depleted B- cells while recent reports have shown that CY is also cytotoxic for T-cells, particularly T-helper and T-suppressor populations (Bash et al., 1976; Milton et al., 1976; Dean et al., 1979b). In the studies described here, immunosuppressive doses of CY were used to refine, validate and determine the sensitivity of certain host susceptibility assays prior to applying them to assess the immunotoxicity of selected chemicals.

Diethylstilbestrol (DES) is a synthetic nonsteroidal chemical with potent estrogenic activity. DES was of interest to us because of its association with human cancer following *in utero* exposure (Herbst, 1971; Cutler et al. 1972), its widespread distribution in the human food chain (McMartin et al., 1978) and recent reports of immunologic alterations following *in utero* (Luster et al., 1979), neonatal (Kalland and Fosberg, 1978; Kalland et al., 1978, 1980; Kalland 1980a,b) or adult exposure of mice (Luster et al., 1980).

The host resistance assays selected were also used to examine mice exposed *in utero* and postnatally to 2,3,7,8-tetrachlordibenzo-*p*-dioxin (TCDD). Pre/postnatal exposure of mice to TCDD at similar dosages employed in the present study causes severe thymus atrophy, increased sensitivity to bacterial endotoxin, depression of cell-mediated and humoral mediated immunity (Vos and Moore, 1974; Thomas and Hinsdill, 1979; Luster et al., 1980) and reduced host resistance to challenge with *Salmonella Bern* in exposed adults (Thigpen et al., 1975).

Thus, the goals of these studies were two-fold: 1) to refine and validate tumor susceptibility assays for altered host resistance using CY, and 2) to apply a series of host resistance assays using mice exposed to chemicals of environmental concern with known immunologic effects including DES and TCDD.

MATERIALS AND METHODS

Mice

Female $B_6C_3F_1$ (C57BL/6N × C_3H) and male inbred BALB/c weighing 18 to 22 g were obtained from the production contracts of the National Institutes of Health (Fort Detrick, MD) and used throughout the studies.

Chemicals and Exposure Regimen

Cycloposphamide (CY) was obtained from Mead Johnson and Company (Evansville, IN) and was dissolved in sterile saline immediately prior to use. Animals were injected intraperitoneally once with a total dose of 1.8-180 mg/kg body weight given.

Diethylstilbestrol (DES) was obtained from Sigma Chemical Company (St. Louis, MO). Adult female $B_6C_3F_1$ mice were injected subcutaneously (sc) with DES in corn oil at 8, 2 or 0.2 mg/kg body weight in corn oil on 5 successive days. Controls were simultaneously injected with corn oil alone (0.1 ml).

2,3,7,8-Tetrachlorodibenzo-*p*-dioxin (TCDD), greater than 99% purity was synthesized by the Environmental Chemistry Laboratory, NIEHS. TCDD was dissolved in reagent-grade acetone and subsequently diluted with corn oil. TCDD exposure was accomplished through maternal dosing and was administered by gavage to randomly distributed pregnant mice as previously described (Luster et al., 1980). Mothers were administered TCDD at day 14 of gestation and again on day 1, 7 and 14 following birth at dosages of 1.0 or 5.0 μg/kg body weight. Control animals received 0.1 ml of corn oil. Litters were standardized to contain 6 neonates/litter on postnatal day 4. Neonates from different litters were randomly selected from each of the host resistance assays studied.

Tumors

BALB/c mice were challenged subcutaneously (sc) with the mKSA-TU5 tumor cell line obtained from primary BALB/c kidney cells transformed with Simian virus-40. $B_6C_3F_1$ mice were challenged subsutaneously with PYB6 sarcoma, a polyoma virus induced tumor of C57BL/6 mice. Both tumor lines have been maintained in our laboratory in parental strains by *in vivo* serial passage. A challenge dose of 5×10^2 to 5×10^3 cells produces tumors in 10-20% (TD_{10-20}) of unimmunized, nontreated mice, while higher doses (1×10^5) produce tumors and deaths in 100% of the animals challenged.

Madison 109 lung tumor was kindly provided by Mr. Fred Vieria (Litton Bionetics) and maintained in C57BL/6 mice by biweekly passes of an intramuscular injection in the right hip of 1×10^4 tumor cells.

Lewis lung tumor was kindly provided by Mr. Mike Chirigos (National Cancer Institute) and passed in BALB/c mice at biweekly intervals by the same procedure as used for Madison 109 tumor.

Tumor Susceptibility Assay

The tumor susceptibility procedure was performed as described previously (Dean et al., 1979). Briefly, BALB/c mice were exposed to graded doses of CY (1.8-180 mg/kg body weight) 2-7 days prior to sc challenge with 5×10^2 to 5×10^3 mKSA-TU5 ascites tumor cells (Figure 1). Normal and chemically exposed $B_6C_3F_1$ mice were challenged sc with 5×10^3 PYB6 tumor cells 2-3 days following their last CY or DES exposure or 12 weeks after birth in TCDD treated mice. Untreated control mice challenged with this tumor cell dose had tumors in only 10-20 %

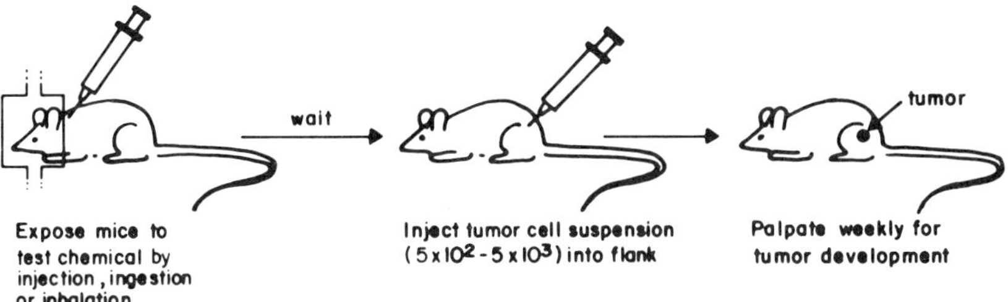

Fig. 1. Demonstrates the methodology of the tumor susceptibility assay to assess chemical-induced immunotoxicity.

(TD_{10-20}) of those animals. Animals were weighed and palpated twice weekly for 60 days to assess the development of tumors. Data were expressed as: 1) the number of mice with palpable tumors/number of mice inoculated; and 2) the mean latency in days to tumor detection ($\geqslant$ 5mm tumor).

[125]IUDR Assay for Determining Lung Tumor Mass

Treated and control mice were challenged intravenously (iv) with a single cell suspension of Lewis lung (5×10^3-5×10^4) tumor cells or Madison 109 (5×10^3) 2-3 days following chemical exposure. Eight-14 days later control and treated mice received 1 mg/kg of FUDR by intraperitoneal (ip) injection followed in 1 hour by 1×10^6 CPM ($\sim 1\mu$Ci) of [125]IUDR (ip) to quantitate tumor mass as diagrammed in Fig. 2. The mice were sacrificed 22-24 hours later and the lungs were removed and profused with saline. The lungs were placed in Gamma counting tube and counted to preset error of 1% or for 10 minutes in a PRIAS model Gamma counter (Packard Instrument Co.).

Wexler assays (Wexler, 1966) employing India ink were used to visualize tumor colonies in the lung in parallel with some [125]IUDR assays to determine comparability of these two methods.

Listeria Monocytogenes Susceptibility Assay

The bacterium *L. monocytogenes* (strain L242/73 Type 4B) from a naturally infected mouse was used from the same frozen stock throughout the study (Figure 3). Organisms were grown overnight at 37°C on Trypticase soy agar containing 5% sheep blood. Colonies were selected

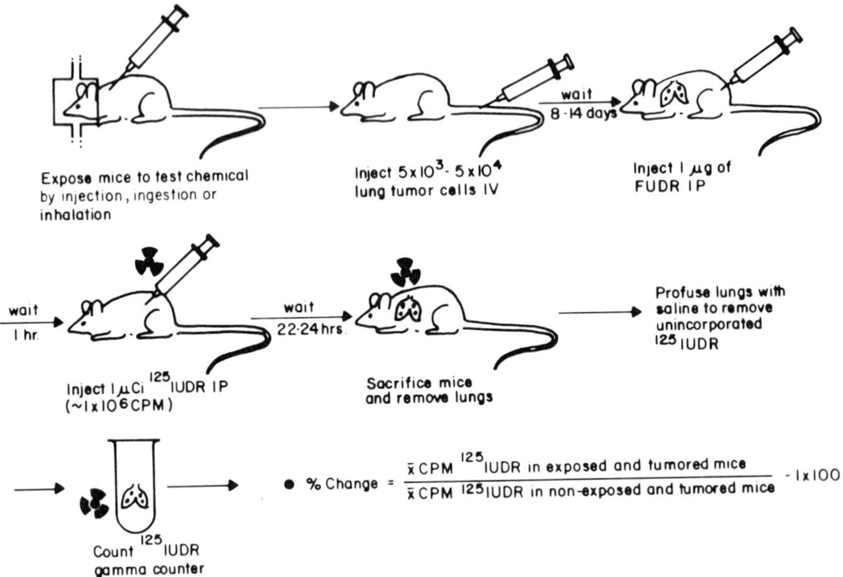

$$\bullet \ \% \ \text{Change} = \frac{\bar{x} \ \text{CPM} \ ^{125}\text{IUDR in exposed and tumored mice}}{\bar{x} \ \text{CPM} \ ^{125}\text{IUDR in non-exposed and tumored mice}} - 1 \times 100$$

Fig. 2.   Diagram of the ¹²⁵IUDR incorporation assay to estimate lung tumor mass following an intravenous challenge of lung tumor cells in mice exposed to an immunosuppressive chemical.

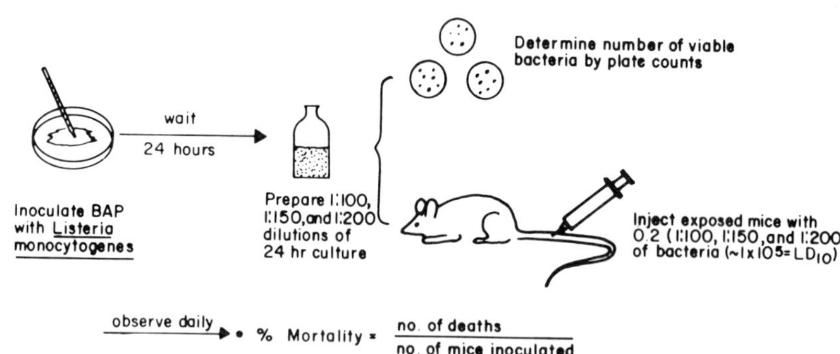

$$\bullet \ \% \ \text{Mortality} = \frac{\text{no. of deaths}}{\text{no. of mice inoculated}}$$

Fig. 3.   Demonstrates the *Listeria monocytogenes* susceptibility assay procedure to measure alterations of host resistance following chemical or drug treatment.

and a stock suspension was prepared in sterile physiological saline. The number of bacteria was quantitated turbidimetrically in a Coleman model 6/12 spectrophotometer at 540 μm. Dilutions of 1:100, 1:150 and 1:200 were prepared for injection. The number of viable bacteria in all dilutions used for animal inoculations was confirmed by conventional plate count procedures and approximated $1\text{-}4 \times 10^5$ ml. Mice, in groups of 10, received 0.2 ml of the selected dilutions intravenously and were monitored daily for 14 days for death.

Trichinella Spiralis Infection Procedure

The method of Larsh and Kent (1949) as modified by Weatherly (1970) was used to produce infection in experimental and stock $B_6C_3F_1$ mice. Briefly, larvae were obtained by digestion of stock infected mice in artifical gastric juice (1% HC1, 0.7% pepsin) at a rate of 1L per skinned, eviscerated carcass. Sedimented larvae were added to 37° nutrient broth with 5% gelatin in a Kolmer 30 ml centrifuge tube and mixed using a 1 ml glass tuberculin syringe fitted with an 18 gauge lavage needle. Next, 0.05 ml aliquots were streaked onto glass slides for larvae count. During standardization and injection procedure, larvae and larval suspension were kept in a 37° H_2O bath to help maintain viability. Larvae suspensions were adjusted until repeated counts contained one fourth the number of larvae to be given to recipients (approximately 200/mouse). Mice were infected by lavage with 0.2 ml of the larvae suspension. A group of infected, non-treated controls were included in all experiments and were killed at 7 days post- infection for adult worm counts (infection control) which generally approximates 50-80% of the infecting dose larvae count. DES treated and control mice were infected with larvae by lavage and sacrificed at day 14. The number of adult worms remaining in the gut of control and DES treated mice were enumerated by the method described in detail by Larsh and Kent (1949).

Endotoxin Hypersensitivity

$B_6C_3F_1$ mice were challenged intravenously with *Escherichia coli* 055:B5, lippolysaccharide (LPS), (Difco Laboratories, Detroit, MI), extracted by the Westphal process. Dosage levels (600 μg/mouse) were selected which kill 20% or less of the control mice (LD_{20}). Ten mice per group were first exposed to the chemical under study and then challenged with LPS. Mortality was recorded at 24 and 48 hours.

Table 1.   Promotion of Tumor Growth with Cyclophosphamide.

CHALLENGE LEVEL OF mKSA TUMOR CELLS	DOSE OF CYCLOPHOS- PHAMIDE [1] (MG/KG)	NO. OF MICE DEVELOPING TUMORS NO. OF MICE INOCULATED	%	MEAN LATENCY (DAYS)
5×10^4	0	8/10	(80%)	10
	180	10/10	(100%)	8
5×10^3	0	2/10	(20%)	21
	180	9/10	(90%)*	10
5×10^2	0	1/10	(10%)	30
	180	8/10	(80%)*	19
5×10^1	0	0/10		—
	180	0/10		—

[1] Mice were given a single injection of CY 2 days prior to tumor challenge.
* Significantly different from controls by Chi-square analysis with Yate's correction.

RESULTS

Increased Susceptibility to mKSA Tumor Cells Following Cyclophosphamide

Validation studies for tumor development in mice treated with an immuno-suppressive dose of CY (180 mg/kg) and then challenged with graded doses of tumor cells (mKSA-TU5) are summarized in Table 1. At doses of mKSA cells which produced 10-20% tumors (TD_{10-20}) in control mice, a significant increase ($p < 0.05$) in tumor frequency (80-90%) was observed in CY treated mice. The mean latency to tumor detection increased in a dose-dependent manner as the challenge cell level decreased and was significantly shortened by CY exposure.

Table 2 summarizes further validation studies and demonstrates the effects of graded doses of CY susceptibility to a TD_{10} of mKSA-TU5 tumor cells. This dose curve was constructed to define the minimal dose of CY which significantly altered host resistance to tumor cell challenge. A single exposure between 14 and 180 mg/kg of CY significantly en-hanced ($p < 0.05$) the frequency of tumors (50-80%) which occurred following a challenge dose of 5×10^2 (TD_{10}) mKSA tumor cells. The mean latency to tumor development was likewise significantly shortened in CY treated mice even at the 14 mg/kg dose.

Table 2. **Effects of Graded Doses of Cyclophosphamide on Host Resistance to A Low Challenge Level of mKSA Tumor Cells.**

DOSE OF CYCLOPHOSPHAMIDE (MG/KG) ON DAY-2	NUMBER OF MICE DEVELOPING TUMORS / NUMBER OF MICE INOCULATED [1]	% TUMOR TAKES	MEAN LATENCY (DAYS)
0	2/20	10%	17
180	8/10 *	80%	13 †
108	6/10 *	60%	13 †
39	6/10 *	60%	11 †
14	5/10 *	50%	9 †
5	3/10	30%	14
1.8	1/10	10%	16

[1] Mice were challenged subcutaneously with 5×10^2 mKSA tumor cells.
*Significantly different from tumor frequency in control mice at $p < 0.05$ by Chi-square analysis with Yates correction.
† Significantly different from controls at $p < 0.05$ by Student's t-test.

Increased Susceptibility of PYB6 Tumor Cells Following DES Exposure

The next phase of study examined the application of tumor susceptibility models of host resistance following exposure to a chemical of environmental concern. Figure 4 demonstrates the tumor frequency in $B_6C_3F_1$ mice challenged with a TD_{10} of syngeneic PYB6 tumor cells following a subchronic low-level exposure to DES at 0.2, 2.0 and 8.0 mg/kg of body weight administered daily in corn oil for 5 days. There was a significantly greater ($p < 0.05$) frequency of tumor takes (80-90%) in mice which received 8.0 and 2.0 mg/kg of DES and tumor challenge when compared to mice dosed with corn oil alone (10%). Animals receiving the low DES had a trend for more tumors which was not significant. The mean latency in days to tumor detection was unaltered in DES exposed mice as was the mean tumor volume indicating that residual DES did not have a stimulatory effect on tumor cell growth.

Validation of [125]IUDR Assay for Quantitating Lung Tumor Mass

Table 3 demonstrates a pairwise comparison of the [125]IUDR and Wexler assays for estimating Madison 109 tumor foci and mass on days 4-14

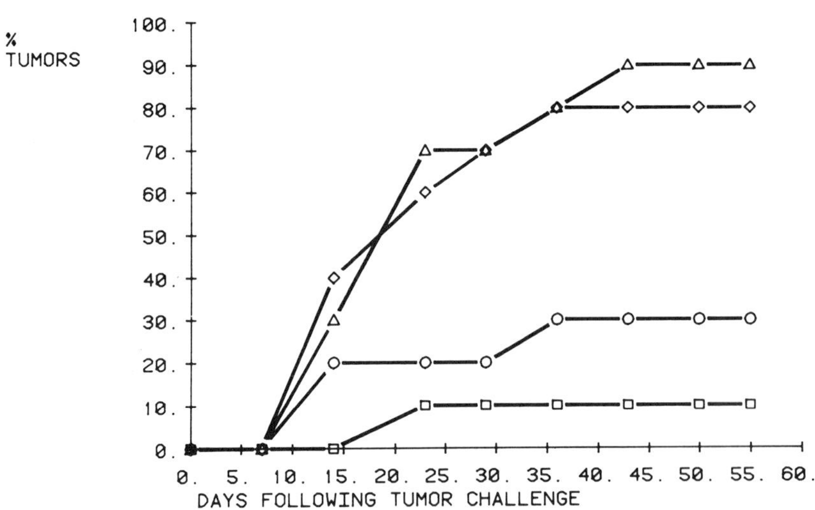

Fig. 4. Demonstrates the effect of DES exposure on the tumor frequency in B[6]C[3]F[1] mice challenged with TD_{10} (5×10^3) of PYB6 cells on day 3 following DES treatment. Animals were palpated twice weekly for 60 days and tumor measurements were recorded. Three groups exposed to DES (8 mg/kg, △; 2 mg/kg, □; and 0.2 mg/kg, ●) as well as a corn oil control (O) were examined.

Table 3. Comparison of Wexler and ^{125}IUDR Incorporation Assays for Estimating Lung Tumor Mass.

DAYS FOLLOWING IV CHALLENGE WITH MADISON-109 [1]	MEAN NUMBER OF VISIBLE TUMOR FOCI/MOUSE [1]	MEAN CPM ($\pm$SEM) OF ^{125}IUDR		% CHANGE
		CONTROL LUNGS	TUMOR LUNGS	
4	0	2,256 ($\pm$112)	4,525* ($\pm$280)	100%
8	19	2,238 ($\pm$138)	7,437** ($\pm$385)	232%
10	56	2,008 ($\pm$98)	12,952** ($\pm$812)	544%
14	56	3,132 ($\pm$180)	36,832** ($\pm$2,208)	1,075%

[1] BALB/c mice were challenged with 5×10^3 Madison-109 tumor cells intravenously on day 0. Foci number and CPM of ^{125}IUDR incorporation represent mean of six animals per group, with separate groups for Wexler and ^{125}IUDR assays. Values of ^{125}IUDR incorporation were significantly different from mean CPM of control nontumored mice at $p < 0.05$ (*) and $P < 0.01$ (**).

following an iv challenge with 5×10^3 tumor cells. With the Wexler assay the foci were too small to quantitate on day 4 and gave similar values on days 10 and 14, even though the tumor foci were rapidly proliferating between these two assay points. Significant ^{125}IUDR incorporation ($p < 0.05$) between tumored and control mice was observed within 4 days following challenge and increased logarithmically through day 14. Thus, the ^{125}IUDR assay appears more sensitive and quantitative for estimating the amount of lung tumor following an iv challenge than does the Wexler procedure.

Table 4 summarizes validation studies in BALB/c mice challenged with 1×10^4 Madison 109 lung tumor cells 2 days following a single injection of graded doses of cyclophosphamide. Mice exposed to CY at 65 and 23 mg/kg had a significantly greater ($p < 0.05$) incorporation of ^{125}IUDR when compared to untreated control mice challenged with tumors. Data from two separate experiments (Table 4) are presented and demonstrate that systemic CY exposure enhanced the development and growth of Madison 109 lung tumor cells.

Increased Mortality Following Lewis Lung Tumor Challenge in DES Exposed Mice

Table 5 summarizes a mortality study in $B_6C_3F_1$ mice exposed to DES and then challenged iv with 5×10^3 Lewis lung tumor cells. These

Table 4. Effects of CY on Tumor Cell Foci and Tumor Mass Following IV Challenge with Madison-109 Tumor Cells.

| | DOSE OF CYCLOPHOSPHAMIDE (MG/KG) ON DAY-2 | MEAN CPM OF [125]IUDR (+SEM)[1] | | % CHANGE |
		CONTROL	TUMOR	
Experiment I	0	3,311 (±383)	4,055 (±724)	22%↑
	8	3,104 (±174)	3,679 (±1,016)	18%↑
	23	3,112 (±270)	7,942 * (±528)	155%↑
	65	3,047 (±214)	7,728 * (±621)	154%↑
Experiment II	0	3,263 (±883)	3,908 (±546)	20%↑
	8	3,908 (±546)	4,634 (±593)	19%↑
	23	2,814 (±111)	4,820 * (±708)	71%↑
	65	3,290 (±398)	6,119 * (±808)	86%↑

[1] BALB/c mice (six/group) were challenged intravenously with Madison-109 (1×10^4) on day 0 and sacrificed on day 8.
* Significantly different from controls at $p < 0.05$ by Student's t-test.

Table 5. Effects of DES Treatment on Mortality Following Challenge with Lewis Lung Tumor Cells.

DES CONCENTRATION (MG/KG)	NUMBER DEAD / NUMBER CHALLENGED	% MORTALITY	MEAN LATENCY TO DEATH (DAYS)
0	0/9	0	—
0.2	0/9 *	0	—
2.0	6/9 *	67%	14
8.0	7/9 *	78%	14

$B_6C_3F_1$ mice were dosed with DES in corn oil daily × 5 and challenged intravenously with 5×10^3 Lewis lung cells 3 days following the last dose. Mice were observed daily for 21 days. Significance was determined by Chi square analysis using Yates correction at $p < 0.05(*)$.

animals died with a mean latency of 14 days. Mortality was significantly enhanced in the groups which got the medium (67%) and high (78%) DES dose at day 21. Thus, DES exposure followed by challenge with 5,000 Lewis lung tumor cells resulted in decreased latency to death and increased mortality. [125]IUDR studies are in progress.

Alteration of Other Host Resistance Parameters
Following DES Exposure

Table 6 summarizes challenge studies with *Listeria monocytogenes,* gram negative bacteria endotoxin and the nematode *Trichinella spiralis* in mice following DES exposure. Mice from all DES exposure groups demonstrated a significantly reduced ($p < 0.01$) resistance to *Listeria* (i.e. 100% mortality) to a challenge dose of organisms that killed only 20% of the corn-oil treated control group. The mean latency in days to death was likewise reduced in the DES exposure group with an average latency of from 4.8-5.4 days as compared to 8.0 days in the control group.

DES exposed animals were also significantly ($p < 0.01$) more sensitive to gram negative endotoxin than were normal mice (Table 6) although a dose-response pattern was not observed since the high DES dose demonstrated less endotoxin mortality than did the middle or low dose.

When mice are infected with *T. spiralis* larvae, the animals develop immunity which rids the infected host of the adult parasite through expulsion from the gut in about 14 days. The presence of an increased number of adult parasites in the gut at day 14 indicates impaired host resistance and was observed following DES exposure (Table 6). DES treated mice had a significantly greater number of adult worms ($p < 0.05$) in their gut at 14 days than did non-exposed mice.

Table 7 summarizes studies of lymphocyte mitogen responses and host resistance parameters following pre/postnatal exposure to the environmental chemical TCDD. The PHA responses, but not LPS response, was significantly impaired ($p < 0.05$) at the 5 mg/kg dose of TCDD, but not the 1 mg/kg dose. In addition, mortality following *Listeria* challenge was increased at both the 1 mg/kg level (40%) and became significantly different from the control at the 5 mg/kg level (73%). Likewise, susceptibility to a small challenge dose of PYB6 tumor cells was enhanced at both TCDD dosages. The correlation should be noted between suppressed T-cell responses to PHA and increased susceptibility to both bacteria and tumor cell challenge.

Table 6. Effects of DES Exposure on Other Host Resistance Parameters.

| DES MG/KG | LISTERIA MONOCYTOGENES | | | ENDOTOXIN SENSITIVITY | | TRICHINELLA EXPULSION |
| | MORTALITY [1] | | MEAN LATENCY TO DEATH | MORTALITY [2] | | NO. ADULT WORMS [3] |
	NO. CHALLENGED	(%)	(DAYS)	NO. CHALLENGED	(%)	AT DAY 14 $\pm$ SEM
0	2/10	(20%)	8.0	0/10		5.5 $\pm$ 1.9
0.2	10/10**	(100%)	5.4	6/9**	(67%)	43.0 $\pm$ 13.8*
2.0	10/10**	(100%)	5.4	9/10**	(90%)	ND
8.0	8/8*	(100%)	4.8	4/9	(44%)	104 $\pm$ 12.6**

[1] Mortality to *L. monocytogenes* scored for 14 days following an IV injection of 1.1×10^5 viable bacteria/mouse.
[2] Mortality within 48 hours following challenge with 600 μg/ mouse of *Escherichia coli* lipopolysaccharide.
[3] Adult worm counts $\pm$ SEM in mouse intestine (7 mice/group) at day 14 following infection. Significantly different from control group at $p < 0.05$ (*) and $p < 0.01$ (**) by Chi-square analysis or Student's t-test.
ND Not done.

Table 7. Correlation of Lymphoproliferative Responses and Susceptibility to *Listeria Monocytogenes* and PYB6 Tumor Cells in TCDD Pre/Postnatal Exposed Mice.

DOSE OF TCDD (μG/KG)	CPM $\times$ 10^{-3} ^{3}H-TdR (% CHANGE)		L. MONOCYTOGENES MORTALITY/NO. CHALLENGED (%)	PYB6 TUMORS NO. TUMORS/NO. INOCULATED (%)
	PHA	LPS		
0	31	3.8	7/25 (28%)	4/18 (22%)
1.0	36 (14%↑)	4.3 (21%↑)	6/15 (20%)	6/10 (60%)†
5.0	15 (52%↓)*	3.1 (18%↓)	11/15 (73%)†	4/9 (44%)

* p $<$ 0.05 vs control by Student's T-test.
† p $<$ 0.05 vs control by Chi-square analysis.

DISCUSSION

Tumor susceptibility studies reported here have demonstrated that BALB/c or $B_6C_3F_1$ mice with normal unimpaired host resistance can resist a challenge dose of 500-5,000 syngeneic tumor cells mKSA-TU5 or PYB6 with a frequency of 80-90% (i.e., TD_{10-20}). The mechanism by which the unimmunized host resists this rather large challenge dose of viable tumor cells is thought to involve an immune mechanism probably requiring immunocompetent T-cell macrophages (MØ). This aspect of host resistance has been termed "immune surveillance" by Burnet (1970) Following exposure of these mice to a non-lethal dose of the known immunosuppressive agent cyclophosphamide, host resistance was severely impaired resulting in a high frequency of tumor takes in CY treated mice. The immune alterations induced by CY appear to also affect the number of Madison-109 lung tumor cells which grow into tumor foci in the lungs following an iv challenge of lung tumor cells, as measured by incorporation of ^{125}IUDR into rapidly proliferating tumor cells. These studies validate the sensitivity and reproducibility of the tumor susceptibility assay described by Dean (1979). Furthermore, the assay can be successfully applied for detecting immune dysfunction and altered host resistance following exposure to known immunosuppressive drugs and environmental chemicals suspect of altering host resistance The sensitivity of the assay is exemplified by the fact that even small doses of CY (14 mg/kg) which produce marginal immunological alterations when assayed by *in vitro* CMI assays produced a significant increase in the frequency of tumors following a TD_{10} challenge dose of mKSA tumor cells. High dose CY exposure, because of its selective cytoreductive action on rapidly proliferating cells, produces a spectrum of immune dysfunction resulting from a depletion of lymphocytes (Stockman et al., 1973), functional impairment of remaining lymphoid cells (Dean et al., 1979), and activation or elimination of suppressor or regulatory cells (Turk et al., 1972; Spears et al., 1979) depending on when the antigen was administered relative to the dose of CY. This assay has the advantage of not requiring the additional observation time needed for spontaneous tumor development (28 weeks) such as in the Shimkin assay procedure used to screen for chemicals with potential as carcinogens or immunosuppressants (Shimkin and Grady, 1940).

To validate our assays, DES, a chemical of immense environmental concern, was studied because of its widespread distribution (McLachlan and Dixon, 1977) and its association with cancer in humans (Herbst et al., 1971). DES was found to significantly promote tumor development when $B_6C_3F_1$ mice were exposed to multiple, but therapeutically relevant levels of DES (8-0.2 μg/kg) prior to challenge with PYB6 or Lewis lung tumor cells. This was an unexpected observation since DES is a recognized and potent stimulant of the reticuloendothelial system, reportedly producing increased Kuppfer cell activity (Kelly, 1962) and either increased (Steven and Snook, 1975) or decreased (Slijivic and Warr, 1973) phagocytic activity in splenic macrophages. The enhanced tumor susceptibility observed following adult DES exposure using 2 different tumor models, may result from either a T-dependent lymphocyte dysfunction or impaired MØ cytolytic activity reported in a companion paper (Luster et al., 1980).

A previous report from this laboratory (Luster et al., 1979) indicated that prenatal exposure on day 16 of gestation to DES resulted in abnormal thymus development in both male and female mice and altered CMI and humoral immune parameters in adult life. Similar observations were found by Kalland (1980a, 1980b) who found that neonatal exposure on days 1-5 after birth to 5.0 μg doses of DES resulted in a persistent depression of Con A and LPS induced blastogenic responses. In an earlier paper by this group (Kalland et al., 1978) similar neonatal exposures to DES resulted in a pronounced degeneration of thymus cortex with reduced mitotic rates and depressed peripheral mononuclear cell counts. Severely altered thymus cortex development (Greeman et al., 1972) and concomitant depressed bone marrow progenitor cells have been consistent findings in this laboratory even following adult exposure to DES (Boorman et al., 1980). Similar adult exposure (Luster et al., 1980) resulted in severely impaired lymphoproliferative responses to mitogens and alloantigens in one-way mixed leukocyte cultures, depressed delayed cutaneous hypersensitivity to recall antigens, depressed antibody PFC to T-cell dependent and independent antigens and altered MØ function characterized by increased phagoctosis proliferation and tumor cell cytostasis.

The alteration in susceptibility to challenge with an LD_{10} of *Listeria monocytogenes* was striking following DES exposure. This may be related to an impaired ability of the MØ's to affect intracellular killing or bacterial replication. Alternatively, increased susceptibility may result from the T-cell dysfunction by preventing development of T-cell immunity to assist the MØ's in controlling the intracellular replication of the bacterium (Mackness, 1969). The altered tumor and bacterial susceptibility were inconsistent with previously observed increased macrophage phagocytic and tumor cell cytostatic activity (Luster et al., 1980; Boorman et al., 1980). Studies on the ability of MØ's from DES exposed mice to demonstrate tumor cell cytolytic and bactericidal activity *in vitro* are currently in progress and should provide data to support or refute the hypothesis that DES activated MØ's have impaired cytolytic and bactericidal potential, even though other parameters of MØ function are activated including increased phagocytosis and proliferation, which may or may not be protective to the host. Conversely, the activation of suppressor adherent cells may interfere with the establishment of primary immunity to *Listeria.*

The increased sensitivity to gram negative bacterial endotoxin observed following DES exposure further substantiates impairment of MØ function as being central to the problem of increased bacterial susceptibility since endotoxin is prinicpally detoxified by the hepatic MØ's (Braude et al., 1955). Increased susceptibility to endotoxin has been observed following administration of known RES activants such as glucan (Crafton and DiLuzio, 1969), yeast (Benaceraff et al., 1959) and intravenous BCG (Suter, 1958) and after exposure to some chemicals of environmental concern which alter immune function (Vos, 1977). Thus, the increased endotoxin sensitivity observed in this study following DES exposure is consistent with what is known about other agents which alter endotoxin sensitivity and increase macrophage activity.

A recent observation by Seaman and associates (1979) of loss of natural killer cell (NK) activity following a 6 week exposure to 17 β-estradiol might also be considered as a possible explanation for the increased tumor cell susceptibility we observed *in vitro* following exposure to a more potent synthetic estrogen such as DES. Kalland and associates (1980b) have recently observed that neonatal DES exposure has a persistant depressive effect on NK activity. Since NK was not directly examined in the present study, we can only speculate that NK activity would also be impaired following adult exposures to DES. Although the role of NK activity in immune surveillance against tumor cells *in vivo* is only postulated (Herberman and Holden, 1978), it is interesting to speculate that the increased susceptibility to the transplantation of a limited number of syngeneic tumor cells might result from a dysfunction of NK surveillance mechanisms. Alternatively, the impairment of T-lymphocyte function, reported by this laboratory in DES treated mice (Luster et al., 1979), might in itself account for this defect in tumor resistance since proliferative and alloantigen recognition responses are impaired *in vitro*. This would indicate impaired ability of the host to expand the memory cell population against these antigenically foreign tumor cells. A slight defect in T-cell recognition may also be compounded by the moderate to weakly antigenic nature of both these tumor lines.

It is clearly established, that *in utero* DES exposure results in hyperplastic changes in genital tract tissues of mice (McLachlan & Dixon, 1976) and a high frequency of vaginal clear cell (Herbst, 1971) and squamous cell cancers (Cutler et al., 1972) in humans. A role of the immunologic alterations reported accompanying DES exposure in mice (Luster et al., 1979, 1980; Kalland et al., 1978, 1980; Kalland, 1980a, b) in increasing the carcinogenic potential of DES in laboratory animals as well as humans is suggested although documentation of altered immune function in humans following DES exposure awaits study.

T-lymphocyte dysfunction could also be invoked to explain impaired expulsion of *Trichinella spiralis* following DES exposure. The expulsion of adult worms from the intestinal tract of mice has previously been shown to require immunocompetent T-lymphocyte as determined by sensitivity to treatment with antilymphocyte sera (Ruitenberg, 1974) and impairment in nude mice (Ruitenberg, 1976). The reduced expulsion of adult worms observed in the present study is consistent with the impaired T-lymphocyte function observed in DES exposed mice (Luster et al., companion paper).

Mice treated pre- and postnatally with TCDD were also studied to further validate our host resistance assays and to correlate these data with depressed lymphoproliferative responses to PHA, but not LPS. Pre/ postnatal exposure to TCDD reduced host resistance to challenge with PYB6 tumor cells and *Listeria*. TCDD exposure has previously been shown to cause severe thymus atrophy characterized by depletion of lymphocytes from cortical areas and depression of cell-mediated immunity in mice (Vos and Moore, 1974; Thomas and Hinsdill, 1979; Luster et al., 1980). TCDD exposure has also been shown to depress host resistance in mice to *Salmonella bern* infections (Thigpen et al., 1975). The observations reported here extend these earlier studies and include increased susceptibility in pre/postnatally TCDD exposed mice to syngeneic transplantable tumor cells and gram postive intracellular bacteria (i.e., *Listeria monocytogenes*). The accompanying depressed lymphoproliferative response to T-cell mitogens observed following TCDD exposure (Luster et al., in press) as well as DES (Luster et al., 1980, Dean et al., 1979) are believed to be central to the reduced host resistance observed. Host susceptibility parameters appear to provide sensitive and meaningful endpoints for further studies in animals exposed to chemicals and drugs with suspect immunological effects. Extrapolation of significance to humans, occupationally or inadvertently exposed to environmental chemicals, awaits further documentation.

SUMMARY

Mice were exposed to the non-lethal doses of the known immunosuppressive drug cyclophosphamide to refine and substantiate the validity of tumor and bacterial susceptibility assays as endpoints for altered host resistance and immune dysfunction. These assays were shown to be reproducible, sensitive and relevant endpoints for assessing changes in host resistance. Studies to apply host resistance assays to examine chemicals of environmental concern such as DES and TCDD, previously shown to alter immune function, further validated the sensitivity of these endpoints and assay systems for detecting altered host resistance accompanying documented immune dysfunctions. Correlations were found between depressed lymphoproliferative responses to T-cell mitogens and reduced host resistance parameters that awaits further definition.

REFERENCES

Allen, J. C. Infection Complicating Neoplastic Disease and Cytotoxic Therapy. *In: Infection and the Compromised Host.* J. C. Allen (Ed.), Williams and Williams Co., Baltimore, MD, 151-171 (1976).

Bash, J. A., Singer, A. M., and Waksman, B. H. Suppressive effect of Immunization on the proliferative response of rat T-cell *in vitro*. II. Abrogation of antigen-induced suppression by selective cytotoxic agents. J. Immunology, *116*:1350-1353 (1976).

Bekesi, J. G., Holland, J. F., Anderson, H. A., Fischbein, A. S., Rom, W., Wolff, M. S., and Selikoff, I. J. Lymphocyte function of Michigan dairy farmers exposed to poly-brominated biphenyls. Science, *199*:1207 (1978).

Benacerraf, B.. Thorbecke, G. J., and Jacoby, D. Effect of zymoran on endotoxin toxicity in mice. Proc. Soc Exp. Biol. Med., *100*:796-799 (1955).

Boorman, G. A., Luster, M. I., Dean, J. H., and Wilson, R. E. The effect of adult exposure to diethylstilbestrol in the mouse. Alteration in macrophage function and number (in preparation).

Braude, A. I., Carey. F. J.. and Zalesky, M. Studies with radioactive endotoxin. J. Clin. Invest., *34*:858-866 (1955).

Brook. N., and Hohorst. H. J. Metabolism of cyclophosphamide. Cancer, *20*:900-904 (1967).

Burnet. F. M. The concept of immunological surveillance. Prog. Exp. Tumor Res.. *13*:1-27 (1970).

Crafton, C. G., and DiLuzio, N. R. Relationship of reticuloendothelial functional activity of endotoxin lethality. Am. J. Physiol. *217*:736-742 (1969).

Cutler, B. S., Forbes, A. P., Ingersoll, F. M., and Scully, R. E. Endometrial carcinoma after stilbestrol therapy in gonodal dysgenesis. N. Eng. J. Med., *287*:628-631 (1972).

Dean, J. H., Padarathsingh, M. L., and Jerrells, T. R. Application of immuno-competence assays for defining immunosuppression. Ann. New York Acad. Sci., *320*:579-590 (1979a).

Dean, J. H., Padarathsingh, M. L., Jerrells, T. R., Keys, L., and Northing, J. W. Assessment of immunobiological effects induced by chemicals, drugs or food additives. II. Studies with cyclophosphamide. Drug Chem. Tox., *2*(1 × 2):133-153 (1979b).

Fairchild, G.A., Roan, J., and McCarroll, J. Atmospheric pollutants and the pathogenesis of viral respiratory infection. Arch. Environ. Health,*25*:174-182 (1972).

Faith, R. E., and Moore, J. A. Impairment of thymus-dependent immune function by exposure of the developing immune system and 2,3,7,8-TCDD. J. Toxicol. Environ. Health., *3*:451 (1977).

Friend, M., and Trainer, D. O. Polychlorinated biphenyl: Interaction with duck hepatitis virus. Science, *170*:1314 (1970).

Gainer, J. J., and Pry, T. W. Effect of arsenicals on viral infections in mice. Am. J. Vet. Res., *33*:2299-2307 (1972).

Goodman, L. S., and Gilman, A. 1975. The Pharmacological Basis of Therapeutics. MacMillan Publishing Co., New York, 1262-1487 (1975).

Greenman, D. L., Dooley, K., and Breeden, C. R. Strain differences in the response of the mouse to diethylstilbestrol. J. Toxicol. Environ. Health., *3*:589 (1977).

Hemphill, F. E., Kaeberle, M. L., and Buck, W. B. Lead suppression of mouse resistance to *Salmonella typhimurium*. Science, *172*:1031-1032 (1971).

Herberman, R. B., and Holden, H. T. Natural cell-mediated immunity. Adv. Cancer Res., *27*:305-377 (1978).

Herbst, A. L., Ulfelderand, H., and Poskanzer, D. C. Adenocarcinoma of the vagina; association of maternal stilbestrol therapy with tumor appearance in young women. *N*. Eng. J. Med., *284*:878-881 (1971).

Kalland, T. Alterations of antibody response in female mice after neonatal exposure to DES. *J*. Immunol. (1980a, in press).

Kalland, T. Reduced natural killer activity in female mice after neonatal exposure to DES. J. Immunol. (1980b, in press).

Kalland T., and Forsberg, J. G. Delayed hypersensitivity response to oxazolone in neonatally estrogenized mice. Cancer Letters, *4*:141-146 (1978).

Kalland, T., Forsberg, T. M., Forsberg, J. G. Effects of estrogen and corticosterone on the lymphoid system in neonatal mice. Exp. Mol. Path., *28*:76-95 (1978).

Kalland, T., Strand, O., and Forsberg, J. Long term effects of neonatal estrogen treatment on mitogen responsiveness of mouse spleen lymphocytes. J. Natl. Cancer Inst. (1980, in press).

Kelly, L. S., Brown, B. A., and Dobson, E. L. Cell division and phagocytic activity in liver reticuloendothelial cells. Proc. Soc. Exp. Biol. Med., *110*:555–563 (1962).

Koller, L. D. Some immunological effects of lead, cadmium and methyl mercury. Drug Chem. Tox. 2:99-110 (1979).

Law, L. W., and Ting, I. C. Immunologic competence and induction of neoplasms by polyoma virus. Proc. Soc. Exp. Biol. Med., *119*:823-830 (1965).

Loose, L. D., Silksworth, J. B., Pittman, K. A., Benitz, K. F., and Mueller, W. Impaired host resistance to endotoxin and malaria in polychlorinated biphenyl and hexachlorobenzene-treated mice. Infect. Immunity, *20*:30-35 (1978).

Luster, M. I., Boorman, G. A., Dean, J. H., Harris, M. W., Luebke, R. W., Thigpen, J. E., Padarathsingh, M. L., and Moore, J. A. Examination of bone marrow immunological and host susceptibility parameters following pre- and postnatal exposure to TCDD. *Int*. J. Immunopharm. (1980, in press).

Luster, M. I., Dean, J. H., and Moore, J. A. Methods in Immunotoxicology. *In: Methods In Toxicology*. A. W. Hayes (Ed.). Raven Press, New York (1979, in press).

Luster, M. I., Faith, R. E., McLachlan, J. A., and Clark, G. C. Effects of *in utero* exposure to diethylstilbestrol on the immune response in mice. Toxicol. Appl. Pharmacol.,*47*:279-285 (1979).

MacKaness, G. B. The influence of immunologically committed lymphoid cells on macrophage activity *in vivo*. J. Exp. Med., *129*:973-992 (1969).

Mansour, A., and Nelson, D. S. Effect of cyclophosphamide treatment on the response of rat peripheral blood lymphocytes to phytohemagglutinin. Cell. Immunol., *30*:272 (1977).

Milton, J. D., Carpenter, C. B., and Addison, I. E. Depressed T-cell reactivity and suppressor activity of lymphoid cells from cyclophosphamide treated mice. Cellular Immunol., *24*:308-317 (1976).

McMartin, K. E., Kennedy, K. A., Greenspan, P., Alam, S. N., Greener P., and Yam, J. Diethylstilbestrol: A review of its toxicity and use as a growth promotant in food-producing animals. J. Environ. Path. and Toxicol., *1*:297 (1978).

Penn, I. Development of cancer in transplant patients. Adv. in Surgery, *12*:155-191 (1978).

Seaman, W. E., Gindhart, T. D., Greenspan, J. S., Blackman, M. A., and Talal, N. Natural killer cells, bone, and the bone marrow: Studies in estrogen-treated mice and in congenitally osteopetrotic (mi/mi) mice. J. Immunol. *112*:2541-2547 (1979).

Shimkin, M. B., and Grady, H. G. Carcinogenic potency of stilbestrol and estrone in strain C³H mice. J. Natl. Cancer Inst., *1*:119-128 (1940).

Sljivic, V. S., and Warr, G. W. Activity of the reticuloendothelial system and the anitbody response. II. Effect of stilbestrol on the immune response to sheep erythrocytes in the mouse. Br. J. Exp. Path., *54*:69 (1973).

Speirs, R. S., Benson, R. W., Knowles, B. J., and Roberts, D. Models for assessing the effect of toxicants on immunocompetence in mice. II. Effects of cyclophosphamide on the antibody responses to Type III pneumococcal polysaccharide and tetanus toxoid in BALB/c female mice. J. Environ. Path. Tox.,*1*:791-812 (1979).

Steven, W. M., and Snook, T. The stimulatory effects of diethylstilbestrol and reticuloendothelial cells of the rat spleen, Am. J. Anat., *144*:339-360 (1975).

Stockman, G. D., Hein, L. R., South, M. A., and Trentin, J. T. Differential effects of cyclophosphamide on the B and T cell compartment of adult mice. J. Immunol., *110*:227 (1973).

Suter, C., Ulman, E. G., and Hoffman, R. G. Sensitivity of mice to endotoxin after vaccination with *Bacillus calmette-guerin*. Proc. Soc. Biol. Med., *99*:167 (1958).

Thiss, J. C., Shimkin, M. B., and Poirier, L. A. Interaction of pulmonary adenomas in strain of mice by substituted organohalides. Cancer Res., *39*:391-395 (1979).

Thigpen, J. E., Faith, R. E., McConnell, E. E., and Moore, J. A. Increased susceptibility to bacterial infection as a sequela of exposure to 2,3,7,8-tetrachlorodibenzo-p-dioxin. Infection and Immunity.,*12*:1319-1324 (1975).

Thomas, P. T., and Hinsdill, R. D. The effect of prenatal exposure to tetrachlorodibenzo-p-dioxin on the immune response of young mice. Drug Chem. Tox., *2*:77-97 (1979).

Turk, J. L., and Poulter, L. W. Selective depletion of lymphoid tissue by cyclophosphamide. Clin. Exp. Immunol., *10*:296 (1972).

Vos, J. G. Immune suppression as related to toxicology. CRC Critical Reviews in Toxicology., *5*:67-101 (1977).

Vos, J. G., and Moore, J. A. Suppression of cellular immunity in rats and mice by maternal treatment with 2,3,7,8-tetrachlorodibenzo-p-dioxin. Inter. Arch. Allergy Appl. Immun., *47*:777-794 (1974).

Willers, J. M., and Sluis, E. The influence of cyclophosphamide on antibody formation in the mouse. Ann. Immunol. Paris., *126*:267-279 (1977).

DISCUSSION

HADDEN: I congratulate you on looking at resistance models as a way to interpret the significance of drugs which may be toxic to the immune system. I would like to add some nuances, however, to the interpretation of your model system.

Where it's evident in animals infected with Listeria monocytogenes that T-cell–related responses are critical to the handling of disease, in survival models it would appear that issues, perhaps independent of T-cells and related to natural kill, may be involved. Natural kill and related resistance mechanisms may be the primary determinant very early as to whether an animal develops disease. In an attempt to interpret these models, rather than frequency of disease, longevity with disease may be the more critical function that relates to T cells. For both these issues, selection of the strain of mouse is critical to whether they develop disease and how they handle it.

The use of the nude mouse with, of course, its well known T-cell defects or the beige mouse with its NK cell defect, may allow one to test systems to determine to what extent T cells or natural killer cells may be involved in the resistance that's being examined.

Concerning the reproducibility of the Listeria system, if you passage Listeria in mice, using not an LD-10 but a lower dose, you will maintain high virulence, and may be able to make a more reproducible system.

DEAN: I agree and think that possibly we should be looking at mice immunized against Listeria. The animals might first be immunized with a low dose of Listeria, next exposed to chemicals, and then challenged with a higher dose of Listeria. Dr. Hadden, would you think this might provide a more sensitive model?

HADDEN: I've not used it, but certainly within the context of conventional dogma, resistance to facultative intracellular pathogens would be a test of T-cell and macrophage function, i.e., classic cell-mediated immunity.

DEAN: Some of our more recent findings suggest the Listeria model may be much more complex than once thought. There appear to be alternative non-T pathways operative following the primary challenge of Listeria. Would you agree with that, Dr. Hadden?

HADDEN: Yes, I would agree with that. Experiments with nude mice infected with Listeria have been published which show evidence of resistance to challenge. Again, dose of challenge is critical in determining that.

Nude mice don't accept low doses of tumors, but one can override their natural resistance by increasing the dosage of tumors, and then one indeed confronts the T-cell defect.

DEAN: Yes, I am aware of these studies. There's another point that should be brought up. Most people are probably aware of Dr. Stuttman's very fine paper examining the tumor induction with MCA in DBA nude mice. DBA nude mice have the same frequency of MCA-induced tumors as does the parental animal. He invokes non-alternative, T pathways to provide this resistance.

MUNSON: There could be another alternative explanation to your results with the Madison 109 and the Lewis lung carcinoma. First of all, the Madison 109 does have fairly strong tumor-associated antigens, while the Lewis lung is quite weak; yet your results look somewhat similar. Intravenous injections of tumor cells cause the cells to lodge almost completely in the lung during the first pass. If DES alters electrolyte balance, increases edema, or anything that would alter pulmonary capillary flow, it might enhance the number of cells that lodge in the lung. This could result in what you are seeing and have nothing to do with the immunity.

On the 125 IuDR assay, we haven't had much luck. Your data look very good. One thing I think we have to keep in mind in using this assay in the future is the following. If the chemical—particularly when administered by inhalation—causes any inflammatory response in the lung, which it usually will, the background level and variation may be such that it's going to be difficult to interpret your data. This is what we have found with agents that alter pulmonary functions. The Wexler technique provides backup. This is of particular importance when we start to look at long-term exposures. When one has committed oneself to a minimum of a three-month study and all assay systems must go at that particular time, one can end up with a log data that is difficult, if not impossible, to interpret.

This carries over to the Listeria model. We have been working with this for a number of years and have found that it requires commitment of a large number of animals so that an LD-10 dose can be calculated. One can do everything to predict an LD-10 dose but, when it comes right down to it, one may come up with nothing. This becomes an even greater problem in thinking about chronic exposure.

DEAN: Let me agree with some of your comments. I, too, think we need better bacterial models. Since, with Listeria, it is difficult to reproducibly get an LD-10. I think the bottom line for immune dysfunction following chemical exposure is alteration of host resistance. To my surprise, most of these models have been used for some time and are really not very well worked out. In reference to Lewis lung (125 IuDR), I'm convinced, from repeated experiments, that systemic immune suppression does alter host resistance in the lung. I do not think inflammatory or traffic problems are a concern in this study since administration of the chemical preceded the 125 IuDR by approximately two weeks. Your concerns are valid precautions.

FISH: I would like to comment on and support your use of measuring the animal's resistance to challenge as the final test in all model systems for studying effects on the immune system. In the course of our studies on immunoprevention of transplantable tumors in the rat, we had to correct our protection results for the "tumor dormant state." Therefore, I appreciate the fact that you were held up with your I^{125} and had to go to a lethal assay.

What we find in challenging rats is that the control animals will come down with essentially 100 percent tumors in our system within 14 days. We used to run the assay to an endpoint of 28 days and then record animals with tumors or without as protected or not. In the course of following the animals for longer periods of time, we found that we really had to go 45 days before all the animals that were going to come down with tumor actually came down with tumor. We then followed them for a year to make sure that this was true. The major point of this is that, if one is only going to record tumor takes at some point in time and compare this to control values as a measure of protection, one may get a much different answer by waiting a longer time. Anyone who is going to do this assay should really consider following the animals through an extended period of time to avoid prejudicing the data by failing to account for the tumor dormant state which translates to a non-protected animal.

BICE: I was very curious about your inhalation exposures.

DEAN: We haven't started inhalation exposure yet.

BICE: Well, I thought you indicated on one side that inhalation was the exposure route. So you haven't actually done that yet?

DEAN: No. In validation of the lung tumor model, we started with systemic treatment. We have only developed the lung model for exposure.

KERMAN: Dr. Dean, in reporting your mitogen studies, did you titrate the mitogens?

DEAN: Yes, the mitogens were titrated; three levels of mitogen were used in all tests.

KERMAN: So this was a reflection of the titration.

DEAN: That's correct.

GHAFFER: Just a comment on your observations on resistance to bacteria. When we are choosing a model we have to be careful about the bacteria because our interpretation, whether it is a T-cell or B-cell macrophage, may be clouded by the fact that certain bacteria activate alternate pathways of complement; this recruits a whole new system. Once again, we must be careful in interpreting our results.

DEAN: I agree with you. However, if we wait until the model is fully defined and worry about all the possible nuances, we might never do host-resistant assays. I think that's why these types of studies haven't been done. That is to say we don't totally understand the immunologic mechanism responsible for host resistance.

17
Influence of Xenobiotics on Host Defense

Leland D. Loose,
W. Müller, F. Blumenstock, and T. Charbonneau

Institute of Comparative and Human Toxicology,
Albany Medical College, Albany, New York

INTRODUCTION

Accidental exposure incidences and laboratory studies have demonstrated an influence of environmental chemical contaminants on immune responses including host defense to microbial pathogens. These studies have been quite diverse using organohalides, organophosphates, carbamates and heavy metals as representative xenobiotics. The extensive laboratory studies which have been conducted subsequent to the environmental or industrial exposure incidences have examined a wide range of humoral and cellular immune responses and, in some instances, host responses to microbes. In general, the test chemicals have been shown to be immnuosuppressive but adequate dose-response studies have not been conducted nor have environmentally relevant levels been used (Vos, 1977). However, the converse may also occur in single exposure paradigms, that is, an immunostimulation may result if the timing of the antigen exposure relative to the chemical exposure incident is appropriate.

Although most studies have examined the influence of the chemical on the host, the influence of the host macrophage-lymphoid elements on the chemical via altered pharmacokinetics and metabolism must be considered. Since the fixed tissue macrophages contain aryl hydrocarbon hydroxylase (AHH) the metabolic status of the macrophage, i.e., resting versus activated, may be an important consideration in xenobiotic metabolism (Authrup et al., 1978). In addition, the very nature of the xenobiotic may render it immunogenic which, if an autoimmune response to the xenobiotic (hapten): tissue macromolecule complex is elicited, could result in an immunopathologic manifestation which may be incorrectly attributed to direct chemical toxicity.

Previous studies have demonstrated that Aroclor 1242, polychlorinated biphenyl (PCB) and hexachlorobenzene (HCB) induce a significant humoral immunosuppression in the presence of high chemical levels but in the absence of histopathologic changes (Loose et al., 1977). Further studies revealed a significant increase in endotoxin sensitivity and susceptibility to a malaria infection (Loose et al., 1978) in mice receiving a dietary administration of PCB_{1242} or HCB. Cell-mediated immune parameters were not remarkably altered (Silkworth and Loose, 1979).

Since macrophage function is an integral component of the immune parameters previously evaluated, subsequent experiments have been conducted to determine their ability to respond to a chemotactic agent and their spontaneous spreading activity. In addition, to extend our studies on host defense the susceptibility to an ascites-type tumor (mKSA) was evaluated. An essential part of all of these parameters are membrane-mediated events and for this reason serum fibronectin, a cell surface-binding glycoprotein, was quantitated.

MATERIALS AND METHODS

Animals

Male Balb/c mice 18–20 g were used throughout the experiments. They received powdered Wayne lab diet (with or without test chemicals) and water *ad libitum* and were on a 12:12 day:night photo period.

Chemicals

Polychlorinated biphenyl (PCB) Aroclor 1242 (Monsanto) and hexachlorobenzene (HCB) (Eastman Chemical Co.) were mixed in the diet at a concentration of 5 and 100 ppm. Dieldrin (Shell) was mixed in the diet at a concentration of 1 and 5 ppm. Control animals received the normal diet without chemicals.

Cell Isolation

Elicited peritoneal macrophages (PM) were obtained from the peritoneal cavity by saline lavage 4 days after i.p. injection of 1 ml of 6% Na+ caseinate in 0.9% sterile saline. Polymorphonuclear neutrophils (PMNs) were obtained in the same fashion but elicitation was 18 hr prior to cell harvest. Cells were washed 2X in M199 (1X, Gibco) without phenol red. Cell counts and viability (as determined by trypan blue dye exclusion) were measured and cell suspensions adjusted to the desired concentration.

Chemotaxis and Spontaneous Migration

The method for measuring PNM chemotaxis was that reported by Nelson et al., (1975). Briefly, 1.2% agarose [in M199 with 10% fetal calf serum (FCS)] plates were made 24 hours prior to the test and stored inverted at 4°C. Wells were cut into the plates using a template and a small bore cutter (2.4 mm) Removal of the agarose plug was accomplished with a capillary tube and light suction. Then 10 μl of control media (M199 with 10% FCS) was added to the inner most wells. These wells served to measure spontaneous migration. To the wells were added 10 μl of chemoattractant (zymosan treated FCS), which was used to measure chemotaxis. In the middle wells was added 10 μl of PMNs suspended in M199 with 10% FCS at a concentration of 2.5×10^7 cells/ml. Each test sample was run in triplicate and the average of the 3 readings constituted one data point. The plates were incubated at 37°C in a 5% CO_2 humidified atmosphere for 2 hours. Plates were examined using the 4X objective of a Nomarsky interference contrast microscope (Zeiss) fitted with an ocular micrometer for measuring the distance of cell migration. Modifications for measuring PM chemotaxis were described by Dohlman and Goetzl (1978). Gelatin was added to the agarose plates so that the final concentration of gelatin was 0.25% in 2% agarose. This eliminated the necessity of adding FCS to the cell suspensions. Also, PM chemotaxis was best quantified after a 3-hour incubation.

    Measurements and Calculations:
A. Chemotaxis = Cell migration from the middle well towards the chemoattractant well (outermost).
B. Spontaneous Migration = Cell migration from middle well toward the control well (innermost).
C. Chemotactic Differential = Chemotaxis − spontaneous migration. (A − B = Chemotactic differential).

Spontaneous Cell Spreading

The method for quantitating cell spreading was an adapation of the method of Fauve and Dekaris (1971). The test cell suspension, whether PM or PMN, was adjusted to a concentration of 2.0×10^6 cells/ml in M199 with 2% bovine serum albumin (BSA) and 5 μ heparin/ml. This

1.0 ml cell suspension was gassed with 5% CO_2 and then tightly closed in plastic culture tubes and incubated in a 37°C waterbath for 30 min. The cell suspension was agitated and an aliquot was placed in one chamber of a hemacytometer slide. The slides were placed into petri dishes which were used as moisture chambers and incubated at 37°C in a 5% CO_2 humidified atmosphere for 30 min. Slides were then examined under the 16X objective of a phase-contrast microscope.

Measurements and Calculations: The number of cells in 1 mm^3 were counted, noting the number that were spread, not spread and dead. Cell types such as erythrocytes which appear discoid in shape and lymphocytes which are either large or small with a homogenous cytoplasm were disregarded.

Total Cell = Number of spread, not spread and dead, phagocytes in 1 mm^3.

$$\text{Spread Cells/ml} = \text{Number of spread cells/mm}^3 \times 10^4.$$

$$\%\ \text{Spread Cells} = \frac{\text{Number of spread cells/mm}^3}{\text{Total Cells}} \times 100.$$

$$\%\ \text{Spread Cells/animals} = \frac{\text{Spread cells/ml}}{\text{Cells harvested/animal}}$$

Tumor Susceptibility Study

SV40-transformed mouse kidney (mKSA) cells were obtained from Dr. J. Dean, Litton Bionetics, Kensington, Maryland and were used as the tumor challenge cells. They were maintained by serial passage *in vivo* in male Balb/c mice; 1.0×10^7 tumor cells/ml were injected i.p. and 7 days later cells were harvested by peritoneal lavage with 5 ml of 0.9% saline. Cells were suspended in saline at a concentration of 1.0×10^7/ml and a 0.5 ml i.p. injection was given to each control or test animal. Daily checks were made and the cumulative percent dead for each day was noted. The Litchfield (1949) test was used for an analysis of time *vs* effect and linear regression analysis was used to compute the mean survival time.

Quantitation of Immunoreactive Fibronectin (Opsonic α_2SB Glycoprotein)

Electroimmunoassay or "rocket" immunoelectrophoresis was used to quantitate plasma fibronectin or opsonic protein levels as previously described (Blumenstock et al., 1977; Saba et al., 1978). Experimental serum was assayed for immunoreactive fibronectin. Blood samples obtained from the abdominal vena cava were allowed to clot for 60 min at 29°C prior to centrifugation to obtain serum. It is recognized that the serum concentration of circulating fibronectin (Opsonic glycoprotein) is consistently less than that of plasma due to the incorporation or covalent binding of plasma fibronectin to fibrin in the presence of Factor XIII (Mosher, 1976). This difference is minimal if the blood is allowed to clot at room temperature prior to collection of serum (Mosesson, 1977). All samples for analysis were carefully handled under such constant conditions so that serum could be the test media used for the immuno-assay as previously standardized (Blumenstock et al., 1977). The serum was diluted to 10% and 10 μl was added to each well cut into the solidified agarose-antiserum solution layer on the glass plate (5 $\times$ 10 inch) used in the electroimmunoassay. The samples were then moved electrophoretically toward the anode at a voltage of 7.5 V/cm at 4°C for 22 hr using an LKB multiphore system. The plates were washed overnight, pressed and dried, and subsequently stained (Blumenstock et al., 1977). Rocket heights were used as a quantitative index of immunoreactive opsonic α_2SB glycoprotein concentration. Rocket heights were recorded in millimeter and a double reciprocal standard plot (1/mm vs 1/μg opsonic or 1/mm vs 1% serum) was defined with a DEC-10 computer using protein standards at varying concentrations. This standard curve was used to determine serum immunoreactive opsonic α_2SB glycoprotein in μg/ml (Saba et al., 1978).

RESULTS

The yield of elevated PMNs and peritoneal macrophages from the PCB_{1242}, HCB or dieldrin treated mice was essentially unchanged following either 3, 6 or 18 weeks dietary administration of the chemicals (Table 1 and 2). However, a significant increase in spontaneous cell spreading of PMNs, but not macrophages, was demonstrated at the 18-week test interval (Tables 1 and 2). In contrast to the increased spontaneous cell spreading there was a significant decrease in spontaneous migration of PMNs and macrophages at 18 weeks which did not appear to be dose-related. Concomitant alterations in the chemotactic differential were not observed (Tables 3 and 4), suggesting that the response to a chemotactic agent was not changed.

A modulator of cell surface activity, i.e., fibronectin, a surface binding glycoprotein, was measured and was found to be significantly decreased, primarily at the 18-week test period (Table 5). In general, an approximate 40% reduction, below control values, was observed in the fibronectin

Table 1.   Spontaneous Spreading of Elicited Peritoneal Macrophages from Mice Fed PCB$_{1242}$, HCB or Dieldrin.[1]

TREATMENT	CELL YIELD $\times 10^6$			% SPREAD CELLS			TOTAL SPREAD CELLS/ANIMAL		
	3 WK	6 WK	18 WK	3 WK	6 WK	18 WK	3 WK	6 WK	18 WK
Control	6 ± 0.6	9 ± 0.7	10 ± 1.6	51 ± 4.6	32 ± 11	38 ± 8.8	5 ± 0.3	5 ± 0.3	4 ± 1.3
PCB 5 ppm	6 ± 0.6	5 ± 1.0*	8 ± 0.8	53 ± 5.2	58 ± 2	33 ± 3.1	7 ± 1.3	15 ± 2.9*	5 ± 1.9
PCB 100 ppm	5 ± 0	7 ± 0.5	11 ± 1.8	57 ± 3.2	57 ± 8	30 ± 9.6	9 ± 1.9	7 ± 1.7	6 ± 4.1
HCB 5 ppm	6 ± 0.5	7 ± 0.9	9 ± 0.8	45 ± 2.5	61 ± 7	41 ± 4.2	5 ± 1.1	10 ± 2.1*	5 ± 2.3
HCB 100 ppm	6 ± 0.5	7 ± 0.6*	10 ± 2.5	59 ± 8.8	52 ± 7	28 ± 3.1	7 ± 1.4	14 ± 3.5*	6 ± 2.5
Dieldrin 1 ppm [2]	12 ± 1.3	9 ± 1.1	8 ± 0	45 ± 5.6	50 ± 1.9	54 ± 6.6	4 ± 0.6	9 ± 1.2	9 ± 2.3
Dieldrin 5 ppm	5 ± 0	9 ± 1.6	11 ± 1.0	66 ± 2.5*	68 ± 6 *	33 ± 4.1	9 ± 1.7*	7 ± 4.6	5 ± 2.1

[1] PCB$_{1242}$, HCB or dieldrin were administered in the diet for 3, 6 or 18 weeks at the stated levels. All data are presented as the mean ± standard error with an asterisk (*) denoting significance at p $<$ .05; n = 4–5 for all data points. Peritoneal macrophages were harvested by saline lavage 4 days after an i.p. injection of 6 ml of 6% Na+ caseinate. Controls received saline.
[2] Dieldrin (1 ppm) group was run independently and significance is based on its own control group.

Table 2. Spontaneous Spreading of Elicited Polymorphonuclear Leukocytes (PMNs) from Mice Fed PCB$_{1242}$, HCB or Dieldrin.[1]

TREATMENT	CELL YIELD $\times 10^6$			% SPREAD CELLS			TOTAL SPREAD CELLS/ANIMAL		
	3 WK	6 WK	18 WK	3 WK	6 WK	18 WK	3 WK	6 WK	18 WK
Control	10 ± 1.4	8 ± 2.4	11 ± 3.0	74 ± 3.0	67 ± 6.0	47 ± 11.9	13 ± 3.1	14 ± 2.8	4 ± 1.2
PCB 5 ppm	12 ± 2.1	9 ± 0.6	14 ± 1.5	71 ± 2.8	63 ± 2.1	76 ± 1.8*	20 ± 8.3	26 ± 7.3	5 ± 1.2
PCB 100 ppm	8 ± 0.8	10 ± 0.5	15 ± 1.6	67 ± 2.7	68 ± 3.0	76 ± 3.3*	20 ± 3.1	18 ± 2.5	12 ± 2.3*
HCB 5 ppm	12 ± 2.6	13 ± 1.8	15 ± 1.6	69 ± 2.6	67 ± 4.3	60 ± 13.9	19 ± 5.6	19 ± 4.9	11 ± 2.8
HCB 100 ppm	9 ± 1.6	10 ± 0	22 ± 5.2	72 ± 3.5	72 ± 5.7	76 ± 2.9*	23 ± 7.0	23 ± 4.3	5 ± 0.8
Dieldrin 1 ppm [2]	16 ± 2.2*	19 ± 3.5	17 ± 1.3	61 ± 3.7	76 ± 2.7	77 ± 2.3*	16 ± 2.3	5 ± 1.2	6 ± 0.4
Dieldrin 5 ppm	12 ± 2.2	9 ± 0.6	17 ± 3.0	67 ± 1.1	65 ± 3.4	74 ± 2.9*	21 ± 7.1	19 ± 3.0	9 ± 1.1*

[1] PCB$_{1242}$, HCB or dieldrin were administered in the diet for 3, 6 or 18 weeks at the stated levels. All data are presented as the mean ± standard error with an asterisk (*) denoting significance at p <.05; n = 4–5 for each data point. Peritoneal PMNs were harvested by saline lavage 18 hours after an i.p. injection of 6 ml of 6% Na+ caseinate. Controls received saline.
[2] Dieldrin (1 ppm) group was run independently and significance is based on its own control group.

Table 3. Chemotaxis and Spontaneous Migration of Elicited Peritoneal Macrophages from Mice Fed PCB$_{1242}$, HCB or Dieldrin.[1]

TREATMENT	CHEMOTAXIS			SPONTANEOUS MIGRATION			CHEMOTACTIC DIFFERENTIAL		
	3 WK	6 WK	18 WK	3 WK	6 WK	18 WK	3 WK	6 WK	18 WK
Control	81 ± 5	55 ± 11	71 ± 5.8	7 ± 1.9	8 ± 3.0	20 ± 1.7	74 ± 4.5	47 ± 11	51 ± 7.2
PCB 5 ppm	82 ± 5	55 ± 7	76 ± 2.4	6 ± 1.2	8 ± 2.3	12 ± 1.5*	77 ± 4.4	48 ± 8	64 ± 3.9
PCB 100 ppm	84 ± 4	61 ± 10	76 ± 1.5	5 ± 1.7	8 ± 1.8	20 ± 7.9	78 ± 4.6	53 ± 9	57 ± 6.7
HCB 5 ppm	83 ± 3.6	62 ± 7	81 ± 5.3	8 ± 1.4	8 ± 1.1	15 ± 4.9	75 ± 4.9	54 ± 8	67 ± 3.8
HCB 100 ppm	70 ± 6.8	62 ± 9	74 ± 6.8	8 ± 1.8	11 ± 2.0	10 ± 3.2*	63 ± 5.9	52 ± 9	64 ± 9.2
Dieldrin 1 ppm [2]	39 ± 2.9	38 ± 4.3	18 ± 1.9	2.3 ± 0.8	7 ± 0.9	5 ± 0	36 ± 3.1	31 ± 4.2	13 ± 1.9
Dieldrin 5 ppm	74 ± 6.7	63 ± 4	83 ± 11.6	5 ± 0.6	11 ± 1.6	21 ± 1.5	70 ± 7.3	52 ± 4	62 ± 12.4

[1] PCB$_{1242}$, HCB or dieldrin were administered in the diet for 3, 6 or 18 weeks at the stated levels. All data are presented as the mean ± standard error with an asterisk (*) denoting significance at p < .05; n = 4–5 for all data points. Peritoneal macrophages were harvested by saline lavage 4 days after an i.p. injection of 6 ml of 6% Na+ caseinate. Controls received saline.
[2] Dieldrin (1 ppm) group was run independently and significance is based on its own control group.

Table 4. Chemotaxis and Spontaneous Migration of Elicited Polymorphonuclear Leukocytes (PMNs) from Mice Fed PCB_{1242}, HCB or Dieldrin.[1]

TREATMENT	CHEMOTAXIS			SPONTANEOUS MIGRATION			CHEMOTACTIC DIFFERENTIAL		
	3 WK	6 WK	18 WK	3 WK	6 WK	18 WK	3 WK	6 WK	18 WK
Control	63 ± 17	61 ± 8	54 ± 7.9	7 ± 2.2	5 ± 0.8	19 ± 4.8	54 ± 16.6	56 ± 8	29 ± 2.2
PCB 5 ppm	73 ± 12	71 ± 11	45 ± 6.8	17 ± 8.2	5 ± 1.2	9 ± 1.8	56 ± 10.8	66 ± 10	28 ± 2.8
PCB 100 ppm	84 ± 14	71 ± 10	53 ± 10.3	12 ± 4.9	6 ± 1.7	7 ± 1.0*	73 ± 11.1	65 ± 8	36 ± 4.2
HCB 5 ppm	65 ± 6	60 ± 11	42 ± 2.9	8 ± 1.9	5 ± 1.3	7 ± 0.8*	57 ± 4.0	55 ± 10	38 ± 4.6
HCB 100 ppm	69 ± 6	71 ± 11	47 ± 3.1	5 ± 1.3	5 ± 0.4	19 ± 3.3	64 ± 5.3	66 ± 11	27 ± 4.7
Dieldrin 1 ppm [2]	61 ± 8.4	27 ± 2.6	53 ± 3.2	6 ± 1.1	5 ± 1.0	6 ± 0.3*	55 ± 7.9	22 ± 1.7	46 ± 3.2
Dieldrin 5 ppm	77 ± 9	73 ± 13	48 ± 3.5	4.2± 1.2	9 ± 4.1	25 ± 5.3	73 ± 8.5	64 ± 11	35 ± 11.6

[1] PCB_{1242}, HCB or dieldrin were administered in the diet for 3, 6 or 18 weeks at the stated levels. All data are presented as the mean ± standard error with an asterisk (*) denoting significance at $p < .05$; $n = 4$–5 for each data point. Peritoneal PMNs were harvested by saline lavage 18 hours after an i.p. injection of 6 ml of 6% Na+ caseinate. Controls received saline.
[2] Dieldrin (1 ppm) group was run independently and significance is based on its own control group.

Table 5.   Serum Fibronectin Concentrations in Mice Fed PCB$_{1242}$, HCB or Dieldrin [1]

	FIBRONECTIN CONCENTRATION (% OF CONTROL)		
	3 WK	6 WK	18 WK
PCB 5 ppm	139	83	40*
PCB 100 ppm	99	78*	45*
HCB 5 ppm	115	72	74
HCB 100 ppm	92	70*	52*
Dieldrin 1 ppm [2]	42*	131	86
Dieldrin 5 ppm	107	100	51*

[1] Presented as % of control mean with an asterisk (*) denoting significance at p $<$ 0.05; n $=$ 7–10 for each group.
[2] Dieldrin (1 ppm) study was conducted independently and significance is based on its own control group.

levels in the chemical-treated mice following 18 weeks of dietary administration of the chemicals. Coincident with the decrease in serum fibronectin was a significant increase in the susceptibility of the chemical-treated mice to a challenge of mKSA ascites tumor cells (Table 6). This increase was most marked at the 18-week test period.

Table 6.   Mean Survival Time in Mice Fed PCB$_{1242}$, HCB or Dieldrin and Challenged with mKSA Tumor Cells.[1]

	MEAN SURVIVAL TIME (DAYS)		
	3 WK	6 WK	18 WK
Control	19.8	17.0	21.3
PCB 5 ppm	19.2	19.2	20.0
PCB 100 ppm	17.6	16.1	16.0*
HCB 5 ppm	19.8	18.8	18.5*
HCB 100 ppm	20.6	17.0	18.0*
Dieldrin 1 ppm [2]	24.0	19.4	14.3
Dieldrin 5 ppm	17.4	18.2	17.2*

[1] Ascites tumor cells mKSA-Tu5 (1.0×10^7/ml) were injected intraperitoneally in 0.5 ml sterile isotonic saline. The percent cumulative mortality was recorded and the mean survival time was determined. Asterisk (*) denotes significance at p $<$ 0.05; n $=$ 7–10 for each group.
[2] Dieldrin (1 ppm) study was conducted independently and significance is based on its own control group.

DISCUSSION

The conceptual framework as to the possible interactions of environmental chemical contaminants with the immune system is depicted in Figure 1. The majority of studies cited in the immunotoxicology literature have dealt primarily with the immunosuppressive activity of the xenobiotics; however, this may be a dose phenomenon and a possible immune stimulation may occur if a dose *vs* time of immunization study would be conducted, such results would be more applicable to acute rather than chronic exposures incidences.

The immunohemolytic anemia induced by dieldrin (Hamilton et al., 1978) further emphasizes the need for concern regarding the haptenic/antigenic nature of the xenobiotics. In this regard, such a host response to the xenobiotic may result in a classical autoimmune event which could induce a pathologic condition which may be incorrectly attributed to a direct chemical toxicity.

In the present study, an extension of previously reported decreases in host responses to malaria and endotoxin (Loose et al., 1978) revealed a significant depression in mean survival time of mice which received a dietary administration of PCB (100 ppm), HCB (5 and 100 ppm) or dieldrin (5 ppm) for 18 weeks and were then challenged with 1×10^7 mKSA tumor cells. No significant alterations in survival time following tumor challenge were noted following 3 or 6 weeks administration of the chemicals or at 18 weeks in mice receiving 5 ppm of PCB or 1 ppm of dieldrin (Table 6).

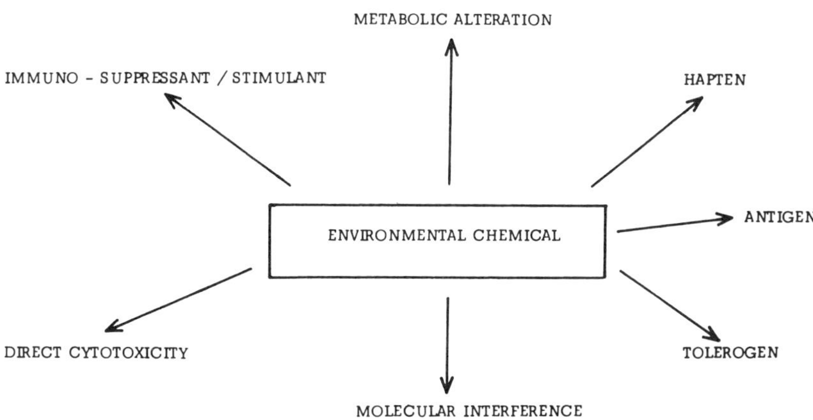

Figure 1. Possible modes of action of environmental chemical contaminants and their relation to immune processes.

Since Synderman et al. (1974) previously reported a deficit in monocyte chemotactic activity in cancer patients, the macrophages and PMN chemotactic activity were evaluated. Although no alteration in either PMN or marophage chemotactic differential were noted at 18 weeks, at a time when the sensitivity to tumor challenge was the greatest, a decrease in the spontaneous migration was observed. The decrease in PMN migration was most marked in the high dose PCB (100 ppm) and low dose HCB (5 ppm) and low dose dieldrin (1 ppm). No dieldrin-induced macrophage migration was observed, however, low dose PCB (5 ppm) and high dose HCB (100 ppm) significantly reduced the spontaneous migration (Tables III and IV).

Concurrent with the decreased spontaneous migration of PMNs at 18 weeks was a significant increase in their spontaneous spreading (Table II). Similar results were not observed with the elicited peritoneal macrophages (Table 1). Although Matossian-Rogers (1979) related cell spreading to cell activation and since Dekaris et al. (1969) suggested that cell spreading inhibition is a correlate of delayed hypersensitivity the present results suggest that this may be correlated with a specific cell population. Of considerable interest is the almost inverse relationship between the increased sensitivity to the tumor challenge and the decreased serum fibronectin levels (Table 5).

Any statement as to the cause and significance of the decreased levels of plasma fibronectin found in this study can only be speculative. Several possibilities could be suggested such as the fact that dieldrin and PCB mediated depression of RNA synthesis could lead ultimately to enhanced uptake of the protein from the blood by the RES phagocytic cells. The most probable explanation for the decreased levels of plasma fibronectin in these studies may be that since blood levels of lysosomal proteases increase there is enhanced degradation of the plasma fibronectin which has been shown to be exquisitely sensitive to any sort of proteolytic digestion. Whatever the cause, however, the fact that decreased plasma fibronectin is associated with depressed host defense mechanisms helps explain some observations concerning the increased susceptibility of PCB and HCB treated animals to infection and tumor growth.

CONCLUSION

Modulation of the immune response by xenobiotics is of increasing concern. Using two common environmental chemical contaminants, polychlorinated biphenyl (PCB) (Aroclor 1242) and hexachlorobenzene (HCB), we previously demonstrated a profound humoral immunosuppression with a concurrent endotoxin hypersensitivity and impaired host resistance to a test pathogen, i.e., *Plasmodium berghei* (NYU-2). Graft-vs-host reactivity, mitogen-induced lymphocyte blastogenesis and mixed lymphocyte culture activity were not as severely compromised. Further studies have been conducted to determine host resistance to a tumor (mKSA) cell injection and to quantitate discrete macrophage functions, e.g., spontaneous cell spreading and response to a chemoattractant (zymosan activated serum). Since these are classical membrane mediated events a concurrent measurement of the serum levels of the surface binding glycoprotein, fibronectin, was made· These studies demonstrated a time and dose related sensitivity to the ascites tumor mKSA in PCB, HCB and dieldrin treated mice. An inverse relationship between serum fibronectin and spontaneous cell (phagocyte) spreading was observed, i.e., as fibronectin levels decreased cell spreading increased. Changes in chemotactic activity were not remarkable.

ACKNOWLEDGMENTS

Supported, in part, by a joint program between the Gesellschaft f. Strahlen- und Umweltforschung mbH, Munich, Germany, and the Institute of Comparative and Human Toxicology, Albany Medical College, Albany, New York 12208.

REFERENCES

Authrup, H., Harris, C. C., Stoner, G. D., Selkirk, J. K., Schafer, P. W. and Trump, B. F.: Metabolism of[³H] benzo[a] pyrene by cultured human bronchus and cultured human pulmonary alveolar macrophages. Lab. Invest., *38(3)*:217-224 (1978).

Blumenstock, F. A., Weber, P., Saba, T. M. and Laffin, R.: Electroimmunoassay of alpha-2-opsonic protein during reticuloendothelial blockade. Am. J. Physiol., *232*:80-87 (1977).

Dean, J. H., Lewis, D. D., Padarathsingh, M. L., McCoy, J. L., Northing, J. W., Natori, T. and Law, L. W.: Cellular immunity to SV-40-induced tumor cells and solubilized tumor-associated antigens in immune mice using an isotopic footpad assay. Int. J. Cancer, *20*:951-959 (1977).

Dekaris, D., Fauve, R. M. and Raynaud, M.: Delayed hypersensitivity and inhibition of macrophage spreading: *In vivo* and *in vitro* studies of tuberculin and streptococcal hypersensitivities in guinea pigs. J. Immunol., *103*:1-5 (1969).

Dohlman, J. G. and Goetzl, J.: Unique determinants of alveolar macrophage spontaneous and chemokinetically stimulated migration. Cell. Immunol., *39*:36-46 (1978).

Fauve, R. M. and Dekaris, D.: An *in vitro* test for delayed hypersensitivity: Macrophage spreading inhibition (M. S. I.). *In Vitro Methods in Cell Mediated*

Immunity (B. R. Bloom and P. R. Glade, eds.), pp. 313, New York: Academic Press (1971).

Hamilton, H. E., Morgan, D. P. and Simmons, A.: A pesticide (Dieldrin)-induced immunohemolytic anemia. Environ. Res., *17*:155-164 (1978).

Litchfield, J. T., Jr.: A method for graphic solution of time-percent effect curves. J. Pharmacol. Exp. Ther., *49*:399-408 (1949).

Loose, L. D., Pittman, K. A., Benitz, K. F. and Silkworth, J. B.: Polychlorinated biphenyl and hexachlorobenzene induced humoral immunosuppression. J. Reticuloendothel. Soc., *22*:253-271 (1977).

Loose, L. D., Silkworth, J. B., Pittman, K. A., Benitz, K. F. and Mueller, W.: Impaired host resistance to endotoxin and malaria in polychlorinated biphenyl (PCB) and hexachlorobenzene (HCB) treated mice. Infect. Immun., *20*:30-35 (1978).

Matossian-Rogers, A.: Specificity of the macrophage spreading test with reference to *Leishmania* antigens and correlation with delayed hypersensitivity. Clin. Exp. Immunol., *36*:38-45 (1979).

Mosher, D. F.: Action of fibrin-stabilizing factor in cold-insoluble globulin and α_2 macroglobulin in clotting plasma. J. Biol. Chem., *251*:1639-1645 (1976).

Mosesson, M. W.: Cold-insoluble globulin (CIg): A circulating cell surface protein. Thrombosis and Hemostatis, *38*:742-750 (1977).

Nelson, R. D., Quie, P. G. and Simmons, R. L.: Chemotaxis under agarose: A new and simple method for measuring chemotaxis and spontaneous migration of human polymorphonuclear leukocytes and monocytes. J. Immunol., *115*:1650-1656 (1975).

Saba, T. M., Blumenstock, F. A., Scovill, W. A. and Bernard, H.: Cryoprecipitate reversal of opsonic α_2 surface binding glycoprotein deficiency in septic surgical and trauma patients. Science, *201*:622-624 (1978).

Silkworth, J. B. and Loose, L. D.: Environmental chemical-induced modification of cell mediated immune responses. Adv. Exp. Med. Biol. (in press) (1979).

Synderman, R., Dickson, J., Meadows, L. and Pike, M.: Deficient monocyte chemotactic responsiveness in humans with cancer. Clin. Res., *22*:430-437 (1974).

Vos, J. G.: Immune suppression as related to toxicology. CRC Critical Reviews in Toxicology, *5(1)*:67-101 (1977).

DISCUSSION

KERMAN: What happens to these parameters after the animals are off the diets? What happens to the animals? In many instances you show no change and, in those instances or in those parameters that changed, they were out 10 weeks, 16 weeks, and so forth. What happens if you stop that diet and then measure those parameters 1, 3, or 12 weeks out?

LOOSE: We have done that with the previously published endotoxin and malaria studies. We've studied them after they had been on diet for six weeks. We've taken them off diet for six weeks and challenged them again with endotoxin and malaria, and they recoup their deficits.

KERMAN: So what's the relevance to the fact that while on exposure there are some parameters of increased susceptibility. For instance, if a group of individuals are at risk and they move from Wisconsin to Houston, do they lose that risk? Is this a transient thing? What do you think the significance is?

LOOSE: Well, I would like to think that it's a transient event, and I think your question raises a good point. What component or phase of the immune system is most sensitive. I think what some people have begun to assess, primarily with TCCD, is developing phases of the neonatal immune systems versus an aging immune system. I think these are more critical.

To get back to your clinical relevance statement, I think if you take people out of the exposure environment and assess them away from that compound, if they turn over that body burden, they may recoup the deficit.

MOORE: With regard to your last statement, do you know that the body doesn't clear PCB? It might clear some isomers, but the half-life of 2,4,5-2,4,5 for example, is infinite and that's a major constituent of PCB.

LOOSE: Yes. I think there are pools, Dr. Moore, that you are talking about. As long as it stays in adipose tissue, I don't think you have anything to worry about. I think it's the circulating and/or the lymphoid pool that's deleterious. That's what you want to get out.

LaVIA: I would like to hear you comment at greater length concerning precisely the effect on developing immune systems versus aging immune systems. Has any work been done? Do you have any data on animals of varying ages, and how do they relate, for example, to the question you raised at the beginning of possible release of fat deposits upon dieting? Are these questions being addressed?

LOOSE: We haven't done aging studies but they are being planned. Have you, Dr. Moore? I think you have; do you want to address yourself to that?

MOORE: The only aging studies that we did were with TCCD and, along with other studies, these data suggest that the developing immune system seems to be at greater risk to immunotoxicity than does the adult immune system. However, if you follow these compromised neonates, impaired in their immunologic competence at birth or weaning, the effect is reversible. Only after 150 or 160 days (9 months) does the conversion back to normal occur.

SIGEL: Would you consider an experiment with your mice aimed at their losing weight in the expectation that they would become more vulnerable to the chemical which is stored in adipose tissue and thereby show greater suppression of immune response? I'm assuming that the reason they are not showing too much loss of competence is that the toxic agents are kept in adipose tissue. Have you compared the immunologic competence in normal and malnourished mice carrying the same burden of agent?

LOOSE: No, we have not. Good suggestion, though.

MOORE: Without looking at immune parameters with compounds like that, there has been work done with DDT. I think Wasserman, a number of years ago, as well as recent studies done with a different arachlor, showed that one builds a body burden during a four-to-six months' exposure. When taken off the diet and put on a calorie-deprived diet which forced mobilization of fat, the animals were more susceptible to toxicity. I know of no immune parameters that were assessed during these studies.

LOOSE: There were similar studies done with dieldrin, but not immunological studies.

NEWELL: I want to remind the previous discussants that you cannot necessarily assume those kinds of parameters are always going to be meaningful, that is, inducing stress by diet restriction but maintaining a high physical workload so that lipid reserves are called upon. You may remember studies done with prisoners who had very high levels of chlorinated hydrocarbons in their adipose tissues. They were put on a starvation regimen and made to work rockpiles: they showed no adverse effects whatsoever. So be cautious, rather than jump to conclusions.

LUSTER: There is one study that has been done by Glick with Mirex and Kepone which showed that there was no immunologic effect until he put them on a fasting diet.

McCOY: I just want to commend the previous speaker for the way he presented the overall picture. I think many of us get caught up in looking only for immune suppression. The fact that there may be no immediately observable effects does not mean that autoimmune phenomena may not occur later. He pointed this out very nicely.

18
Effects of Environmental Chemicals on Host Defense Responses of the Lung

Donald E. Gardner

*Inhalation Toxicology Branch, Health Effects Research Laboratory,
Environmental Protection Agency,
Research Triangle Park, N.C.*

INTRODUCTION

The growing complexity of atmospheric pollutants with the continuous influx of new chemicals makes it vitally important to develop reliable, sensitive, and inexpensive screening approaches that can aid toxicologists in making decisions concerning the relative potential health hazards resulting from exposure to these environmental chemicals. It is important to be able to detect how the host will respond to these chemicals assaults. Rarely can one expect the host response to environmental injury to be a simple one-to-one cause/effect relationship, but instead the organism will exhibit a wide diversity of responses. Although there are numerous methods presently available specifically designed to measure individually these diverse responses, the host must be capable of coping with the total injury, and it is the summation of these assaults that the toxicologists must seek to understand since these ultimately will determine the overall health of the individual.

The traditional toxicologist often measures biological responses by simply increasing the concentration of the test substance and by examining for specific physiological, biochemical or morphological effects. Although toxicological studies conducted at unrealistic concentrations may have some value to the individual researcher's goals, such grossly toxic levels often produce data in which much difficulty can be encountered in separating the overt toxic effect from more meaningful subtle effects. In addition, the potential exists for concentrations possibly resulting in false estimations of health consequences at ambient concentrations. The environmentalist should be more restricted in his investigations and must design and perform his studies using more realistic concentrations in order that his laboratory exposures more nearly mimic those exposures found in the urban environment. However, at these lower levels of exposure, numerous subtle trends may often be observed which are not, in themselves, statistically significant and are therefore often overlooked. These subtle effects may or may not be significant to the host. It is the responsibility of the investigator to make this decision. However, to fully understand such environmental insults depends upon the existence of the appropriate animal model. Such an animal model system should permit the occupational and environmental toxicologist to perform meaningful dose-response studies, at realistic concentrations which mimic those found in the ambient environment.

There is ample evidence in the literature that infectious diseases are rarely entirely attributed to a single entity, but are instead the result of a primary stress and one or more secondary factors that interfere with homeostasis and the ability of the host to cope with the primary etiologic assult. Any suppression in the host's body defenses by environmental chemicals would be expected to result in prolonged microbial viability and enhanced multiplication thus increasing the risk of the individual to infection. Utilizing this principle of multiple causality it becomes possible to measure subtle defects in an individual's total defenses by testing the host's capability and efficiency in defending itself against a laboratory induced infection that the unexposed animals could normally control. This model system would then reflect the summation of all of the various deleterious changes within the host which may include immunosuppression, cellular and acellular dysfunction, inflammation as well as various physiological alterations.

The studies to be described here are a brief review of our investigation utilizing this infectivity model system to assess the health effects of various gaseous and particulate environmental chemicals on the susceptibility to infections.

THE MODEL SYSTEM

A great amount of evidence exists in the literature that illustrates the relationship between an increased susceptibility to viral, fungal or bacterial infections and the suppression in various host's defenses. Measurement of the competency of the host's anti-microbial mechanisms can best be tested by challenging both the toxic-exposed and the clean air control animals to an aerosol of viable microorganisms. If the test substance had any adverse influences on the efficiency of any of the host's many protective mechanisms, i.e., mechanical clearance via the mucociliary escalator, biological clearance mediated through macrophages, and associated cellular and humoral immunological events, that would normally function in defending the host against this microbe, the organism, in its attempt to survive, would take advantage of these weaknesses. In these cases, one can easily measure, by the use of appropriate microbiological techniques, the actual increase in number of microorganisms in the host, and by following the pathogenesis of the disease, one can estimate the severity of the toxic effect. A detailed description of this infectivity model has been published elsewhere (Gardner et al., 1977a; Coffin and Gardner, 1972; Ehrlich, 1979).

Many problems, both technical and practical, beset the toxicologist who is trying to carefully develop and select an appropriate animal model for his research objectives. There are certain criteria that this animal model should meet if the data collected are to be relevant for regulatory purpose. These include that the model system sould be (1) valid across species; (2) allow for reproducible data; (3) sensitive for a wide range of gaseous and particulate pollutants as well as complex mixtures; (4) supported by mechanistic studies; and finally (5) it should be applicable for human studies.

To be effective in this model system the infectious agent must also fulfill certain criteria: (1) small variations in dose or virulence should not greatly influence mortality rate; (2) the organisms must be able to multiply within and infect susceptible tissue; (3) the natural mortality or rate of infection must be low in experimental animals not exposed to the pollutant; (4) a method must be available for quantifying the bacterial dose; and finally (5) if the route of infection is via inhalation, the microbes must be able to withstand the trauma of being aerosolized.

A wide range of infectious agents have been employed successfully by various investigators using various modifications of this model. These include *Streptococcus pyogenes, Escherichia coli, Diplococcus pneumoniae, Klebsiella pneumoniae, Salmonella typhimurium, Mycoplasma pneumoniae* and influenza virus. A variety of animal species has also been employed which includes the squirrel monkey, rat, hamster, guinea pig, and mouse (Henry et al., 1970; Fairchild et al., 1972; Ehrlich, 1975).

GASEOUS ENVIRONMENTAL CHEMICALS

In reviewing the available literature on the health effects of toxic chemicals, it becomes abundantly apparent that there is a significant lack of information concerning the pulmonary and extrapulmonary responses observed when test substances are introduced into body via the inhalation route, even though the lungs represent the largest exposed surface area, nearly 70 m^2, of the total body. In addition, after coming into contact with the various tissues of the respiratory tract, the chemicals or their reactive by-product, "ultimate toxicants," may then pass into the circulation, which transport them to other target sites throughout the body.

Inhalation of noxious gases, such as photochemical oxidants has been shown to adversely affect the host's defense system resulting in an enhancement in susceptibility to respiratory infection (Miller et al., 1978; Gardner and Graham, 1976). Mice which have been exposed for durations of 6 mins to one year to nitrogen dioxide (NO_2) concentrations ranging from $0.94 - 52.6$ mg/m^3 (0.5 to 28 ppm) showed at each concentration tested excess mortality for the pollutant exposed test group as compared to clean air controls, that received only the infectious agent. Table 1 lists the number of mice exposed to each concentration, the exposure duration in hrs. and the percent excess in mortality (NO_2 $-$ control).

The family of curves (Figure 1) that can be generated from these data shows how the toxic effect is related to the duration of a continuous exposure to NO_2 at different concentrations. The linear dose response data generated from this study indicated that mortality increases with time and also with increasing concentrations (Gardner et al., 1977b).

Ozone exposure either following or preceding exposure to the pathogenic bacteria also significantly enhances the mortality in mice. These effects were evident after only a 3 hr exposure to O_3 concentrations as low as 0.196 μg/m^3 (0.1 ppm) (Miller et al., 1978).

Not all gaseous pollutants affect the ability of the host to fend off infectious challenge at such low concentrations. A three hr exposure to the oxidant peroxy acetyl nitrate (PAN) produced a significant enhancement of respiratory pneumonia only after exposure to 14.8 to 28.4 mg/m^3 (Ehrlich, personal communication). Concentrations as high as 13.1 mg/m^3 (5.0 ppm) of SO_2 failed to have any effect on resistance to streptococcal pneumonia as measured by changes in mortality rates even after a 3 mo continuous exposure (Ehrlich, 1979).

**Table 1. Differences in Percent Mortality from Control for Mice
Exposed to Various NO_2 Concentrations for Various Durations
of Exposure and Then Challenged with An Aerosol
of an Infectious Agent.**

NO_2 CONCENTRATION (PPM)	EXPOSURE DURATION (HR)	TOTAL NO. ANIMALS		% MORTALITY (NO_2—CONTROL)
		CONTROL DEAD/TOTAL	EXPOSED DEAD/TOTAL	
0.5	168.0	187/280	189/280	0.8
	336.0	81/180	92/180	5.1
	720.0	49/120	55/120	5.0
	1440.0	34/50	78/100	10.0
	2160.0	72/180	127/210	19.9
	4320.0	51/110	84/120	23.7
	6480.0	52/90	63/90	12.3
	8760.0	19/30	26/30	23.4
1.5	2.0	45/90	51/90	6.7
	8.0	45/90	67/90	24.4
	18.0	4/20	9/20	25.0
	24.0	61/150	90/150	15.6
	96.0	31/120	44/120	10.8
	126.0	4/20	11/20	35.0
	168.0	17/80	37/80	25.0
	222.0	4/20	9/20	25.0
	336.0	18/80	43/80	31.3
	504.0	8/60	35/60	45.0
3.5	0.5	19/100	29/100	10.0
	1.0	37/200	53/200	8.0
	2.0	8/40	13/40	12.5
	3.0	37/200	75/200	19.0
	5.0	8/40	23/40	37.5
	7.0	56/280	152/280	34.3
	14.0	19/80	55/80	45.0
	24.0	29/140	98/140	49.3
	48.0	31/160	121/160	56.3
	96.0	2/20	17/20	75.0
	168.0	2/20	19/20	85.0
	384.0	2/20	15/20	65.0
7.0	0.5	27/120	52/120	20.8
	1.0	27/120	62/120	29.2
	1.5	27/120	61/120	28.3
	2.0	27/120	86/120	49.2
14.0	0.5	13/60	27/60	23.3
	1.0	13/60	36/60	28.3
	1.5	13/60	53/60	66.7
	2.0	13/60	52/60	65.0
28.0	0.1	18/97	60/100	41.6
	0.25	18/97	72/100	53.6
	0.42	18/97	79/100	60.6
	0.58	18/97	92/100	73.6

PARTICULATE ENVIRONMENTAL CHEMICALS

The infectivity model has also been utilized to examine the question of whether inhalation of three common trace metals (cadmium, nickel and manganese) can adversely affect host defenses, thereby increasing susceptibility to respiratory infections. These three metals were chosen since they are industrial and environmental pollutants that are associated with fine mode particulates which are preferentially deposited in the lungs (Lee and Von Lehmden, 1973; Natusch et al., 1974; Miller et al., 1979). In all of these studies, the duration of the exposure to the aerosol was 2 hrs.

There was a significant enhancement in percent mortality due to the 3 metals tested (Figure 2). The ranking of toxicity for these metals were: cadmium > nickle > manganese. There were apparently differences in the mechanisms of action of the metal. Cd and Mn caused an increase in mortality in animals challenged with bacteria immediately after the metal exposure. However, for Ni, mortality was only enhanced when the mice received the microbial aerosol 24 hrs. post-metal exposure. In addition to the dose-response curves shown in Figure 1 for $CdCl_2$, $NiCl_2$, Mn_3O_4 and $MnCl_2$, the sulfate forms of Ni and Cd were also tested to determine the importance of the anion in eliciting the biological response. The data indicate that the effects of $CdSO_4$ were similar to those for $CdCl_2$; how-

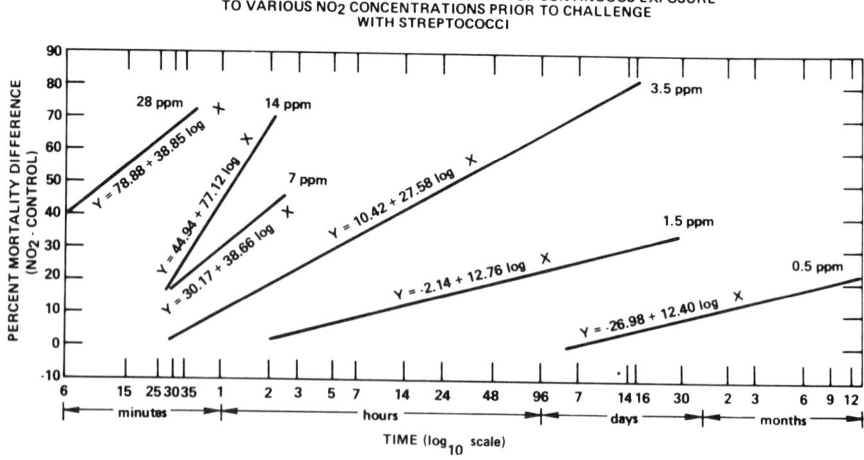

Figure 1.   Increased susceptibility to laboratory induced infections as a result of exposure to NO_2 for various lengths of time.

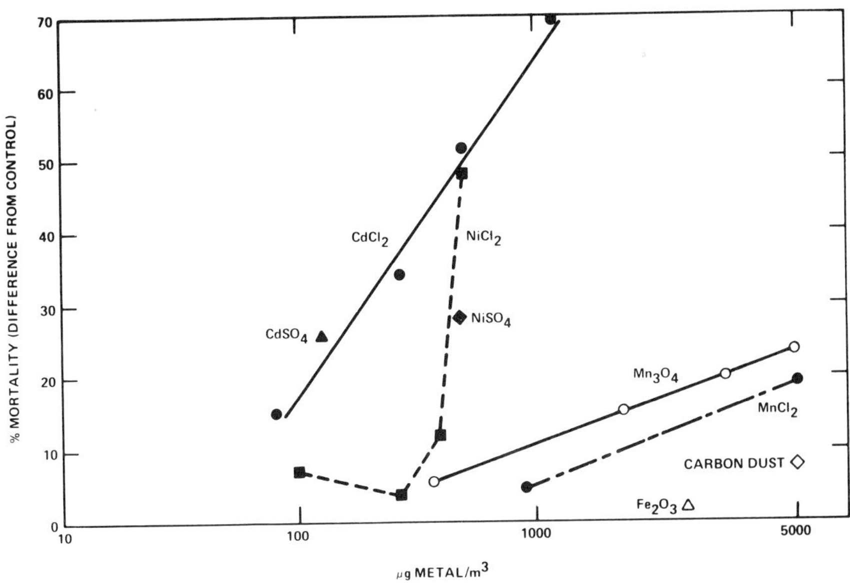

Figure 2.   Percent enhancement in mortality following a 2 hr aerosol exposure to the test substance. The mice exposed to Ni received the bacterial challenge 24 hr after the cessation of the metal exposure. For all other test substances, the bacterial exposure was immediately following the pollutant exposure.

ever, the chloride form of Ni appeared to be more damaging than the corresponding sulfate. To insure that this measured potentiation of respiratory infection can be directly attributed to the effect of the metal itself on the host's defense system rather than through some physical irritation or merely an over-burdening of the defense system with high concentrations of particulates, two other substances, carbon black (5.0 mg/m³) and iron oxide (2.5 mg/m³) were also tested. These particulates did not exhibit any significant effect when compared with the clean air controls.

If the host defense mechanisms are functioning normally, the control animals are capable of rapidly phagocytizing and killing the deposited streptococci; however, with the inhalation of the test chemicals, there is an inhibition of the lung clearance mechanisms, permitting those microbes with pathogenic potential to multiply and produce disease. Figure 3 shows these bacterial growth curves, determined by microbiological plate counts, in the lungs of mice receiving the metal exposure, the ozone exposure, and in the control mice. Similar defects in the bacteriocidal capability of the lung was also found with exposure to other gaseous

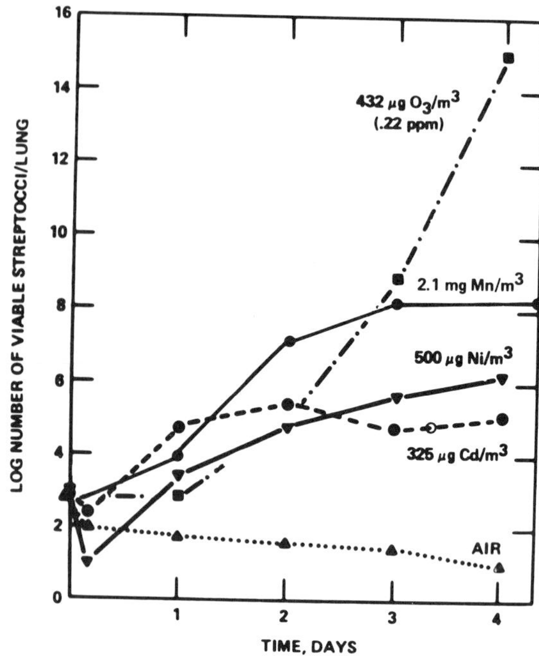

Figure 3.   Comparison of the growth of viable streptococci in the lungs of mice following a 2 hr exposure to the test metal and the control mice that received filtered air.

pollutants (Gardner, 1979). The animals exposed to the test chemicals were unable to cope with the deposited Streptococci. These studies also indicated that when the total number of microorganisms in the lung reaches a critical level of approximately 10^5, the bacteria invade the blood (Gardner et al., 1977). This development of septicemia parallels the mortality rates.

Changes in susceptibility to respiratory infections caused by a single 3 hr. exposure to a number of sulfate aerosols have also been reported (Ehrlich, 1979; Ehrlich, personal communication). The estimated concentration of the compounds which induced a 20% excess mortality (ED_{20}) was 0.2 mg/m³ cadmium sulfate, 0.6 mg/m³ copper sulfate, 1.45 mg/m³ zinc sulfate, 2.2 mg/m³ aluminum sulfate, 2.5 mg/m³ zinc ammonium sulfate and 3.6 mg/m³ magnesium sulfate. Exposure to ammonium sulfate (5.3 mg/m³ ammonium bisulfate (6.7 mg/m³), ammonium nitrate (4.5 mg/m³) and potassium nitrate (4.3 mg/m³) failed to have any effect on susceptibility to infection after a 3 hr. exposure.

Not all investigators used the pulmonary route for exposure to the test substance nor the infectious agents. Cook et al (1975) found that an intravenous administration of an acute dose of lead acetate or cadmium acetate enhanced the susceptibility of rats to intravenous challenge with *E. coli* by approximately 1000 fold.

APPLICABILITY OF MODEL FOR MEASURING IMMUNOLOGICAL TOXICITY

Although the acute infectious disease model has been used only limitedly in assessing the effects of toxic chemicals on immunotoxicity, the potential for extending this model concept is quite good.

The effects of exposure to NO_2 on a few parameters of the immune response have been investigated (Ehrlich et al., 1975). After several weeks of exposure to NO_2, mice were vaccinated with A_2-Taiwan influenza virus vaccine. At two weeks after the vaccination, the serum neutralizing antibody titer and seroconversion rates were depressed. Non-vaccinated mice exposed to NO_2 exhibited, after 12 weeks of exposure, a marked decrease in serum IgA and an increase in IgM, IgG, and IgG_2 immunoglobulins.

These studies were extended by Maigetter et al. (1978) who studied the effects of NO_2 on mitogenic response of lymphocytes involved in humoral and cellular reactions. After 3 mo exposure to NO_2, the lymphocyte response to phytohemagglutinin or lipopolysaccharide was generally depressed when compared with those animals exposed to clean air.

In view of the available evidence that exposure to metals, such as Cd and Ni can significantly alter the function of the host defense mechanisms, as reflected by an enhancement of mortality in the infectivity model system, these studies were expanded to include the examination of the primary humoral immune system following pollutant exposure. Graham et al. (1975, 1978), reported that inhalation of $NiCl_2$ ($\geqslant 250$ μg Ni/m^3) or $CdCl_2$ (190 μg Cd/m^3) for 2 hr resulted in a significant depression in the number of antibody producing spleen cells. A number of other investigators have also found effects of Cd on the immune system (Exon et al., 1975; Koller, 1973; Koller et al., 1976).

Although these studies clearly illustrate that the pollutants that cause an increase in respiratory infection, i.e., NO_2, Cd, Ni, can also alter the host systemic immune system, further studies are still required to directly relate the immune system to the infectivity model. It will be necessary to design experiments to test for pollutant effects on the pulmonary immune system, as it exists as a steady state and also as it can be enhanced by immunization.

The acute infectivity model that has been utilized in the above studies has certain limitations for studying pulmonary immunity. To more completely examine the question of the role of the pulmonary immune system and its interactions between the invading organism and the host respiratory tissue, a chronic infectivity model is being developed. Hu et al., (1979) have recently established such a system using aerosolized *Myco-plasma pneumoniae*. Animals infected with this organism develop a bronchopneumonia which is similar to human disease. Once infected with this microorganism, the number of viable mycoplasmas increases, reaching a plateau after approximately 2 wks. The number of viable organisms is maintained in the host's pulmonary tissue for approximately 6 wks before it starts to decline. All animals ultimately recover from the primary infection and become completely free of the organism. The development of antibodies in the serum follows a time course which appears to be similar to that seen in human patients. In addition, a solid-phase radioimmuno-assay has been developed in our laboratory which would enable us to measure the level of specific antibodies in the lung lavage fluid of animals infected with *M. pneumoniae*. Although the exact mechanisms of the immunological response in the lung is still not clear, it is generally agreed that the local pulmonary immune response plays a greater role than the systemic immunity in the defense of the respiratory tract against infectious agents. Thus, with the establishment of this chronic infectious disease model, we may be able to study how airborne environmental chemicals can affect this pulmonary immune response.

Recently, Dean et al., (1979) have presented a tier testing and screening approach for assessment of immunologic dysfunction following low levels of exposure to test compunds. These tests, in addition to being rapid, simple and inexpensive, should be sensitive to subtle changes following administration of a dose that produces no overt toxicity. Although no single immunologic assay can completely identify and assess the total risk potential, the acute and chronic infectivity model described here may be especially appropriate since it can be used with both acute and chronic studies, it measures changes in the total host defenses, including immunological, and it can offer guidelines for further epidemiological surveys. This model, coupled with various available cell-mediated and humoral immunity tests, will provide the investigator with a scientifically sound data base useful in evaluating the immunobiological effects induced by environmental chemicals.

REFERENCES

Coffin, D. L. and Gardner, D. E.: Interaction of biological agents and chemical air pollutants. Ann. Occup. Hyg., *15*:219-234 (1972).

Cook, J. A., Hoffmann, E. O. and DiLuzio, N. R.: Influence of lead and cadmium on the susceptibility of rats to bacterial challenge. Proc. Soc. for Exp. Biol. Med., *150*:741-747 (1975).

Dean, J. H., Padarathsingh, M. L. and Jerrells, T. R.: Assessment of immunobiological effects induced by chemicals, drugs or food additives. I. Tier testing and screening approach. Drug and chemical Toxicology, *2*:5-19 (1979).

Ehrlich, R.: Personal communication.

Ehrlich, R.: Interaction between nitrogen dioxide and respiratory infection. Scientific Seminar on Automotive Pollutants. EPA Pub. No. 600-9-75-003, Vol. 1, pp. 1-9 (1975).

Ehrlich, R., Silverstein, E., Maigetter, R., Fenters, J. D. and Gardner, D. E.: Immunologic response in vaccinated mice during long-term exposure to nitrogen dioxide. Env. Res., *10*:217-223 (1975).

Ehrlich, R.: Interaction between environmental pollutants and respiratory infections. In Proc. of "Symposium Experimental Models for Pulmonary Research" EPA Publication 600/9-79-022, pp. 145-163 (1979).

Exon, J. H., Patton, N. M. and Koller, L. D.: Hexamitiasis in cadmium exposed mice. Arch. Environ. Health, *30*:463-464 (1975).

Fairchild, G. A., Roan, J. and McCarroll, J.: Effect of SO_2 on the pathogenesis of murine influenza infection. Arch. Environ. Health, *25*:174-182 (1972).

Gardner, D. E. and Graham, J. A.: Increased pulmonary disease mediated through altered bacterial defenses. Proc. 16th Ann. Hanford Biol. Symp., Sept. 27-29 (1976).

Gardner, D. E., Miller, F. J., Illing, J. W. and Kirtz, J. M.: Alterations in bacterial defense mechanisms of the lung induced by inhalation of cadmium. Bull. European de Physiopathologie Resp., *13*:157-174 (1977a).

Gardner, D. E., Coffin, D. L., Pinigin, M. A. and Sidorenko, G. I.: Role of time as a factor in the toxicity of chemical compounds in intermittent and continuous exposures. J. Toxicol. and Environ. Health, *3*:811-820 (1977b).

Gardner, D. E.: Alteration in host-bacteria interaction by environmental chemicals. Proc. of Assessing Toxic Effects of Environmental Pollutants. Ann Arbor Science Publication, pp. 87-103 (1979).

Graham, J. A., Gardner, D. E., Waters, M. D. and Coffin, D. L.: Effect of trace metals on phagocytosis by alveolar macrophages. Infect. and Immun., *11*:1278-1283 (1975).

Graham, J. A., Miller, F. J., Daniels, M. F., Payne, E. A. and Gardner, D. E.: Influence of cadmium, nickel and chromium on primary immunity in mice. Environ. Res., *16*:77-87 (1978).

Henry, M. C., Findlay, J., Spangler, J. Ehrlich, R.: Chronic toxity of NO_2 in squirrel monkeys. Arch. Environ. Health, *20*:566-570 (1970).

Hu, P. C., Kirtz, J. M., Gardner, D. E. and Powell, D. A.: Experimental infection of the respiratory tract with *Mycoplasma pneumoniae*. In Proc. of "Symposium on Experimental Models for Pulmonary Research." EPA Pub. 600/9-79-022, pp. 165-179 (1979).

Koller, L. D.: Immunosuppression produced by lead, cadmium and mercury. Amer. J. Vet. Res., *34*:1457-1458 (1973).

Koller, L. D., Exon, J. H. and Roan, J. G.: Humoral antibody response in mice after single dose exposure to lead and cadmium. Proc. Soc. Exp. Biol. Med., *151*:339-342 (1976).

Lee, R. E., Jr. and Von Lehmden, D. J.: Trace metal pollution in the environment. J. A. P. . A. *23*:853-857 (1973).

Maigetter, R. Z., Fenters, J. D., Findlay, J. C., Ehrlich, R. and Gardner, D. E.: Effect of exposure to nitrogen dioxide on T and B cells in mouse spleen. Tox. Letters, *2*:157-161 (1978).

Miller, F. J., Illing, J. W. and Gardner, D. E.: Effect of urban ozone levels on laboratory induced respiratory infections. Tox. Letters, *2*:163-169 (1978).

Miller, F. J., Gardner, D. E., Graham, J. A., Lee, R. E., Jr., Wilson, W. E. and Backman, J. D.: Size considerations for establishing a standard for inhalable particles. J. A. P. C. A.,*29(6)*:610-615 (1979).

Natusch, D. F. S., Wallace, J. R. and Evans, C.N.: Toxic trace metals: Preferential concentrations in respirable particles. Science, *183*:202-204 (1974).

DISCUSSION

DEAN: Dr. Gardner, I regret that I had to drive 200 miles to hear this wonderful data when we only work a few blocks apart. Have you looked at any cell-mediated immune parameters in this model yet?

GARDNER: No, I have not. We'd like to get involved with you and your staff and start utilizing this model system to better answer some of the important immunological questions that it certainly brings out.

DEAN: It's a very nice model and, hopefully, we can collaborate.

GARDNER: Thank you.

HELLMAN: As I listen to toxicologists I wonder whether experiments are done with sledgehammers, because when one carefully determines the dose of an infectious agent to which an animal is exposed and superimposes exposure to pollutants that are in the environment, one dose not find major or significant differences in pathology due to the pollutant. I worry that in the process of trying to generate data, we will assist in the formulation of legislative road blocks that will never permit us to see the end of the tunnel.

GARDNER: It is important that in these studies the pollutant exposures are done at concentrations routinely found in the polluted ambient atmosphere. In some cases, such as with NO_2 there have been follow-up epidemiological studies, as in Chattanooga, that show the relationship between such gaseous exposure and enhancement of human respiratory infectious disease. In the study with trace metals, we find effects at levels below the TLV standard levels. So we feel it's very important that people in occupational medicine and hygiene recognize these potential health risks.

As long as the experiment was conducted in a scientifically sound manner and at concentrates which are relevant to regulatory needs, these data must be considered in setting standards for environmental chemicals. In setting such standards, human data are used principally but they are substantiated and supported by animal models such as we have presented here.

HELLMAN: Well, all I know is that when you utilize reasonable doses, most of the data would suggest that there is very little risk involved. The things that we're seeing and data that are being published really represent highly magnified exposure doses.

GARDNER: The concentrations we used in our studies are quite relevant and, as was also brought up in the discussion today and yesterday, unless one performs careful dose-response studies utilizing near ambient concentrations, that is, "real world" concentrations, one will have huge gaps in knowledge of the toxicity of these compounds. For this reason, we always try to design our experiments to provide information as to the threshold or no-response level of the pollutant for any measured effect.

19
Approaches for Studying Immunity in Deep Lung and Effects of Corticosteroids

David E. Bice

Inhalation Toxicology Research Institute, Lovelace Biomedical and Environmental Research Institute, Albuquerque, NM

INTRODUCTION

Data have been published from several studies that evaluated immunity after intrapulmonary immunization of dogs with particulate antigen (Kaltreider et al., 1974, 1975; Kaltreider and Turner, 1976; Turner and Kaltreider, 1978). Results of these studies indicated an increase in the number of antigen-specific antibody-forming cells (AFC) in the broncho-alveolar cell population removed from the lung by lavage. In addition, the lung-associated lymph nodes and blood from these dogs also contained AFC. The source of the AFC and antigen-specific antibody in the lavage fluid from the immunized lung was unknown. The immune cells and proteins could have been produced locally by antigen stimulation of lymphoid cells in the alveoli, in the alveolar walls or in bronchus-associated lymphoid tissue (Kaltreider et al., 1975; Daniele et al., 1977). However, it was also possible that the AFC that accumulated in the im-munized lung were produced in the lung-associated lymph nodes, shed into the blood via efferent lymphatics and then migrated from the blood to sites of antigen deposition in the lung. The results described in this paper come from several studies conducted at the Inhalation Toxicology Institute by D. E. Bice, D. H. Harris, J. O. Hill, B. A. Muggenburg, D. G. Brown-stein and C. T. Schnizlein. Our results indicate that an intense immune response is generally restricted to the lung tissues exposed to antigen, and that the lung-associated lymph nodes are probably the sources of the AFC found in immunized lung lobes.

RESULTS AND DISCUSSION

Immune Response in Lung-Associated Lymph Nodes and in Blood

Particulate antigen deposited in the dog lung is translocated to several lung-associated lymph nodes via afferent lymphatics. These lymph nodes are generally bilateral with the tracheobronchial lymph nodes and the mediastinal lymph nodes located on the left and right side of the mediastinum. Because no data were available concerning the clearance of particulate antigen deposited into specific areas of the lung to the lung-associated lymph nodes, and to gain a better understanding of the role played by the lung-associated lymph nodes in antigen recognition and induction of immunity, we immunized individual lung lobes of dogs with sheep red blood cells (SRBC) and evaluated the numbers of AFC in individual lung-associated lymph nodes (Bice et al., 1979b).

Healthy Beagle dogs between the ages of 2 and 3 years were immunized by the deposition of 10^{10} SRBC in 1.0 ml saline in a single airway of the right or left apical lung lobes. A fiberoptic bronchoscope was introduced through an endothracheal tube and was used to locate a selected airway while the dogs were anesthetized by inhalation of 4% halothane in an oxygen and nitrous oxide carrier. The SRBC suspension was instilled through a 1.6 mm diameter polythylene tube that was passed through the bronchoscope into the selected airway. Kaltreider et al., (1974) had previously found that the peak numbers of AFC were found in the lung-associated lymph nodes at 5 days after intrapulmonary immunization. We therefore sacrificed eight dogs that were immunized in either the right or left apical lung lobes at 5 days after immunization. The numbers of AFC in individual tracheobronchial or mediastinal lymph nodes and spleen was determined using the Jerne Plaque assay as modified by Cunningham and Szenberg (1968).

The total numbers of IgM AFC in left or right tracheobronchial and metiastinal lymph nodes are presented in Tables 1 and 2. As suggested by Gottlieb (1974), log transformations of the data were made to stabilize the variance and all AFC data are presented as geometric means. The one-sided, paired t-test was used to determine the statistical significance of the transformed data. These data show that antigen clearance to these lymph nodes was basically ipsilateral with significantly higher numbers of

AFC found in the lymph nodes removed from the side of the lung that was immunized. Data obtained from other dogs immunized in either the left or right diaphragmatic lung lobes were similar and antigen stimulation of the lung-associated lymph nodes was also ipsilateral.

We found few AFC in the spleen at 5 days after immunization ($102 \pm 129/10^6$ lymphoid cells, mean $\pm$ SD) which agreed with earlier observations (Kaltreider et al., 1974). The AFC in the spleen are apparently immune cells that were produced in the lung-associated lymph nodes and which translocate to the spleen via the circulatory system (Kaltreider et al., 1976). An insignificant amount of SRBC antigen is translocated to the spleen after lung immunization (Turner and Kaltreider, 1978), and the AFC observed in the blood are apparently produced in the lung-associated lymph nodes rather than in the spleen.

A separate group of dogs was immunized in either the left or right apical lung lobes and venous blood and lung lavage samples were taken on days 3, 5, 7, 10, 12, 14 and 21 after SRBC exposure (Bice et al., 1979a). The immunized airway and a control airway in the opposite apical lobe were lavaged with 5 saline washes of 10 ml each using the fiberoptic bronchoscope while the dogs were anesthetized. The numbers of IgM and IgG AFC found in the blood of these animals are presented in Figure 1 and 2. The highest concentration of both IgM and IgG AFC occurred in the blood around 7 days after immunization. The time course of the response was rapid with a sharp decline in the number of AFC present after day 7 and few AFC were observed from 12 days through 21 days after immunization. Similar numbers of IgM and IgG AFC were found in the blood after immunization in the left or right apical lung lobes providing further evidence that equal levels of immunity were developed in the lung-associated lymph nodes after immunization of these lung lobes.

Antibody-Forming Cells in Immunized and Nonimmunized Lung

A significant increase in the total number of bronchoalveolar cells was observed in the lavage fluid from the immunized lung lobe when dogs were immunized in the left apical lobe. The highest numbers of cells were seen 10 days after immunization with a mean of 33×10^6 cells. Most of the cells were identified as pulmonary alveolar macrophages (60 percent) and lymphocytes (24 percent). Maximum numbers of polymorphonuclear leukocytes were seen at 3 days after immunization, and constituted 31 percent of the total cells. Although these cell types were all significantly elevated in the left apical immunized lung lobe, no significant increase was observed when right apical lung lobe was immunized.

The numbers of AFC present in the cell population removed from control and immunized airways by localized lung lavage is presented in Figures 1 and 2 (Bice et al., 1979a). These data indicated that after immunization in the left apical lung lobe, an intense immunity with large numbers of both IgM and IgG AFC was found only in the immunized lung lobe. The peak IgM response occurred at 10 days after immunization while the maximum numbers of IgG AFC were found at 12 days. Both IgM and IgG responses were significantly higher than observed in the right apical control lung lobe, and it is important to note that the peak responses at 10 and 12 days after immunization occurred several days later than the maximum response in the blood.

Although Kaltreider and co-workers (Kaltreider et al., 1974; Kaltreider and Turner, 1976; Turner and Kaltreider, 1978) found responses of less than 150 AFC/10^6 lymphoid cells in the bronchoalveolar cell population after intrapulmonary immunizations, the numbers of AFC we found (Figures 1 and 2) were considerably higher. Maximum levels reached over 1000 IgM AFC/10^6 lymphoid cells and over 10,000 IgG AFC/10^6 lymphoid cells. Although there are several explanations for the differences between the present and earlier studies, an important difference is that Kaltreider and co-workers usually measured immune responses at 4-5 days after immunization. The immune responses we observed at 3 and 5 days after immunization were comparable to the responses previously reported (Kaltreider et al., 1974; Kaltreider and Turner, 1976; Turner and Kaltreider, 1978) and significant immunity was observed only at 7 to 14 days after antigen exposure. At 5 days after SRB instillation we found no IgG AFC in the bronchoalveolar cells removed by lung lavage as previously reported (Kaltreider et al., 1974), but large IgG responses were observed at 10 to 14 days after immunization.

The numbers of background AFC in lavage cells from unimmunized dogs are low. The IgM and IgG AFC responses in the unimmunized left and right apical lung lobes at 10 to 14 days after immunization of over 200 AFC/10^6 lymphoid cells therefore represent a significant increase of immune cells in the unexposed lung. Because these tissues were not exposed to antigen, the AFC in the control lung lobes probably represents an accumulation of AFC from the blood to lung tissue. Although the data for the control lung lobes in Figures 1 and 2 were obtained from the right and left apical lung lobes, other studies in our laboratory have shown that similar low responses also are found in unexposed left and right diaphragmatic lung lobes.

The kinetics of the IgM and IgG AFC responses in the immunized right apical lung lobe was the same as observed when the left apical lung lobe was immunized, but the numbers of both IgM and IgG AFC were significantly lower. In dogs immunized in the right apical lung lobe, only the numbers of IgM AFC were significantly higher than levels of IgM AFC observed in the unimmunized lung lobe. The numbers of IgG AFC in immunized and unimmunized lung lobes were the same in these dogs. The immune response observed in the control left apical lung lobe was the same as the response obtained in the immunized right apical lung lobe.

We cannot explain at this time why lower levels of IgM and IgG AFC were recovered from the immunized right apical lung lobe than from the immunized left apical lobe. The numbers of AFC in lung-associated lymph nodes and in the blood were the same regardless of whether the antigen was deposited in the right apical or left apical lobes (Tables 1 and 2 and Figures 1 and 2). We therefore concluded that adequate immunization was induced in regional lymph nodes regardless of the site of immunization. The areas of left or right apical lung lobes exposed to technetium-99m (^{99m}Tc) labeled antigen or to lavage fluid containing ^{99m}Tc labeled colloid particles was visualized with a gamma camera and was found to be the same. In addition, the clearance of ^{99m}Tc labeled SRBC through 24 hours after instillation was identical in both the left and

Table 1.   Calculated Total Numbers of IgM Antibody-Forming Cells in the Tracheobronchial Lymph Nodes 5 Days After Immunization with SRBC.

SITE OF IMMUNIZATION	DOG NUMBER	LEFT TRACHEOBRONCHIAL	RIGHT TRACHEOBRONCHIAL	P VALUE *
Left Apical	1	10 200	0	
	2	29 400	0	p < 0.005
	3	86 700	0	
	4	411 000	1 300	
	Geometric mean	57 200	6	
Right Apical	5	12 200	86 100	
	6	17 100	413 000	p < 0.05
	7	44 200	449 000	
	8	63 300	165 000	
	Geometric mean	27 600	226 000	

* Probability values were determined using one-sided, paired t-tests.

***Table 2.* Calculated Total Numbers of IgM Antibody-Forming Cells in Pools of Mediastinal Lymph Nodes 5 Days After Immunization with SRBC.**

SITE OF IMMUNIZATION	DOG NUMBER	LEFT MEDIASTINAL	RIGHT MEDIASTINAL	P VALUE *
Left Apical	1	14 000	300	
	2	1 300	50	p < 0.01
	3	106 000	74 600	
	4	77 500	700	
	Geometric mean	19 700	1 000	
Right Apical	5	600	24 100	
	6	2 500	75 700	p < 0.01
	7	8 300	342 000	
	8	N.T.†	N.T.†	
	Geometric mean	2 300	85 400	

* Probability values were determined using one-sided, paired *t*-tests.
† Not tested.

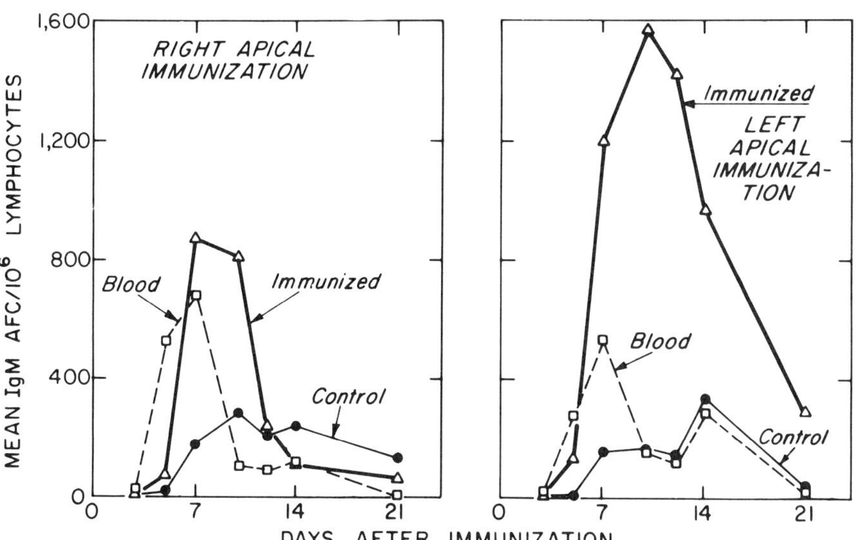

Figure 1.   IgM antibody-forming cells (AFC) in blood, in control lung lobes and in immunized lung lobes after sheep red blood cell immunization in the left apical or right apical lung lobes. Each represents the mean response in four dogs. Redrawn from Chest, 75:249 (1979).

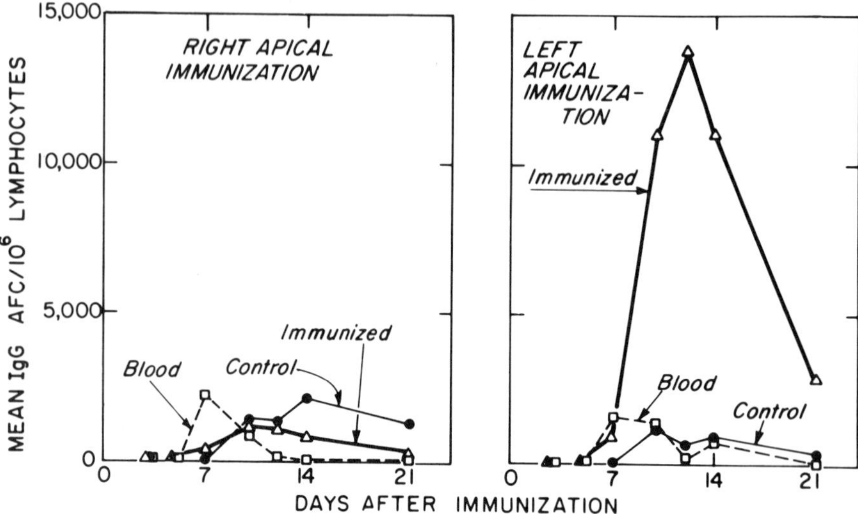

Figure 2.   IgG antibody-forming cells (AFC) in blood, in control lung lobes and in immunized lung lobes after sheep red blood cell immunization in the left apical or right apical lung lobes. Each point represents the mean response in four dogs. Redrawn from Chest, 75:249 (1979).

right apical lobes. Whether the differences we observed in the numbers of AFC in these lung lobes are real or due to artifacts in experimental procedures is not known at this time.

In other studies we have shown that the immune responses in the left and right cardiac lung lobes is similar to the responses observed in the left apical lung lobe. Because the response we observed in the right apical lung lobe is lower than in the other lung lobes of the dog, most of the conclusions in this presentation concerning immunity in the dog lung are based on data obtained by immunization in the left apical lung lobe.

Antigen-Specific Antibody in Immunized and Nonimmunized Lung

We also evaluated the protein and antigen-specific IgM and IgG antibody in lavage fluids from immunized and control lung lobes and in serum (Hill et al., 1979). The immunized lung lobes usually contained more total protein, albumin and IgG than contralateral nonimmunized lung lobes. IgM was rarely detectable. These differences were usually statistically significant when these parameters were compared in dogs immunized in the left apical lung lobe with the right apical lobe used as the control. Right apical immunization rarely resulted in significant increases in total protein.

Antigen-specific antibody evaluated by hemagglutination assays was first detected in the lavage fluid at 7 days after immunization, and reached a peak at 10-12 days after SRBC instillation. As observed with AFC, immunization in the left apical lung lobe resulted in higher anti-SRBC antibody titers than in dogs immunized in the right apical lobe. No significant differences were noted in the antigen-specific antibody levels in lavage fluids from immunized and control lung lobes when the right apical lobe was immunized. The titers in serum were the same after immunization in either the left or right apical lung lobes. Treatment of lavage fluids with mercaptoethanol indicated that most of the antigen-specific antibody present was IgG. Our results also indicated that this antigen-specific IgG was produced by the lymphoid cells in the lung rather than by translocation of antibody from the serum.

Histology of Immune Response in the Lung

It was clear from our studies in the dog that intense immunity was found only in lung lobes that had been exposed to SRBC. However, it was not clear whether the immune cells present in immunized lung lobes were produced *in situ* in local lymphoid tissues, or whether this immune response in the lower respiratory tract was dependent on systemic immunity observed in lung-associated lymph nodes and blood. The presence of AFC in unimmunized lung lobes indicated that AFC were entering the lung from the blood. The results of other publications indicated that AFC could be recruited to immunized tissues that retained small amounts of antigen (Emeson, 1978). This suggested the possibility that the increased number of AFC in the immunized lung lobes was due to the recruitment of antigen-specific lymphoid cells from the blood to lung tissues containing SRBC antigen.

Because an understanding of tissue and cellular changes induced by lung immunization would help answer some of these questions, a separate group of dogs were immunized in the left or right apical lung lobes with 10^{10} SRBC (Brownstein et al., 1979). At 2, 5, 7 and 21 days after immunization, tissues were obtained from lung-associated lymph nodes, immunized lung lobes and control lung lobes. A microscopic examination of tissues from lung-associated lymph nodes draining immunized lung lobes showed cellular changes characteristic of a developing immune response on days 2 and 5. By 7 days after immunization, large germinal centers were present and the medullary cords were distended with large lymphocytes, plasmablasts and plasma cells. The sinuses contained predominantly large lymphocytes and plasmablasts.

Although other species have well developed intrapulmonary lymphoid tissues (Bienenstock and Johnston, 1976; Fournier et al., 1977; Racz et al., 1977) an examination of lung histology of dogs indicated a lack of lymphoid nodules (bronchus-associated lymphoid tissues) in large and medium sized bronchi. Lymphoid-epithelial organs, lymphoid aggregates at the bronchoalveolar junctions, were rarely seen. The exposure of lung tissues to SRBC had no apparent effect on these tissues and they were similar in both immunized and nonimmunized lung tissues.

At 2 days after SRBC immunization an acute inflammatory response was seen in immunized lung lobes, which was resolved by day 5. Numerous venules and small veins within the alveolar septae of immunized lung lobes has perivascular interstitial infiltrates of lymphoid cells by 5 days after SRBC exposure (Figure 3). Most of these lymphoid cells had basophilic, pyroninophilic cytoplasm and central nuclei. Some had characteristics of plasmablasts with eccentric nuclei and prominent perinuclear

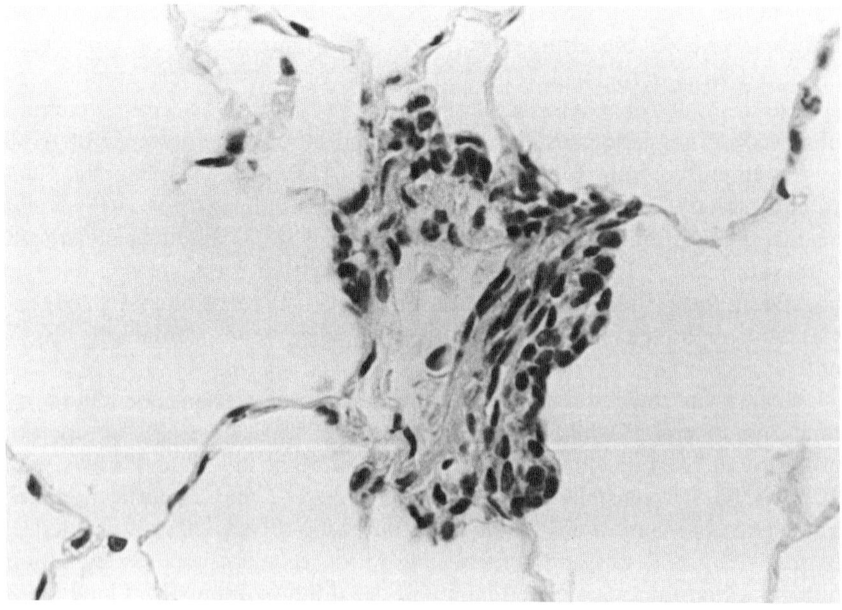

Figure 3. Dog lung lobe 5 days after intrapulmonary instillation of sheep red blood cells. H&E X 460. Pulmonary venule with expansion of perivenular interstitium by activated lymphocytes with basophilic cytoplasm.

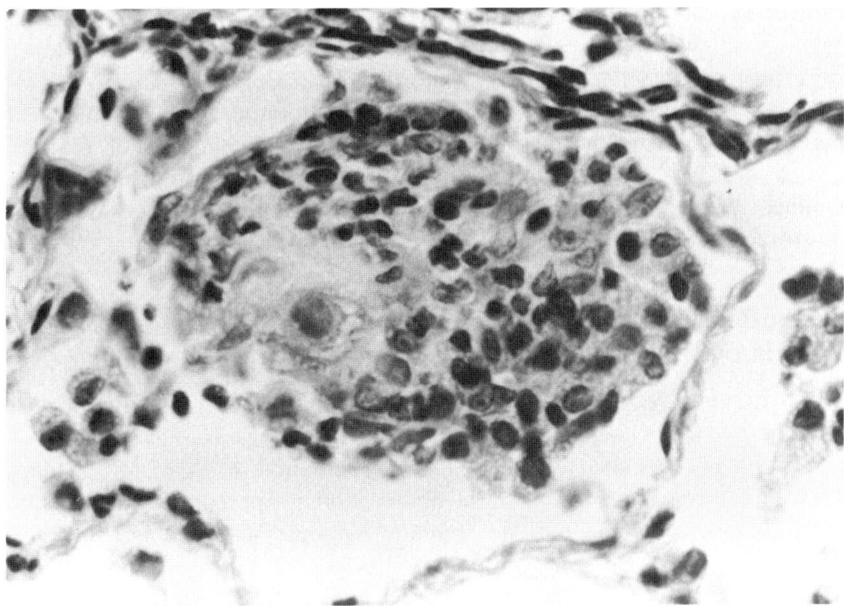

Figure 4. Dog lung lobe 7 days after intrapulmonary instillation of sheep red blood cells. Alveolar macrophages with abundant cytoplasm and indistinct plasma membranes (arrow) and surrounded by activated lymphocytes and macrophages as well as plasma cells. H&E X 460.

clear areas. A few of these interstitial infiltrates had extended into the alveolar spaces by 7 days with immunization and were associated with large mononuclear cells (Figure 4). Some of these large cells had morphological characteristics of activated pulmonary alveolar macrophages, and there appeared to be gradual transitions to bizarre megalocytic mononuclear cells measuring up to 190 μm in diameter. These mixed mononuclear aggregates within the alveolar spaces consisted of pyroninophilic lymphocytes, plasmablasts and plasma cells surrounding or mixed with modified alveolar macrophages. An examination of nonimmunized lung lobes showed similar histologic changes, but fewer venules and veins were affected and no alveolar aggregates were found. By 21 days after antigen exposure the cellular responses in both the lung and lung-associated lymph nodes were largely resolved.

Although we had observed increases in the numbers of macrophages and lymphoid cells in lavage fluid from immunized lung lobes, no cell aggregates were found. We assume that the alveolar aggregates were disrupted by the lavage procedure. A detailed examination of the lung cytology showed that most lymphoid cells from nonimmunized lung lobes were unstimulated lymphocytes, while the remainder were activated lymphocytes. Plasma cells were rarely identified. Immunization resulted in a marked increased in the numbers of activated lymphocytes which reached a peak at 7 days after immunization. Plasma cells began to appear in large numbers 7 days after antigen exposure with maximum numbers occuring at 10 days after immunization.

Conclusions Concerning the Source of Antibody-Forming Cells in the Lung

Based on the above histologic data and on data from the evaluation of AFC in lung-associated lymph nodes, blood and lungs, we have concluded that the lung-associated lymph nodes are the source of AFC in the lung. This conclusion is based on these observations: (1) Histologic evidence showed the development of an immune response in the lung-associated lymph nodes 2 days before lymphoid infiltrates and AFC were found in the lung. (2) The AFC in the blood reached maximum numbers earlier than the AFC in the lung. (3) There were no significant histologic changes in local lymphoid tissues in the lung. (4) The formation of perivascular infiltrates that expanded into alveolar lymphoid aggregates indicates the blood as the source of these cells. Although the mechanisms by which intense immunity is produced in the immunized lung lobes are not known, the retention of small amounts of antigen in immunized lung tissues could be responsible for the recruitment of large numbers of AFC from the blood.

Effects of Immunosuppressive Agents on Lung Immunity

Our investigators at the Inhalation Toxicology Research Institute deal with the effects of inhaled pollutants on lung immunity. Before initiating studies with pollutants, we next evaluated the effects of immunosuppressive treatment on immunity in the lower respiratory tract (Harris et al., 1979). We elected to use the corticosteroid prednisolone and evaluated treatments where the dogs received either systemic or local lung exposure to this corticosteroid. Because of differences observed in immunity in the left and right apical lung lobes, we used the left and right cardiac lung lobes for immunization in this study. In a pilot study we demonstrated that the left and right cardiac lung lobes gave similar immune response that were the same as the level of immunity observed in the apical lung lobe. Dogs treated systemically received daily injections of 20 mg of prednisolone sodium succinate starting 42 days before immunization. These injections continued until 10 days after antigen instillation. To evaluate the effects of local corticosteroid therapy in immunity in deep lung, the left cardiac lung lobes of dogs were treated with a variety of doses ranging between 30 and 60 mg of prednisone around the time of immunization. Treatment with the corticosteroid was made by instillation into specific airways by using the fiberoptic bronchoscope. The right cardiac lung lobes received SRBC only and served as untreated, immunized controls. The left and right apical lung lobes served as untreated nonimmunized controls.

The immune response in the immunized and nonimmunized lung lobes of these dogs was evaluated at 5, 7, 10 and 12 days after immunization. Treatment of dogs with systemic injections of corticosteroids resulted in lowered numbers of circulating lymphocytes and suppressed immune responses in the lower respiratory tract (Table 3). The antigen-specific antibody and numbers of lymphoid cells obtained in lung lavage were also lowered. In contrast, exposure of lung tissue to corticosteroid around the time of immunization resulted in minimal suppression (Table 3). No lymphopenia resulted and the only level that reduced the numbers of AFC in the lung was 30 mg given in 10mg doses at 2 days before immunization, at the time of immunization and 2 days after immunization.

Table 3.   The Effect of Systemic Corticosteroid and Local Lung Corticosteroid on the Number of IgM and IgG Bronchoalveolar Antibody-Forming Cells.

		PEAK $AFC/10^6$ LYMPHOCYTES	
SOURCE OF BRONCHOALVEOLAR LYMPHOCYTES	CORTICOSTEROID TREATMENT	GEOMETRIC MEAN IgM AFC AT 7 DAYS	GEOMETRIC MEAN IgG AFC AT 10 DAYS
Right and left cardiac (immunized)	Systemic prednisolone	2 200	14 400
Right and left cardiac (immunized)	30 mg/prednisolone in right and left cardiac	18 500	92 800
Right cardiac (immunized)	None	29 700	208 000
Right and left apical (nonimmunized)	None	600	4 300

Systemic treatment with corticosteroid also lowered the numbers of AFC and the titer of antigen-specific antibody in the blood, indicating that the immunisuppressive effect was due to an alteration of immunity in the lung-associated lymph nodes. We concluded that there were fewer AFC in blood that could be recruited to the lung. In contrast, treatment of lung tissues with corticosteroid around the time of immunization did not have an effect on the response seen in blood and its only effect appeared to be a slight suppression on the recruitment of AFC into the lung.

CONCLUSION

The results of the studies that are summarized in this chapter have provided additional data important in the understanding of immunity in the dog lung. These data have shown that the lung-associated lymph nodes are the main source of AFC found in the lung, pointing out the importance of these tissues in lung defense. Treatment of dogs with systemic injections of corticosteroid significantly suppressed immunity in the blood and in the lung. It seems possible that if the lung-associated lymph nodes were damaged by inhalation and translocation of inhaled toxic materials to these tissues, that immunity in the deep lung could be compromised.

ACKNOWLEDGMENTS

Research performed under U.S. Department of Energy Contract Number EY–76–C–04–1013 in facilities fully accredited by the American Association for the Accreditation of Laboratory Animal Care.

REFERENCES

Bienenstock, J. and Johnson, N. A.: A morphologic study of rabbit bronchial lymphoid aggregates and lymphoepithelium. Lab. Invest., 35:343-348 (1976).

Bice, D. E., Harris, D. L., Hill, J. O. and Muggenburg, B. A.: Local and systemic immunity following localized deposition of antigen in the lung. Chest, 75:246-248 (1979a).

Bice, D. E., Harris, D. L. and Muggenburg, B. A.: Regional immunologic responses following localized deposition of antigen in the lung. Exp. Lung. Res. (in press) (1979b).

Brownstein, D. G., Rebar, A. H., Bice, D. E., Muggenburg, B. A. and Hill, J. O.: Immunology of the lower respiratory tract: Serial morphologic changes in the lungs and tracheobronchial lymph nodes of dogs after intrapulmonary immunization with sheep erythrocytes. Amer. J. Path. (in press) (1979).

Cunningham, A. J. and Szenberg, A.: Further improvements in the plaque technique for detecting single antibody-forming cells. Immunology, 14:599-601 (1968).

Daniele, R. P., Beacham, C. H. and Gorenberg, D. J.: The bronchoalveolar lymphocytes. Studies on the life history and lymphocyte traffic from blood to the lung. Cell. Immunol., *31*:48-54 (1977).

Emeson, E. E.: Migratory behavior of lymphocytes with specific reactivity to alloantigens. II. Selective recruitment to lymphoid cell allografts and their draining lymph nodes. J. Exp. Med.,*147*:13-24 (1978).

Fournier, M., Vai, F., Derenne, J. P. and Pariente, R.: Bronchial lymphoepithelial nodules in the rat. Morphologic features and uptake and transport of exogenous proteins. Amer. Rev. Resp. Dis., *116*:685-694 (1977).

Gottlieb, C. F.: Application of transformations to normalize the distribution of plaque-forming cells. J. Immunol., *113*:51-57 (1974).

Harris, D. L., Bice, D. E., Muggenburg, B. A. and Hill, J. O.: The effect of corticosteroid therapy on lung immunity following localized deposition of sheep erythrocytes in lungs of beagle dogs. (Submitted for publication) (1979).

Hill, J. O., Bice, D. E., Harris, D. L. and Muggenburg, B. A.: Evaluation of the pulmonary immune response by analysis of bronchoalveolar fluids obtained by serial lung lavage after local immunization (Submitted for publication) (1979).

Kaltreider, H. B., Kyselka, L. and Salmon, S. E.: Immunology of the lower respiratory tract. II. The plaque-forming response of canine lymphoid tissues to sheep erythrocytes after intrapulmonary or intravenous immunizations. J. Clin. Invest., *54*:263-270 (1974).

Kaltreider, H. B., Turner, F. N. and Salmon, S. E.: A canine model for comparative study of respiratory and systemic immunologic reactions. Amer. Rev. Resp. Dis., *111*:257-265 (1975).

Kaltreider, H. B. and Turner, F. N.: Appearance of antibody-forming cells in lymphocytes from the lower respiratory tract of the dog after intrapulmonary or intravenous immunization with sheep erythrocytes. Amer. Rev. Resp. Dis., *113*:613-617 (1976).

Kaltreider, H. B., Turner, F. N., Adam, E. and Chan, M. K.: Bronchoalveolar clearance and immunologic reaction to an organic particulate antigen instilled into alveolar spaces of dog lungs. Chest.,*69*:282-283 (1976).

Rácz, P., Tenner-Rácz, K., Myrvik, Q. N. and Fainter, L. K.: Functional architecture of bronchial associated lymphoid tissue and lymphoepithelium in pulmonary cell-mediated reactions in the rabbit. J. Reticuloendothel. Soc., *22*:59-83 (1977).

Turner, F. N. and Kaltreider, H. B.: Immunology of the lower respiratory tract. III. Concentrations of antigen and of antibody-forming cells in pulmonary and systemic lymphoid tissues of dogs after intrapulmonary or intravenous administration of sheep erythrocytes. Clin. Exp. Immunol., *33*:128-135 (1978).

DISCUSSION

DEAN: Let me ask you a question regarding another possible application of this model. My wife works in pediatric pulmonary allergy, and it seems that pulmonary allergy is a rather major problem in children. Couldn't this type of model be applied to look at allergy? How would you foresee applying this type of a model to dissect allergy in the lung?

BICE: She's looking at asthmatic or IgE responses?

DEAN: Yes, children with cystic fibrosis and other asthma type problems.

BICE: Well, I don't know. We haven't really attempted to use this model in IgE-mediated responses, in fact we have not even looked at IgE. We have evaluated the number of lymphoid cells producing IgA in the deep lung and we find very few. I really do not know if there is a direct application of this model.

DEAN: It might be applicable if antisera to canine IgE becomes available.

BICE: Well, there is no monospecific anti-IgE available. You can induce what appear to be IgE responses in the dog, and of course Dr. Roy Patterson has done that by immunizing with *Ascaris suum* antigens. We have also immunized dogs by inhalation of *Ascaris suum* antigens in an attempt to induce asthmatic responses in the lung of the dog and we, like Dr. Patterson, were partially successful. You can induce asthmatic responses in the dog but these responses do not mimic what you see in humans· The asthmatic responses are very short-lived and, if after you have immunized the dogs and wait six weeks and challenge them again, they have usually lost sensitivity. You have to continually rechallenge to maintain an antibody titer high enough to result in an asthmatic response.

DEAN: I am still convinced that your model may, in the future, lend itself to hypersensitization studies.

BICE: I guess it would. You can repeatedly deposit any antigen you choose in a specific lung lobe and then compare the immune response observed to responses in a control lung lobe.

LaVIA: There's one point that I feel is important about pulmonary allergies, asthma, and so on in children; that is a very large psychological component. It's very hard to compare experimental models to human because of this psychological component, which I'm sure dogs don't have! That's why I'm not very hopeful that this and Dr. Patterson's model may solve anything more than just very simple mechanistic problems.

BICE: I have allergies and I did not know that I had psychological problems!

LaVIA: No. It's important only in childhood asthma. As we age, if we remain asthmatic, that phase is considered secondary.

SIGEL: Dr. Bice, yours was a fascinating story which begins to open up some very interesting possibilities. I would like to ask whether the right apical area, which is less effective in the sense of producing antibody-forming cells (compared to the left apical part), is more enriched in other cells such as alveolar macrophages or natural killer cells, compared to the left side of the lung? Can you relate the very fascinating findings that you showed at the end with the earlier findings, where PFC in the lymph nodes were highly specific and highly restricted to one side with very few cells in the contralateral node; whereas in the opposite direction there was a good deal of spillover? Is there any relationship there?

BICE: Well, we don't really know. Knowledge concerning the lymphatics of the lung is still limited. We have another study that will start soon in which we will deposit insoluble, labeled particles in specific areas of the lung. We will then be able to count the radioactivity that's translocated to individual lymph nodes. When we deposited antigen in the right apical lung lobe, we observed more crossover to the lymph nodes on the opposite side of the lung than when we immunized in the left apical. We do not really understand why.

There are studies that indicate that, if one injects dye into specific lung lobes, nearly all the dye leaves the lung by the right lymphatic duct; very little goes out the left lymphatic duct. If this is true with antigen, then when you deposit antigen in the left apical lung lob, it might tend to cross to the right lung-associated lymph nodes and then exit in the right lymphatic duct.

We have attempted surgically to locate and cannulate the right and left lymphatic ducts of dogs. The left lymphatic duct is almost impossible to cannulate; although the right lymphatic duct can be cannulated. There are techniques available and we are going to do a study to evaluate antibody-forming cells leaving in the lymph from the lung after immunization in specific lung lobes.

GHAFFAR: I heard you mention, I think, that you could not detect any antigen in the spleen of contralateral lymph nodes. Am I correct?

BICE: The studies that were done by Kaltreider using radiolabeled antigen indicated that particulate antigen deposited in the lung did not reach the spleen in measurable quantities. We cannot conclude that antigen was not found in the contralateral lung-associated lymph nodes, because we evaluated an immune response rather than a detecting antigen. We measured the effect of the antigen, rather than detecting the level of antigen specifically, that was present.

There was some crossover to the contralateral lymph nodes. In other words, antigen doesn't all go to ipsilateral lymph nodes, but most of it does.

BELLANTI: I have a question and a comment. First I would like also to congratulate Dr. Bice and his colleagues for a beautiful study.

The question is: Did you look for secretory IgA, since this is the local form of immunoglobulin in which one would certainly be interested?

My comment relates to the question of the model in asthma: I think this has profound significance as a potential look at homocytotropic antibody production, as you suggested; but more importantly perhaps, as a means to look at the production of protective antibody following the use of new vaccine approaches which are currently being tested; e.g., live attenuated viruses and bacteria. I think this makes an excellent model for testing these new vaccines, comparing responses with those that are administered locally with those that are given systemically.

BICE: We have looked for IgA antibody-forming cells, but we haven't really looked for secretory IgA. We don't have the specific antibody to the secretory component necessary to do these studies.

KERMAN: With the differences that you show in terms of right and left cells recovered from the ducts: First, do you know whether, if you remove those cells and put them into a Cunningham system, do they have the same potential?

Second, if it is true that there is this real immune response difference, do you know whether the incidence of malignant tumors in the human lung is geographically more predominant in the right-insides in various lobes similar to, let's say the immune response in the dog?

BICE: Well, the answer to the first question is I don't know. We have not done an *in vitro* immunization study using cells from specific lung lobes.

KERMAN: From the cell duct?

BICE: No, we haven't done that study. The numbers of cells we obtained from the immunized right apical lung lobe were obviously lower. However, we do not know whether their ability to respond to antigen was the same as lymphoid cells from the left apical lung lobe.

The literature available on the number of tumors and/or the infections between the right and left lung lobes is confusing. First of all, there are not many studies comparing tumors in the right with those on the left. Some studies indicate increase of tumors in the right lung, but there are also studies where the number of tumors in the left and right lungs is essentially the same. I guess it really is undecided as to whether or not there really is a difference.

There is a published study in infants that shows the rate of infections in the right apical lung lobes was considerably higher than that in the left apical lung lobes.

KERMAN: It would be interesting if you could establish a model for malignancies in dogs to see where they induce, in which lobes they occur.

BICE: We are looking at tumor induction in dogs on long-term study following inhalation exposure to various radioactive particles. We, of course, are keeping track of the number of tumors that are in the right and left apical lung lobes but so far there is not really a real marked trend either way.

20
A Unifying Model for Immunotoxicology: A Summation Presentation

Joseph A. Bellanti
Nancy J. Balter
Irving Gray

Departments of Pediatrics and Microbiology
International Center for Interdisciplinary Studies of Immunology
Georgetown University School of Medicine
Department of Biology
Georgetown University, Washington, D.C.

INTRODUCTION

Immunity has been classically concerned with *resistance* to infection (Bellanti, 1978). It has long been recognized that following recovery from a specific infectious disease, the individual does not usually succumb to that illness again. It is now apparent that the functions of the immune system are more diverse and embrace not only the functions of defense but also those of *homeostasis* and *surveillance* as well. In order to carry out these diverse functions of immunity, an equally diverse cellular system has evolved within the vertebrates, the *lymphoreticular system*. This consists of a collection of cells which are distributed strategically throughout the body as well as lining the lymphatic and vascular channels. Its cells are housed within the thymus, the lymph nodes and the spleen and also those bodily tracts which are exposed to the external environment and include the respiratory, gastrointestinal, and genitourinary systems.

The prevention of infectious diseases through the effective use of vaccines represents one of immunology's greatest triumphs. Today, the prevention of the most serious health problems facing our nation has to do with the detection and elimination of agents in our environment that induce irreversible progressive forms of *toxicity, hypersensitivity, carcinogenicity, mutagenicity,* and *teratogenicity.* Within the past several decades, a number of procedures has been devised that can detect chemicals that induce mutations by means of a wide variety of biologic assays. Since the correlation between mutagenic and carcinogenic agents is high, the characterization of a chemical as a mutagen in many cases will also identify a carcinogen.

The procedures to detect mutagens are usually carried out in a variety of systems with different degrees of biological complexities. In recent years, a scientific explosion has occurred in the field of immunology which has included the revelation of not only a wide set of cellular and humoral responses but also an increasing awareness that the immunologic system can also sustain injury from toxic substances in the environment.

The term, immunotoxicology, was coined in recent years to describe the harmful effects of environmental agents on various components of the immunologic system (Moore, J. A., 1979). This definition evolved from several reports suggesting that certain environmental drugs, heavy metals, chemicals, herbicides, pesticides and food additives caused immune suppression in both the experimental animal and in the human. The focus of the experimental studies has been primarily the effects of these agents on the immune response to defined antigens, infectious agents or tumors. This type of definition, although important, may be unduly restrictive, however, since it excludes the harmful effects of environmental agents which derive from the immune response to the environmental agent itself as seen in allergic hypersensitivity, autoimmunity or malignancy. Thus, a broader and more contemporary definition of immunotoxicology would be *those harmful effects of the immune response which are mediated either by the effects of the environmental agent on the immunologic system or those triggered by the effects of the immune response to the environmental agent itself.* The importance of the study of immunotoxicology to today's health is seen in the spectrum of diseases which include the well-documented toxic or allergic hypersensitivities as well as a myriad of disease entities of unknown etiology which are probably environmentally induced and whose pathogenesis may derive from immunotoxicologic processes.

The purpose of this presentation is to offer a broad overview of the immune system as a unifying model and to suggest ways in which this information could be useful in the design of future studies concerned with the identification of toxic agents as well as the evaluation of their immunotoxicologic potential.

A Unifying Model for Immunologic Processes

For ease of discussion, we may speak of five components of the host's encounter with foreignness: (1) the environment, (2) the target cell, (3) the phagocytic cells, (4) the mediator cells and the mediator products, and (5) the specific antigen recognition, B-lymphocytes and T-lymphocytes and their specific products.

The Environment

Since most substances that confront and ultimately activate the host's immunologic system arise from the exterior world, the place to begin in

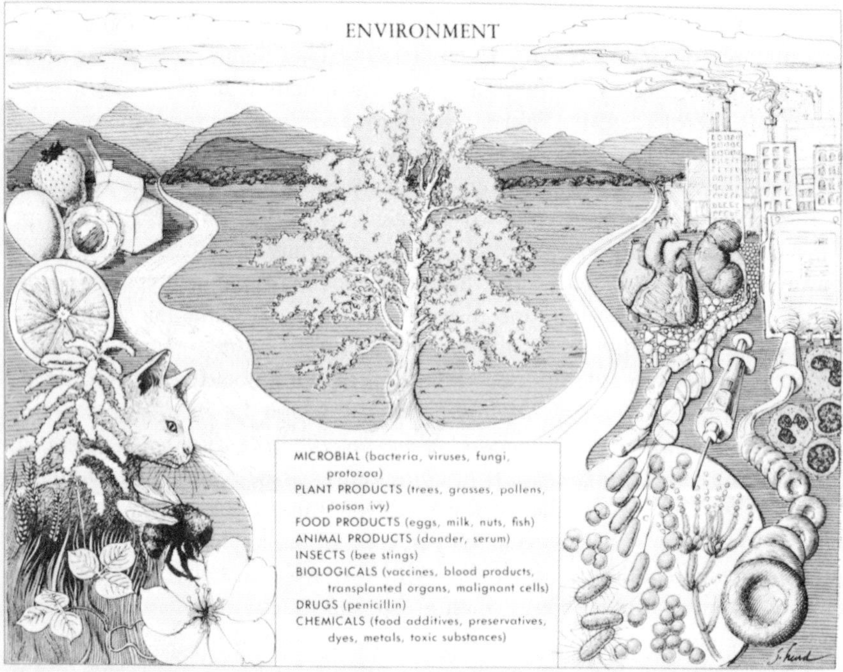

Fig. 1   Examples of environmental agents. (From Bellanti, J. A., 1978, with permission from the publishers).

any discussion is with the external environment (Figure 1). Included within the external environment are the myriad of foreign substances that range from the simplest of low molecular weight chemicals to the most complex microbial agents. It should also be emphasized that the immunologic system may be activated not only for foreign substances that arise in the external environment but also by those that present from the internal environment, e.g., transplanted cells or altered self components (virally transformed or chemically transformed cells). Those substances that have the capacity to evoke immunologic responses are commonly referred to as immunogens or antigens and all share the common characteristic of being recognized as foreign by the host. Occasionally the encounter with a foreign configuration may lead to an inability to respond—a state that is referred to as immunologic tolerance. Such configurations are referred to as tolerogens. Allergens are a specialized class of immunogen and take part in hypersensitivity or allergic reactions. Antigens may be complete and lead to an immune response per se (immunogens) or they may be incomplete (haptens) and require prior attachment to other proteins or cells to become fully immunogenic. As our environment becomes more complex not only does the number of antigens increase but also the potential numbers of chemicals and mutagenic agents to which we are exposed.

Target Cells

The introduction of an environmental agent into a host may have an adverse effect on a target cell. There are a variety of target cells upon which an environmental agent may impact (Figure 2). They vary according to their type and location and the portal of entry of the foreign substance. It is important to emphasize that target cells may be normal host cells that become the adventitious targets of entry by the environmental agent or by immunologic processes referred to above. They may also represent altered host cells that have become modified through the interaction with the environmental substance, e.g., chemical, by infection, e.g., virus, or by malignant transformation, e.g., carcinogen. Alternatively, the target cell may be a foreign cell introduced by transplantation. The target cell may thus sustain direct injury from the environmental agent or indirect injury through immunologic processes. The net effect leads to a disruption of cell function which is commonly referred to as toxicity or cell death with irreversible sequelae. Some of the more common target cells are shown in Table 1.

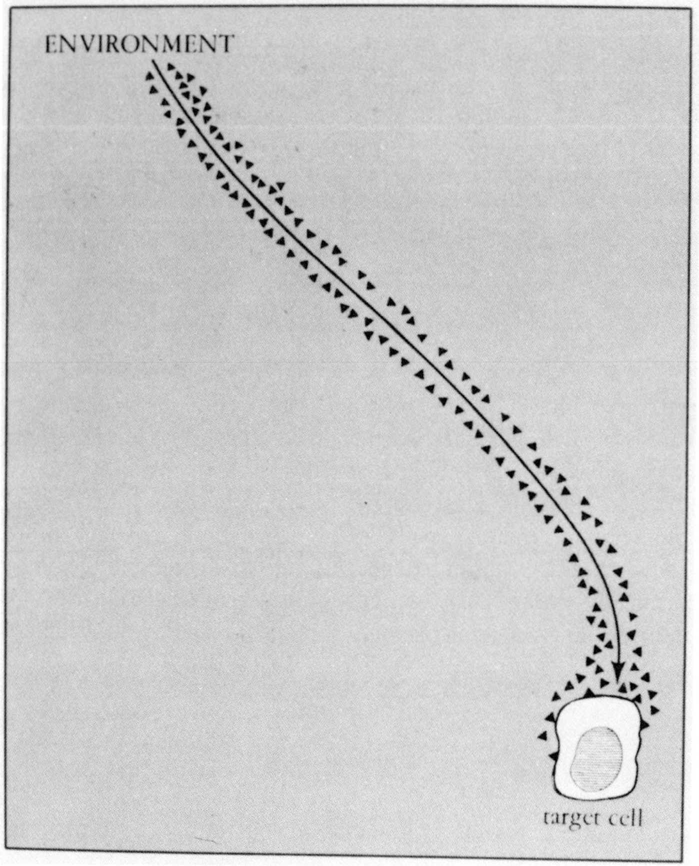

Fig. 2.   Effects of environmental agents on target cells. (From Bellanti, J. A., 1978, with permission from the publishers).

Phagocytic Cells

The phagocytic cells are those elements involved in the process of engulfment and uptake by particles from the external environment. Subsequent digestion of these substances may lead to their elimination. The phagocyte may be considered then as a barrier between the environment and the target cell protecting the target cell from subsequent injury (Figure 3, Table 2). In the human, phagocytosis is carried out primarily by mononuclear phagocytes (macrophages), neutrophils and eosinophils. There are a variety of chemical factors which are generated from the complement

Table 1.   Effects of the Environment on Target Cells.

LOCATION OF TARGET CELL	EXAMPLE OF EFFECT	RESULT
Skin	Disruption of epidermal cells	Dermatitis
Gastrointestinal tract		
Mucosal cell	Destruction	Gastrointestinal bleeding
Smooth muscle	Increased contractility	Diarrhea, vomiting
Glandular cell	Increased secretion	Increased mucus production
Respiratory tract		
Smooth muscle	Increased contraction	Bronchospasm
Glandular cell	Increased secretion	Increased mucus production
Circulatory system		
Endothelial cell	Increased intercellular pore size	Edema
Formed elements	Destruction of erythrocytes	Anemia

system or from lymphocytes which are involved in the mobilization of
these cells. The net effect of these processes is the movement of phagocytic
cells into areas into which their action is required for the protection of
target cells from injury.

Mediator Cells

Certain cells of the body contain macromolecules that have biologic
properties that can amplify the effects of the phagocytic cells or may have

Table 2.   Mobilization Factors and Functions of Phagocytic Cells.

PHAGOCYTIC CELL	AGENTS RESPONSIBLE FOR MOBILIZATION OF CELLS	CELL PRODUCT OR FUNCTION
Macrophages (monocytes)	Chemotactic factors, e.g., migration inhibitory factor (MIF), lymphokines	Processed immunogen, removal of environmental agent
Neutrophils	Chemotactic factors (complement-associated and bacterial factors), lymphokines	Kallikreins (producing kinins), SRS-A, basic peptides, ECF-A
Eosinophils	Identical with neutrophils, specific chemotactic factors, lymphokines	Ingestion of immune complexes, antagonize effects of mediators, e.g., SRS-A

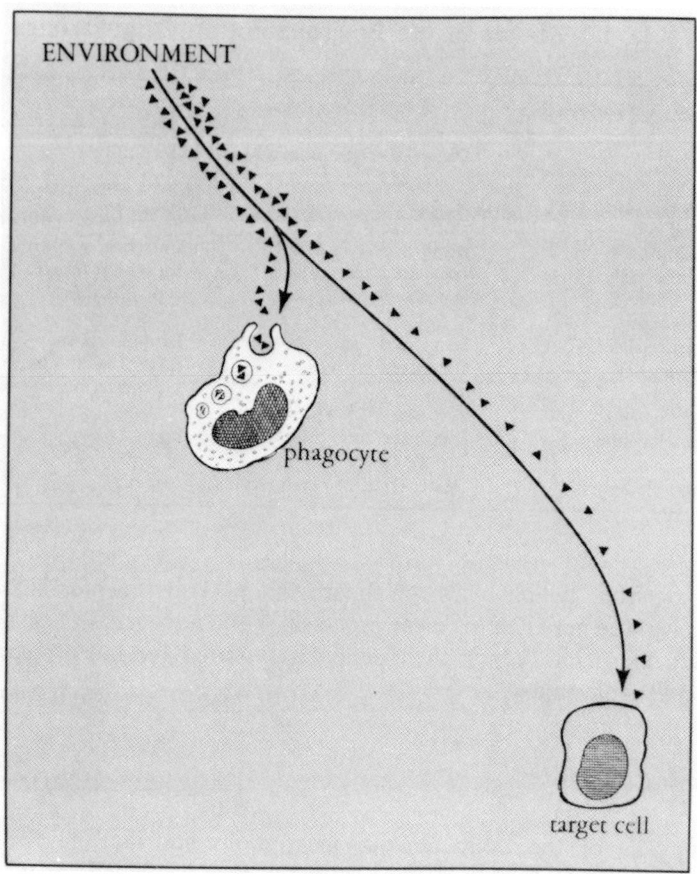

Fig. 3.   Phagocytic cells: Mobilization factors and functions. (From Bellanti, J. A., 1978, with permission from the publishers).

a direct effect on the target cells. These cells are referred to as mediator cells (Figure 4) and their products as mediators. Following their interaction with the environmental agent, these cells perform their function by the release of chemical substances having a wide variety of biologic effects e.g., the increase of vascular permeability or the enhancement of the inflammatory response. The mediator cells, like the target cells, represent a hetergeneous collection of morphologic types that include mast cells, basophils, platelets, enterochromaffin cells and neutrophils. The best studied of these are the mast cells and the basophils. The best studied of the mediator chemical substances are histamine, serotonin, and kinins.

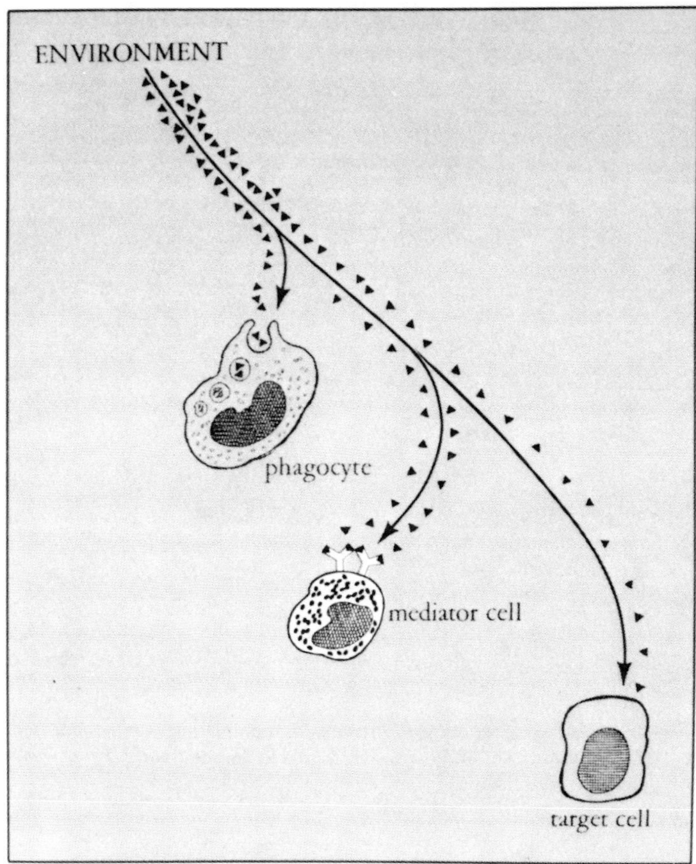

Fig. 4.   Mediator cells: Products (mediators) and functions. (From Bellanti, J. A., 1978, with permission from the publishers).

Cells of the Specific Immunologic System—the Specific Antigen Recognition System

These cells in contrast to those of the non-specific immunologic system interact with the environmental agent in a highly specific way and as described above are carried out primarily by two classes of lymphocytes, the B-lymphocytes and T-lymphocytes. The B-lymphocytes are those cells which ultimately respond to the environmental agent with the production of antibody. There are five classes of immunoglobulins, IgG, IgM, IgA, IgD and IgE each differing in physical, chemical and biologic properties.

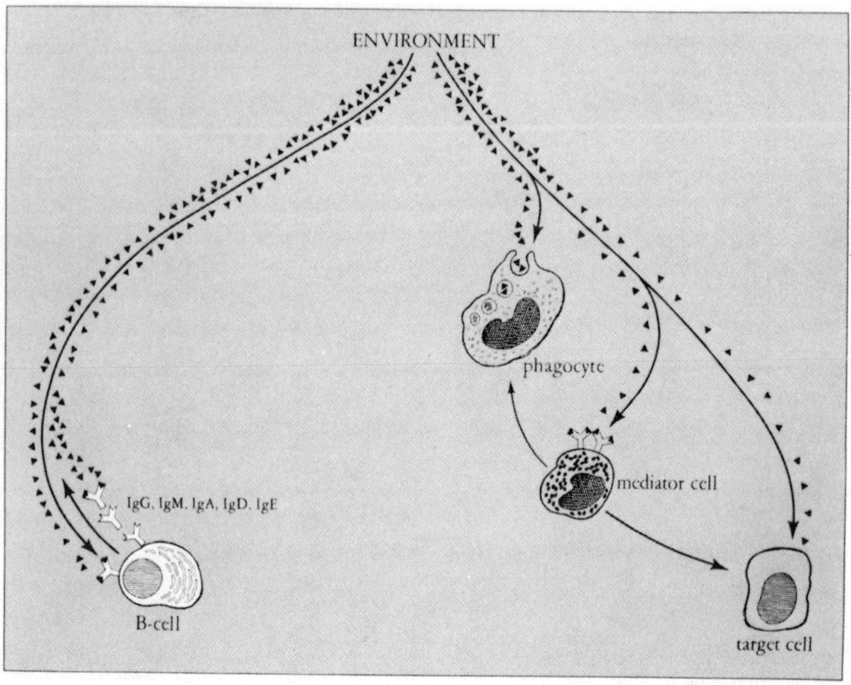

Fig. 5. Reaction of B-lymphocyte to environmental agent through its surface receptor, with resultant antibody production. (From Bellanti, J. A., 1978, with permission from the publishers).

These cell products can either directly interact with the environmental agent (Figure 5), can enhance phagocytosis (Figure 6), can respond with the mediator cells (Figure 7), or directly interact with a modified target cell (Figure 8).

The T-lymphocytes are those cells responsible for cell-mediated immunity and respond to the environmental agent through the interaction of receptors on the cell with the agent (Figure 9). Following the interaction of the environmental agent with the T-cell, a series of morphologic, biologic and biochemical events occur which may cause the cell to function directly or through the elaboration of certain products called the lymphokines. In addition, the T-lymphocyte can participate in the recognition of antigen on the surface of foreign target cells in any of three ways. The cell may participate in direct lymphocyte dependent cytotoxicity (Figure 10). It may respond through the elaboration of cytotoxin and lead to target cell destruction of certain subsets of lymphocytes, the killer or K

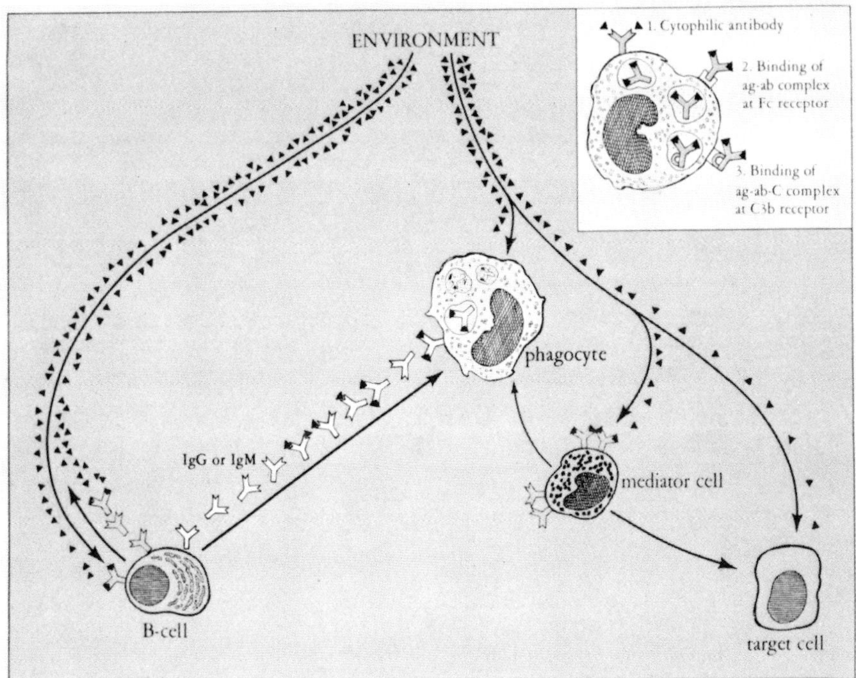

Fig. 6.   Responses of antibody with phagocytic cells. (From Bellanti, J. A., 1978, with permission from the publishers).

cells may lead to target cell destruction through an antibody dependent cytotoxicity (ADCC) reaction. The T-lymphocytes may also interact with the B cells in two ways (Figure 11). One, a subset of T cells, the helper cells, which can interact with B cells to facilitate the production of antibody and, two, another subset, the suppressor cells, which can inhibit the production of antibody. The macrophage may also interact with the T or B-lymphocytes through antigen presentation or processing of antigen or through the elaboration of lymphocyte activating factors (Figure 12).

Thus, the immunologic system may be viewed as a multicellular system involving the interaction of foreign substances with a wide variety of cell types (Figure 13). The immunologic responses may be either helpful or harmful. Those immunologic responses which are concerned with the recognition and disposal of foreignness leading to a beneficial response are termed "immunity". When the interaction of the immunologic components with the environmental agent is ineffective, the target cells may sustain injury as a result of the direct impact of the environmental agent

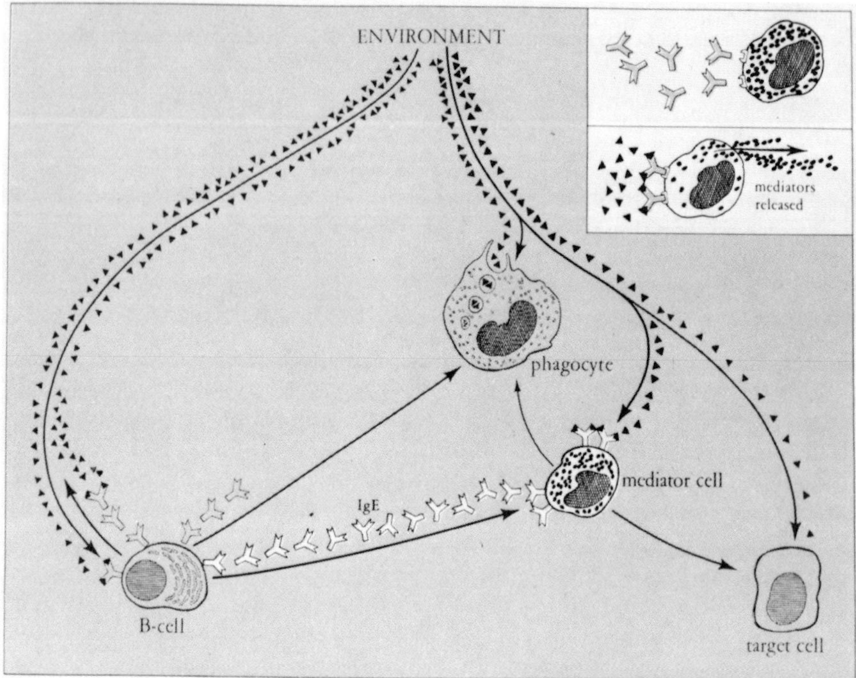

Fig. 7. Responses of antibody with mediator cells with resultant release of mediators (insert). (From Bellanti, J. A., 1978, with permission from the publishers).

in which case we refer to it as toxicity or the target cell may undergo modification with a mutagenic substance resulting in a new phenotypic expression or the environmental agent may serve as a carcinogen resulting in the malignant transformation. In all of these cases, there is the potential for the acquisition of new surface configurations on the altered cells which can be detected by immunologic techniques.

The Interaction of the Target Cell with the Environmental Agent

For ease of discussion, we may speak of two types of environmental agents which can interact with the target cell: (1) an agent which directly interacts with the DNA of the cell and specifies from within new surface configurations on the surface of the cell, and (2) a chemical agent which can modify the cell surface directly.

In the first type of interaction, we may speak of two types of agents:

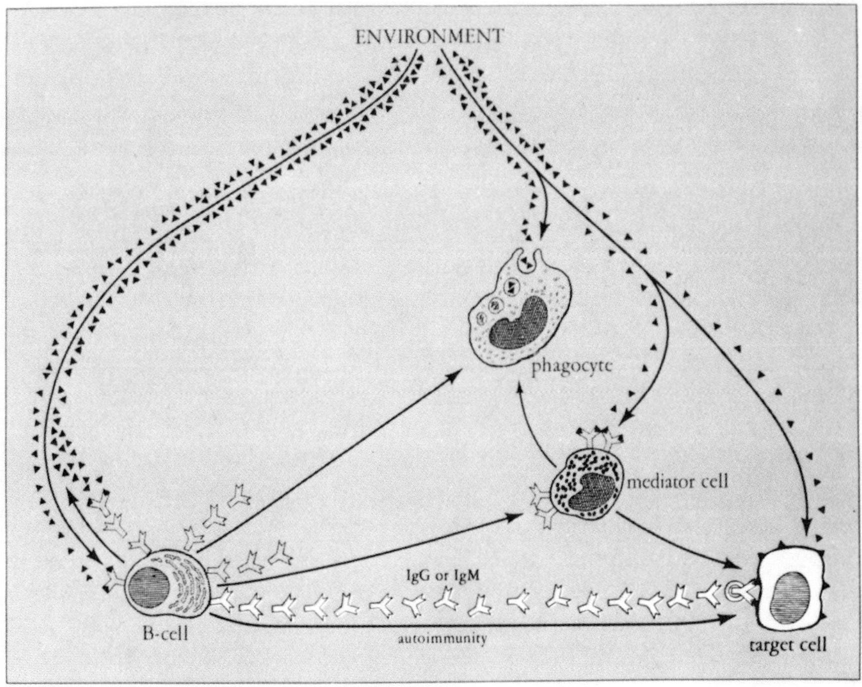

Fig. 8. Effects of antibody on target cells with resultant autoimmunity. (From Bellanti, J. A., 1978, with permission from the publishers).

(a) replicating agents such as viruses, and (b) non-replicating agents such as chemical mutagens or carcinogens. In the case of virus interactions with host cells, the viral DNA or a portion of the viral DNA may be incorporated within the host DNA and specific new viral proteins or non-viral constituents. In either case, the acquisition of surface configurations are the same following infection with a given virus regardless of the morphologic cell type (Figure 14). In contrast, the interaction of a chemical mutagen or carcinogen will vary depending upon the region of DNA in which the interaction occurs resulting in new cell surface configurations (Figure 15). In addition, it is now known that there is the emergence of embryonic antigens following the malignant transformation. This presumably occurs as schematically represented in Figure 16 where normal embryonic antigen produced by a functioning gene is repressed during maturation in the normal adult cell. Following derepression of the gene in a malignant cell upon the interaction with a carcinogenic agent,

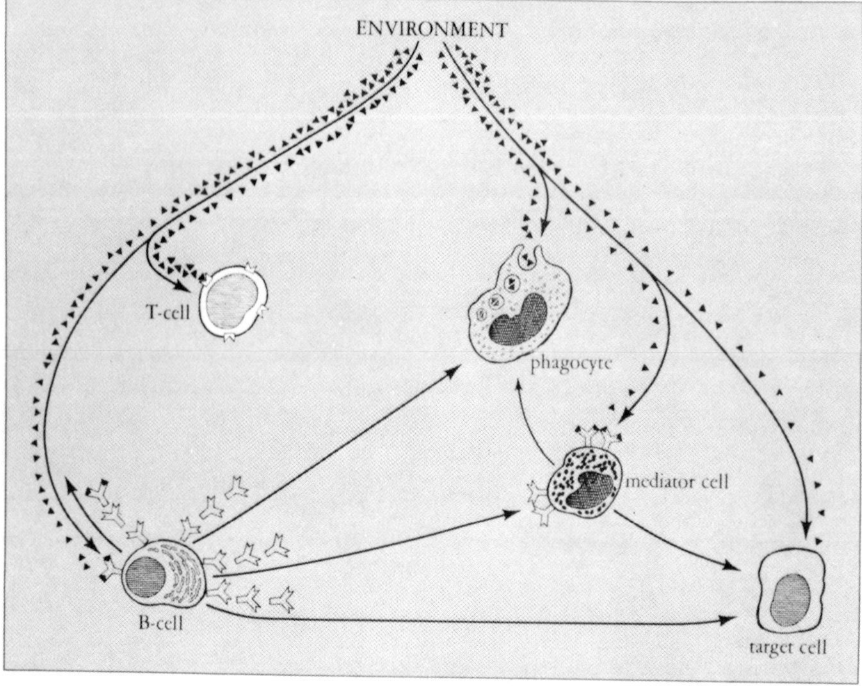

Fig. 9.   Reaction of T-lymphocyte to environmental agent through its surface receptor. (From Bellanti, J. A., 1978, with permission from the publishers).

there is the reappearance of an embryonic antigen on the surface of the cell.

Immunogenetic Studies of the Interaction of the Immune System with Modified Host Cells

As described above, the immune system consists of a highly complex network of components, both cellular and soluble, most of which are specifically encoded by specific gene products. Many genes are therefore involved in the control of cellular interactions within the immune system as well as the interaction with foreign configuration in the environment.

The major histocompatibility complex (MHC) in mammals is a single genetic region that determines the strong transplantation antigens and has a major influence on graft rejection. Not only is this region concerned with histocompatibility but it is now well recognized that certain immune

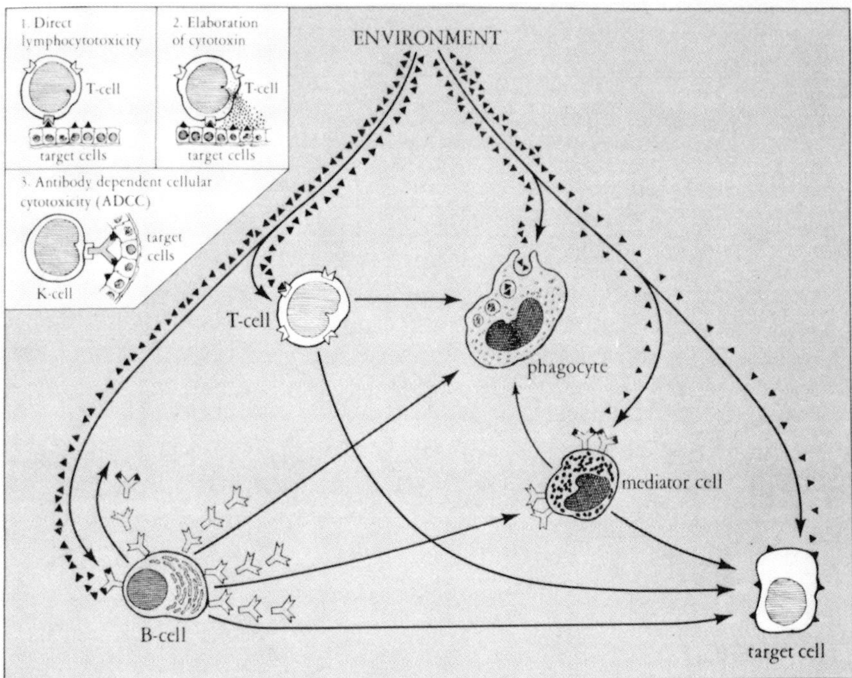

Fig. 10.   Responses of activated T-cells with foreign target cells. (From Bellanti, J. A., 1978, with permission from the publishers).

response genes are also encoded within the MHC regions in both mice and men.

For ease of discussion, the chromosomal fragment controlling immunologic phenomena in the mouse may be visualized as divided into four subregions (Figure 17): the K and D regions encode for surface antigens that are serologically detectible (SD regions) and recognized during graft rejection. The I or immune region appears to encode for antigenic receptors on T-lymphocytes and a group of interaction molecles, the Ia or I region associated molecules, found on the T and B-lymphocytes and a subpopulation of macrophages. The region controls the synthesis of serum complement components (Figure 17). The K and D regions are the regions recognized during graft rejection by cytotoxic T-lymphocytes. Recently, it has been shown that when cells are treated with viruses or chemical haptens, they seem to be specifically associated with the SD regions and cytotoxic T-lymphocytes are lytic only if the target cells that are modified with virus or chemical carry the same modifying antigen and

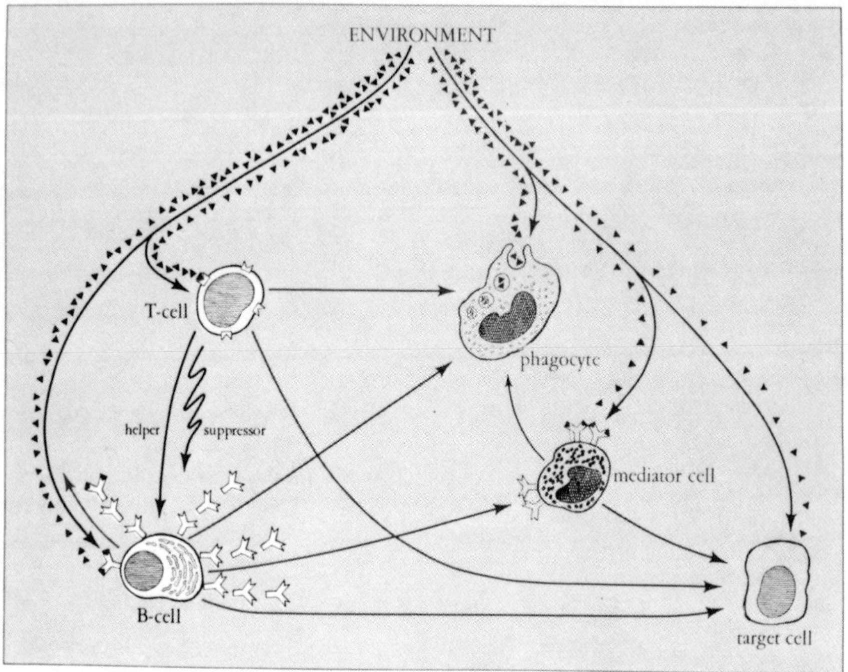

Fig. 11.   Helper and suppressor effects of T-lymphocytes on B-lymphocytes. (From Bellanti, J. A., 1978, with permission from the publishers).

the same K and D region molecules as the original stimulating cells (Figure 18).

In the case of viral infections (Zinkernagel *et al.*, 1977), it has been shown that cytotoxic T-lymphocytes from inbred strains of mice will only kill virus-infected target cells from strains which are genetically identical in the K and/or D regions of the MHC. A similar phenomenon has been observed in the case of chemical substances (Shearer *et al.*, 1977). The modification of autologous cells by the chemical trinitrophenol (TNP) is shown schematically in Figure 19. This scheme shows a two step procedure consisting of (1) the first step of sensitization, and (2) a second stage of the effector phase. In the first stage, following the interaction of responder cell A with stimulating cell A + X, which has been modified to include a viral or chemical product, there is the sensitization of the responder cell A. In the second stage, when the sensitized responder cell is then mixed with a variety of target cells, the reactions shown in the

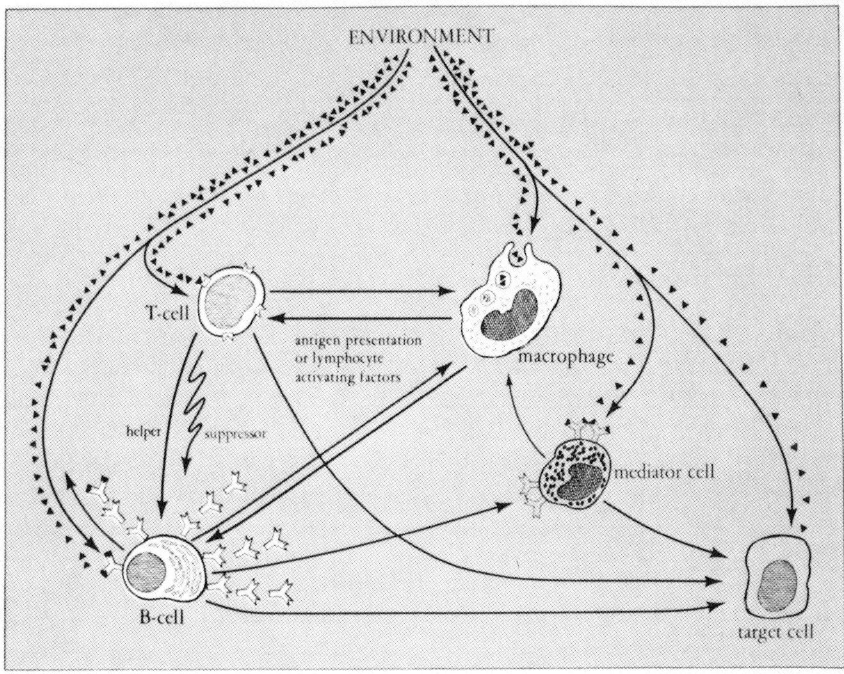

Fig. 12.   Responses of macrophages with T- and B-lymphocytes. (From Bellanti, J. A., 1978, with permission from the publishers).

figure are seen. The conclusions of this experiment are that there is (1) a genetic restriction for cell interaction and destruction, and (2) there is a requirement for an identical determinant which is immunologically specific and sensitive. More recent studies from Shearer's group are quite interesting and demonstrate a dose response relationship between the density of chemical on the cell surface and the genetically controlled ability of effector cells to respond in this reaction. When autologous cells are coated with high densities of hapten or chemical, all congenic strains of mice tested respond to such modified targets via cytolysis. When low densities of hapten are present on autologous cells, however, some congenic strains of mice are responders whereas other strains are non-responders (Shearer *et al.*, 1979). This latter response is under the control of an immune response gene located in the MHC of the mouse. Of major importance is whether a cytolytic response to chemically modified cells is (1) under

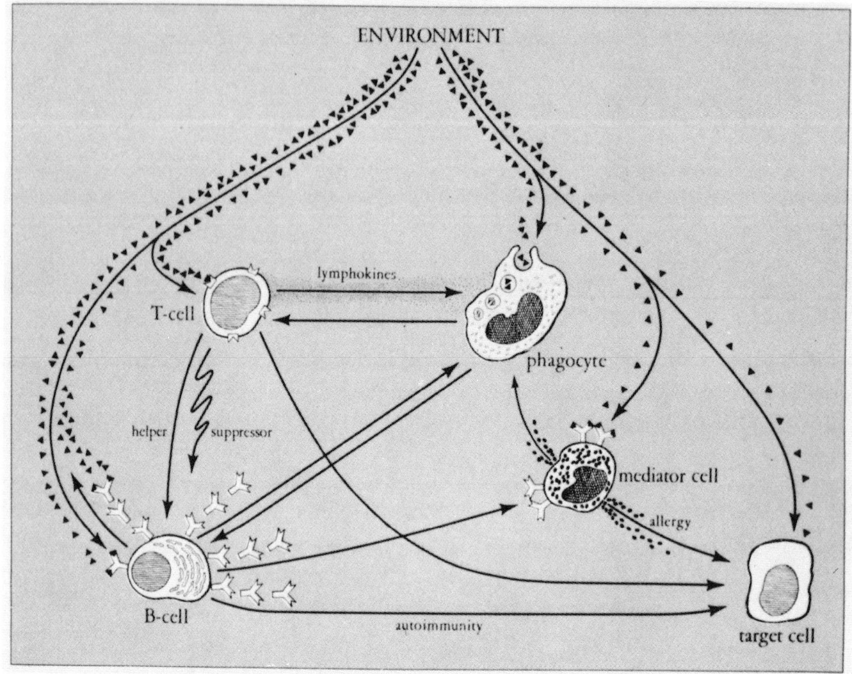

Fig. 13. Total array of immunologic responses to the environment. (From Bellanti, J. A., 1978, with permission from the publishers).

genetic control in the human, and (2) capable of altering the natural course or effect of chemicals on biologic systems (e.g., mutagenesis).

These observations may have profound significance in the design of future studies for the detection of immunotoxic agents as well as for the identification of individuals who may be genetically predisposed to the toxic effects of these agents. This genetic predisposition may be specific for the toxic effect of a given chemical or may represent a more general predisposition toward particular disease entities (e.g., autoimmunity, malignancy) which may be triggered by the exposure to one or more immunotoxic agents. Indeed, this latter possibility may explain the current inability to define the etiology of numerous disease states which are now considered idiopathic or which may masquerade as other disease entities. These may occur in individuals with a genetic predisposition where the disease state has been triggered by exposure to mulitple, rather than single, environmental insults.

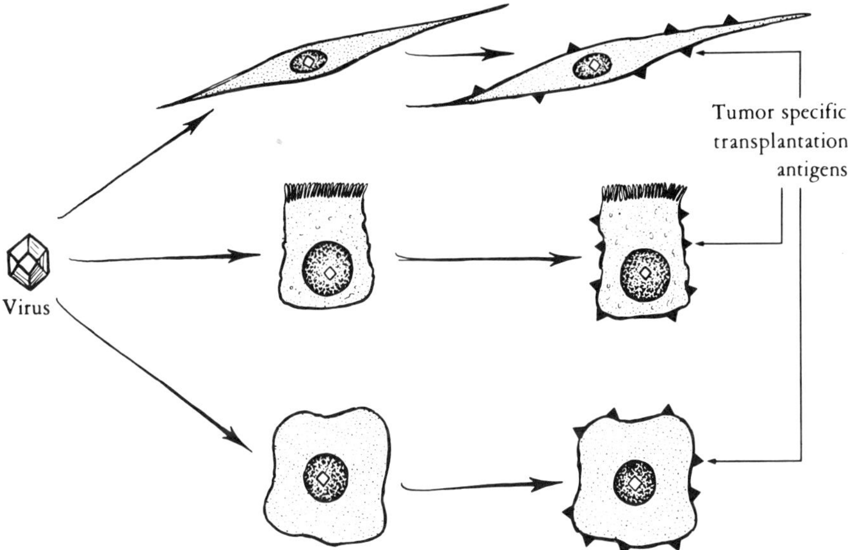

Fig. 14. Schematic representation of the development of tumor-specific antigens (TSA) by a tumor virus. Note that although the morphologic appearance may vary, each tumor induced by a single virus contains the same TSA on the cell surface. (From Bellanti, J. A., 1978, with permission from the publishers).

WORKING HYPOTHESIS OF THE ROLES OF VARIOUS ELEMENTS OF THE IMMUNE RESPONSE IN IMMUNOTOXICOLOGIC PROCESSES

It may now be possible to construct a hypothesis of the interactions of the various elements of the immune response that may be involved in the immunotoxicologic response(s) of the host to environmental substances. The summation of the total immunologic capability of the host to foreign configurations in the environment is shown schematically in Figure 20. There are three types of responses through which all foreign substances can proceed, the progression of which depends upon two factors: (1) the nature of the substance, and (2) the genetic constitution of the host.

The non-specific immune responses, the most primitive type, consist of those ancient responses to first encounter with a foreign configuration, phagocytosis and inflammation. If the substance, e.g., carbon particles, is completely eliminated at this stage, the host response terminates. These responses are not under genetic control and represent primitive endocytic

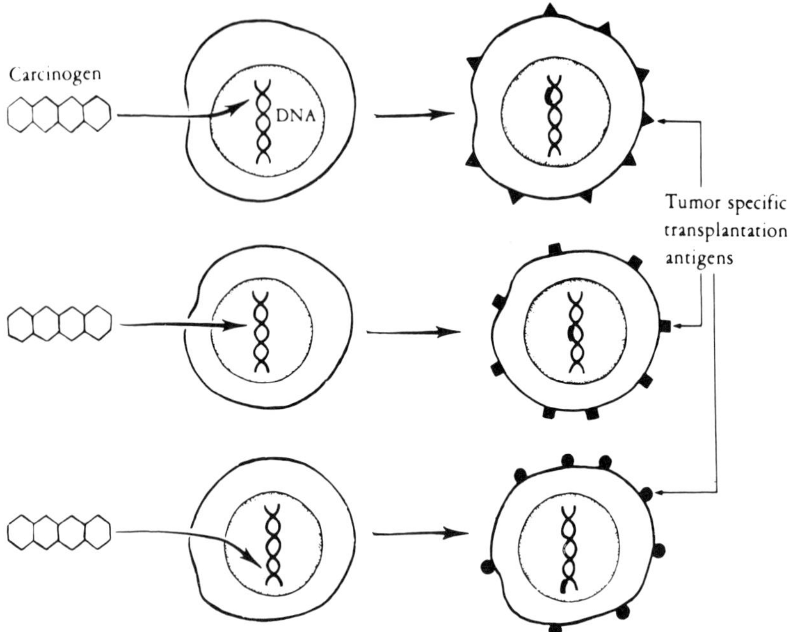

Fig. 15. Schematic representation of development of tumor antigens by a chemical carcinogen. Note that when cells of identical genetic identity are transformed by the same chemical carcinogen, each new tumor has its own unique antigenic specificity regardless of morphologic appearance. (From Bellanti, J. A., 1978, with permission from the publishers).

responses to a foreign configuration. Some substances, however, are not completely eliminated at this stage and may reflect antigen persistence.

If the primary encounter leads to a processed product, e.g., antigen, the specific immune responses are stimulated. These are more sophisticated responses and consist of two possible effector mechanisms: (1) B-lymphocyte mediated humoral immunity with the elaboration of antibody (IgE, IgG, IgM, IgA, IgD), and (2) T-lymphocyte mediated antigen elimination. A sophisticated addition to these mechanisms is the capacity to enhance the immunologic responses through the actions of complement, the coagulation sequence and a bank of memory cells when antigen is reencountered. These responses, in contrast to the non-specific responses are under strict genetic control in their own interaction as well as in their interaction with foreign configurations as will be described

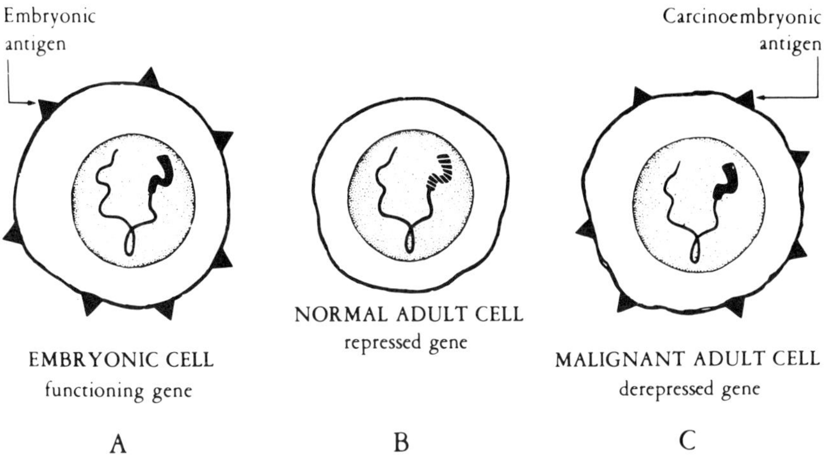

Fig. 16.   Postulated mechanism of emergence of carcinoembryonic antigens. A, A normal embryonic antigen produced by a functioning gene within an embryonic cell. B, Repression of the gene (*dotted line*) with no further elaboration of the embryonic antigen in the adult cell. C, Derepression of the gene in the malignant cell with reappearance of the embryonic antigen (carcinoembryonic antigen) on the surface of the cell. (From Bellanti, J. A., 1978, with permission from the publishers).

below. If antigen is successfully eliminated at this phase, the immunologic response terminates. Normally, most antigens are successfully eliminated at this stage without detriment to the host. If antigen still persists, the tissue damaging responses are called into play. Antigen persistence may result from the nature of the antigen itself or from some genetic defect in antigen elimination. If antigen persists, four types of immunologic interactions can be elicited: types I, II, III, and IV. These responses are no longer beneficial to the host and are manifested as disease phenomena, the immunologically mediated diseases. These may be either temporary or permanent depending upon the efficiency of antigen elimination. If antigen can be removed or eliminated, the tertiary response is terminated with minimal discomfort to the patient. However, if the tertiary response is ineffective, and antigen still persists, the more harmful sequelae of the immune response emerge which represent a maximal deleterious and self-perpetuating attack of an aberrant immune response in which the host sustains injury. These are commonly associated with allergic or the hypersensitivity diseases or with the autoimmune diseases where the immune response is

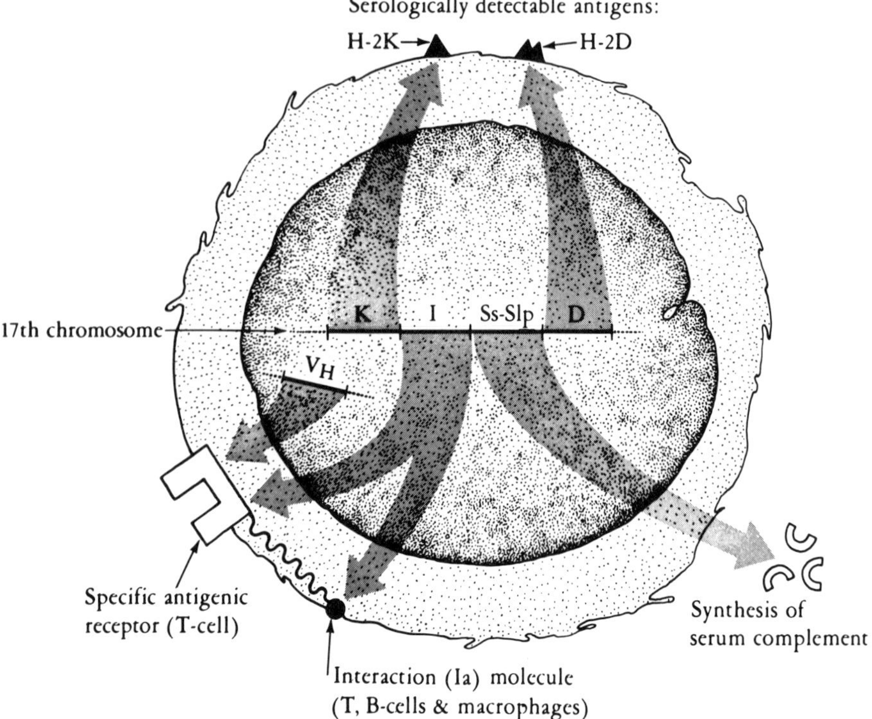

Fig. 17. Schematic representation of the chromosomal sites and gene products of the major histocompatibility complex of the mouse (H-2). (From Bellanti, J. A., 1978, with permission from the publishers).

directed against self. It has also been postulated that a failure in surveillance with persistence of antigen could also be involved in the malignant transformation.

Future Prospects and Concluding Remarks

Immunotoxicology may be defined as the study of the harmful effects of environmental agents on the immunologic system. These include the wide variety of responses resulting from simple chemicals and trace elements to more complex interactions involving pesticides, insecticides, food products and food additives. In addition, we may also begin to direct our attention to the role of these substances in the pathogenesis of allergic

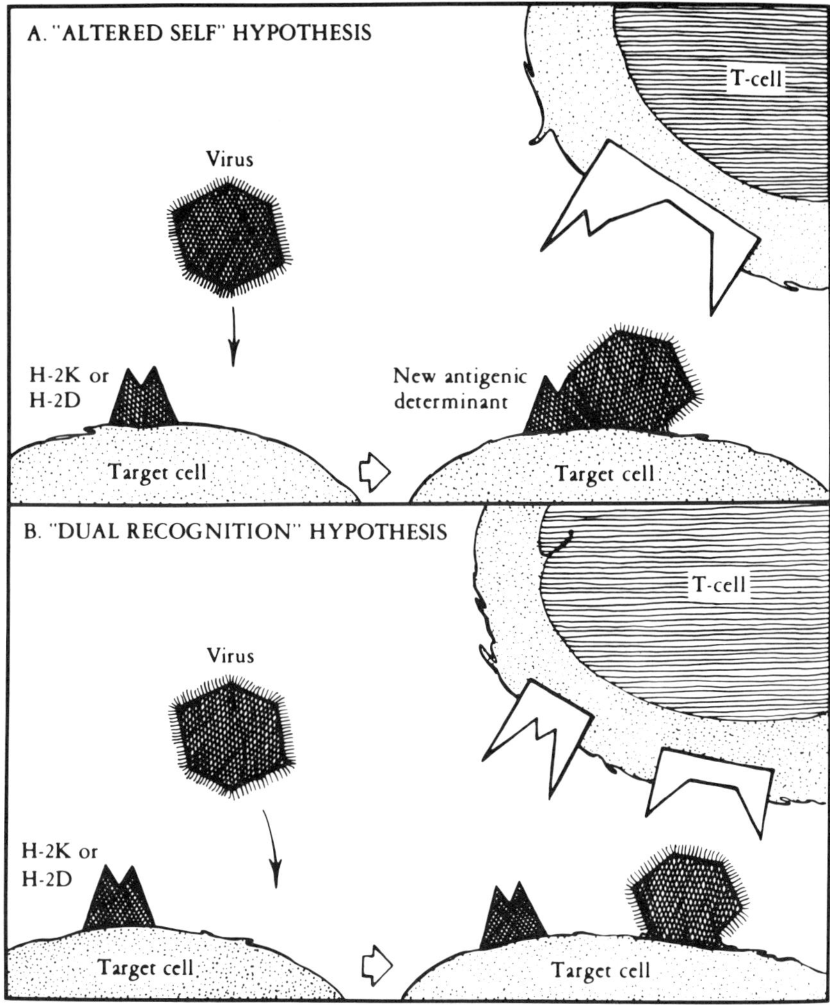

Fig. 18. Schematic representation of two hypotheses of genetic restriction concerned with recognition of virus-infected target cells by cytotoxic lymphocytes. (From Bellanti, J. A., 1978, with permission from the publishers).

and autoimmune disorders and malignancy, long suspected to have an environmental basis.

It is obvious from the discussions of this Conference that the diverse components which comprise immunotoxicology will require the participation of an equally diverse group of a variety of disciplines including the

Step 1 Sensitization	Responder Cell "A"	Stimulatory Cell "A + x" [1]	
Step 2 Effector Phase	Sensitized Responder Cell	Target Cell	Reaction
	A	A	0
	A	A + x	+
	A	B + x	0
	A	A + y	0
	A	A + x′ [2]	0

[1] A + x = Cell of genotype A modified with cell surface viral or chemical determinant, x.
[2] A + x′ = Cell A modified with cross-reacting determinant, x′.

Fig. 19.   Two-step Reaction for Test to Modified Self (after Shearer, *et al.*, 1977).

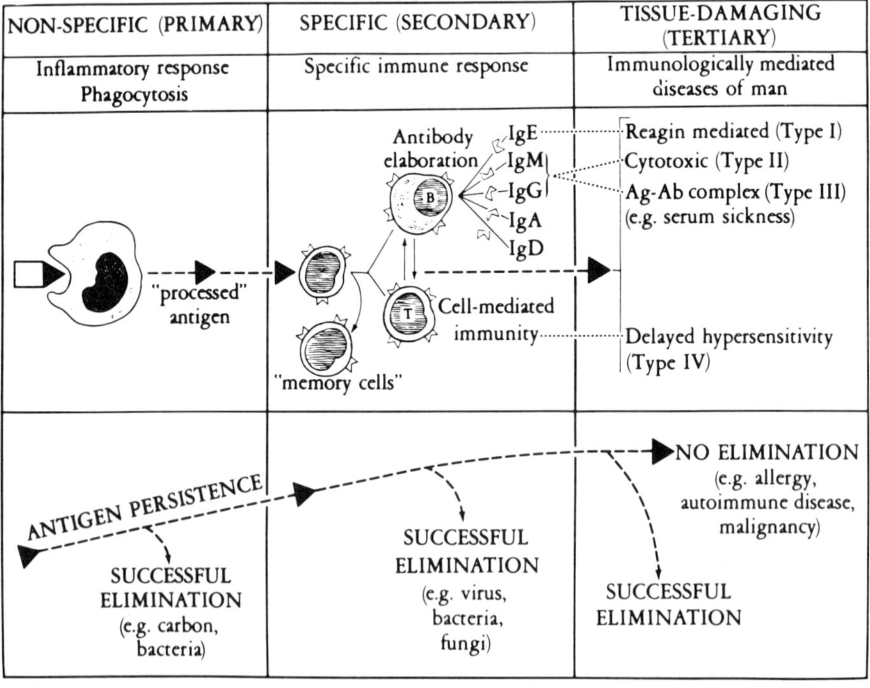

Fig. 20.   Schematic representation of the total immunologic capability of the host based upon efficiency of elimination of foreign matter (From Bellanti, J. A., 1978, with permission from the publishers).

basic sciences of chemistry, biology, pharmacology and toxicology as well as the clinical disciplines of medicine, pediatrics, obstetrics, surgery and veterinary medicine. There will also be a need for more research with a particular emphasis on studies of the developing host because of the great vulnerability of the developing fetus to these toxic substances.

In this particular age when the emphasis is on environmental health and disease prevention, immunotoxicology will be paramount not only in these next decades, but also as we approach the 21st century. The interdisciplinary approach must also involve an effective alliance between the federal agencies with the scientific communities and the public. An effective dialogue must be established which will demonstrate to the nation that science and technology can progress simulaneously under the energizing force of social commitment. Not only will this involve the need for research but an expanded need for innovative training and educational programs for the training of young investigators in this rapidly developing and important field of immunotoxicology.

REFERENCES

1. Bellanti, J. A.: Immunology II. W. B. Saunders, Philadelphia, 1978.
2. Moore, J. A.: The immunotoxicology phenomenon. Drug and Chem. and Toxicol., *2*(1 and 2):1, 1979.
3. Zinkernagel, R., Doherty, P. C., Effres, R. B. and Bennink, J.: Heterogeneity of the cytotoxic response of thymus-derived lymphocytes after immunization with influenza viruses. Proc. Nat. Acad. Sci., *74*:1209, 1977.
4. Shearer, G. M. and Schmitt-Verhulst, A. M.: Major histocompatibility complex restricted cell-mediated immunity. Adv. Immunol.,*25*:55, 1977.
5. Shearer, G. M., Schmitt-Verhulst, A. M., Pettinelli, C. B., Miller, M. W., and Gilheany, P. E.: H-2-linked genetic control of murine T-cell-mediated lympholysis to autologous cells modified with low concentrations of trinitrobenzene sulfonate. J. Exper. Med., *149*:1407, 1979.
6. Bellanti, J. A.: Allergy and clinical immunology: An interdisciplinary concept. Ann. Allergy,*41*:129, 1978.

DISCUSSION

DEAN: I would like to start the discussion by asking for questions or comments from the audience.

BOORMAN: I'd like to make a comment. One thing that was not completely covered in this conference was the subject of progenitor and hemapoietic stem cells. Most scientists, when they illustrate the immune system in overview, include stem cells or progenitor cells; the remainder of their presentation deals only with the mature lymphoid system. I would like to suggest that probably we should also be looking at bone marrow progenitor and stem cells as part of the immune system. I think there are two basic reasons why this would have application to immunotoxicolgy.

First, chemicals can have a direct effect on hemopoietic stem cell and progenitor cells and this may affect the immune system. The second application is that the mature cells of the immune system, primarily the macrophage, play an important role in hematopoiesis. It has been well documented that the macrophage produces both prostaglandins and colony-stimulating factor which have a very nice positive/negative effect on bone marrow hematopoiesis. Mature lymphocytes have also been shown to affect the bone marrow with supressor cells causing anemia.

There is a rapidly growing body of knowledge on clonal growth of progenitor and stem cells. The assays are very easy to perform and can measure macrophage-granulocyte, megakaryocyte, and erythroid progenitors. Both B- and T-lymphocyte colonies can also be grown in culture.

DEAN: Dr. Boorman, would you describe for us chemicals that have shown an effect on bone marrow progenitor cells?

BOORMAN: I think we have done some work in that regard. We have shown that PBB's have very little effect on macrophage-granulocyte progenitors with slight enhancement at the lower dose that also causes mitogen enhancement. With tetrachloro-p-dibenzodioxin (TCDD), we find decreased numbers of both hemopoietic stem cells (CFUS) and macrophage-granulocyte progenitors. Dr. Luster showed some data this morning on the effect of DES on both macrophage–granulocyte progenitors and hemopoietic stem cells.

DEAN: If I remember correctly, wasn't it carbon tetrachloride and some of the sulfa drugs that were found to be bone marrow suppressants?

BOORMAN: Correct.

KERMAN: I am well aware of the alphabet soup that we all generate, but I am not a toxicologist, and I would appreciate definitions of the nomenclature that is being tossed around the table, and has been for the last two days; PBB's and PCB's, and HCB's et cetera? In the ensuing discussion may we please have definitions?

DEAN: Dr. Moore, would you like to comment?

MOORE: PCB's are polychlorinated biphenyls; PBB's, polybrominated biphenyls; TCDD is more correctly called dioxin; you don't want to know the full name! I should like to respond to an earlier comment of mine that apparently puzzled or hypersensitized Dr. Bellanti! I think my comment stems from two facts: One, if you look at hypersensitization as an accepted and well established immune phenomenon, then indeed exposure to certain chemicals leads to hypersensitization. One doesn't have to look very far to find examples that are classically accepted. However, I think immunosuppression as a sequela of environmental chemical exposure, is not well accepted, let alone barely understood. Therefore, the principal reason I omitted hypersensitization from my remarks this morning is that I thought my introductory comments should relate to the presentations before us.

BELLANTI: I wonder if the panel would care to comment on whether, in any forward-moving program involving immunotoxicology, there should be a broader inclusion of cells and cell components and mechanisms to which I alluded?

SIGEL: Dr. Dean, may I respond now as Dr. Bellanti's presentation gives me an excellent point of departure. One is always faced with the dilemma of lumping or splitting, saturating with large doses, or diluting the exposure to small levels of toxicants over long time intervals. There is no doubt that one can cause toxicity by excessive doses of chemicals. Sometimes this is necessary to prove carcinogenicity which would otherwise require years of observation. But if this becomes the sole tactic we may face a lose of credibility. The problem often lies in the methodology which is not sufficiently sensitive to the effects of low doses. It behooves us therefore to look to additional methods which would predict for potential toxicity in a more sensitive way. In developing such methods we should search for criteria and parameters of biological activity evoked by chemical dosage levels representative of those encountered in various environmental situations. This is not to suggest that we do away with dose-response studies or ignore cumlative effects, but rather that we commit more of our resources to ways and means of detecting meaningful effects by low doses brought about by short exposures. The immune mechanism should provide a highly suitable target for such studies provided the workings of its various components to environmental toxicants are identified. There are five unique attributes of the immune system that make it predictively valuable:

1.) Results can be obtained in a matter of days as opposed to the months which are required for standard carcinogenic studies.

2.) Enough is known about the role of various cellular populations and subpopulations of the immune mechanism so that assessment can be made of the impact of chemical agents on T-helper cells, T-suppressor cells, B-cells, or macrophages. You have heard yesterday and today some evidence for this.

3.) There is emerging a precise recognition of different stages of cellular development in immunology, more so than with other types of cells. The participation of these cells and their products in unique functions, both inductive and regulatory, permits a close scrutiny of the action of chemicals on individual or unique stages of differentiation, function, and interaction.

4.) With proper manipulation of the host and the enrichment or depletion of cellular subsets, it is possible to make discriminatory determinations of specific or selective modes of action of chemicals. Immunology is unique in this respect.

5.) The immune response consists of separate steps that were discussed both in the first presentation and in the summation by Dr. Bellanti: Recognition, cell member perturbations, cell proliferation, protein synthesis, effector function. Under proper conditions, it is possible to separate these steps and to determine the action of chemicals on these specific events. Thus, even if a chemical in low dose will not lyse lymphocytes, it may cause subtle changes, e.g., alter expression or configuration of membrane receptors. This alteration may not be grossly visible but may be detected by immunologic fine tuning. Without losing sight of the importance of multiple parameters, immunology must play a key role, in fact a central role, in the creation of a realistic system of recognition and assessment of environmental hazards.

DEAN: Thank you, Dr. Sigel. I think these points are agreed upon by most of us here. Dr. Luster, do you have a comment?

LUSTER: I agree with Dr. Sigel that we should probably emphasize studies with low-level chronic exposures, or even prenatal, postnatal exposures, which are better examples of what may occur in the human situation. I do feel, though, that in some instances the major concern is not what the exposure levels are in general population, but rather what may occur following an inadvertent or occupational exposure, representing therefore an acute exposure. There are many examples of this in large populations, some occurring with PBB's in the Michigan incident, with 245T in the Oregon population or with agent orange in Vietnam veterans. I suppose asbestos would fall in that same category, as well as that to which battery workers have been exposed.

DEAN: Of equal relevance is the problem of bioaccumulation, that is, deposition and concentration of a chemical in tissue. I think Drs. Moore and Bekesi spoke to that problem, at least as it relates to halogenate aeromatic hydrocarbons in which there is an accumulation of the chemical in body fat and then presentation to the immune system. Thus, chronic low-level exposure may lead to bioaccumulation of effective doses of the chemical.

LUSTER: To finish that comment there is one more thing. I think one should look at the toxicologic effects in these studies. One has to be very careful to look at the overt toxicity that's occurring in the animals; because obviously if one sees any overt toxicity, studies on immunocompetence would be relatively meaningless.

ZWILLING: Dr. Dean, I think Dr. Sigel's point is well taken, but I'm afraid we may be missing his point. I think what he's saying is that if the compound is immunologically relevant, it may not take a large dose of that compound to effect an immunological change. It may take a very, very small amount to cause a change, provided one is looking at the right parameter.

KATELEY: Most of the studies reviewed at this meeting were performed in laboratory animals, with the exception of those by Dr. Bekesi. I wonder if he could review for us which immunological studies he believes may be necessary for human immunotoxicity testing. And then perhaps some of the panel members may offer suggestions on other test systems which may be applied.

BEKESI: I don't want to repeat myself. Yesterday I stated that the support for this investigation was initiated during the middle of this year when we were given funds to look in depth into what is truly happening. I can only speculate and I will not do that at this time. I feel at a future meeting I will be able to respond better to that question.

Unfortunately Dr. Selikoff could not come yesterday to give his presentation on asbestos where we have some 7,000 exposed individuals who are at least 25 years old. Some are heavy smokers, other non-smokers. In this group we have a unique opportunity to study both what precedes malignant condition and the malignancy itself. In general, we have seen three well-differentiated groups of mesothelioma patients in terms of immunological competence. Those who, despite massive tumor burden have shown normal immune function and no serum-blocking factors, have the best chance for long-term survival, often without treatment.

KATELEY: To repeat the question: What battery of tests are you using for a human immunotoxicity profile? This is what I want a feeling for. Not your results, but the direction you believe human immunotoxicity testing is going.

BEKESI: We are just beginning to understand the meaning of immunological data in exposed individuals. The battery of *in vitro* immunodiagnostic tests include surface markers for the quantification of lymphocytes, lymphocyte function tests, immunoglobulins and complement tests designed to evaluate the individual's ability to combat infections. *In vivo* immunocompetence is tested by DCH response to five recall antigens.

DEAN: I had proposed this morning, with little resistance, that one of the major end points in assessment of a chemical's effect should be alteration in host resistance. That's the consensus of this group on that subject; what about the correlations or lack thereof between changes in immune parameters and alterations of host resistance? Should host resistance be evaluated as an endpoint for immune alteration? Dr. Roberts, do you have a comment?

ROBERTS: Impaired host resistance to infectious agents is a critical parameter in the assessment of toxic substances. It is essential to keep in mind that, while a substance may cause deflections in various tests of immune function, these changes must be related to adverse health effects to be considered deleterious. Successful resolution of infection involves mobilization of the many cell types involved in immune responses and a delicate balance and appropriate interactions of many factors. These immune responses are important in the context that they mediate defense against bacterial, viral, parasitic, and neoplastic disease. It is quite probable that many immune responses have no clear relationship to protection. Furthermore, impairment in one aspect of immunity may induce or be accompanied by a compensatory protective increase in another immune parameter. I feel that examining the impact of compounds of regulatory concern on host resistance and on the acquisition of immunity is the best way to document important effects on the immune system. Measurement of changes in host resistance to infectious challenge emphasizes those parameters of immunity which are similar in mouse and in man and have importance in the clearly interpretable context of morbidity and mortality If immunotoxicology is to have an important future role, it must compare favorably with carcinogenesis and mutagenesis approaches and be either more sensitive or produce additional useful data regarding adverse health effects. In this context, it is important to recognize that, in contrast to many systems, the immune system is a potential system in which a lesion may go unrecognized in the absence of challenge. I think that many others here would agree with me on the importance of host resistance. Dr. Leland Loose, for one, has said many times that host resistance is the "bottom line" in examining the effect of a toxicant on the well-being of the host.

BELLANTI: I'd like to respond to that question, if I may, Dr. Dean. There is no question that the models that have been presented are well-established; they are very fine models for measuring resistance to infection and, when there is significant impairment of the immune system, exposure to viruses or bacteria, there will be increased susceptibility to infection.

I come back again to the over-all human situation, and I don't mean to minimize the 7,000 Americans who have been exposed to asbestos, which I abhor and feel is a tragedy. However, I am also concerned about the 35 million, or perhaps 50 million Americans, who suffer from other kinds of immunologically mediated diseases, which may not be so life-threatening, but which may lead to significant morbidity, human suffering, absenteeism, and recurrent acute infections. I don't know if this is true, but if the data that I've heard from Dr. Archer and others of additives and various substances in the environment that can significantly reduce human immune responses, the question is: Is there a disease that these individuals are suffering from? Otherwise we come back to the era of "echoviruses," viruses in search of a disease. I know that these are tips of the iceberg; that we are familiar with these acute exposures. My appeal is for more knowledge about these other kinds of exposures leading to significant disease. Only with this information can we develop the models in tandem. Otherwise we end up generating lots and lots of data, which we are all capable of doing, but what is the significance of that data?

KATELEY: I would like to make a comment at this time. In the hospital we see many patients with immunological problems which makes me think about the animal models for autoimmune disease, IgE-mediated responses. In addition to the normals that have been studied in the last few years, it seems to me that perhaps someone should study the effect of chemical exposure on these potentially immunologically altered animal models to see if it exacerbates these responses or exactly what happens.

McCOY: Let me raise the question right now which I think needs to be posed, and that is: Are we willing to make a commitment to perform the basic studies, long-term studies, and studies of the autoimmune and allergy phenomenon that are being pointed out as critical issues of investigation? The people to make those potential commitments are here today and I think that we have to ask ourselves: Is the timing right; are we at the point where we can make such research commitments? If we are, can we methodically and scientifically design the studies so as to get the task done properly? I think that is the crucial issue coming out of this meeting.

DEAN: I would agree with what Dr. McCoy said regarding a need for basic studies and I would then ask Dr. Bellanti if he considers many of the diseases he sees in the clinics to be environmentally related.

BELLANTI: That's the question. I happen to believe that that they are. We are currently involved in studies to prove this possibility. By the way, I'm not trying to minimize basic studies. I think two approaches need to be done. One is the predictive approach, i.e., the building-block type of approach; the other is the phenomenologic, i.e., the clinical investigation of environmentally induced disease in the human or the experimental animal. I think both approaches should be used in tandem. Based on my experience in dealing with allergists and with patients, the magnitude of the real or perceived problems with food additives in this country is unbelievable. Hyperactivity and other problems are perceived to occur from chemicals. I'm making a plea for more research without trying to minimize the studies of autoimmune disease or malignancy which have emotional appeal. I'm talking about studies in addition to these, not substituting for them. Look for other kinds of more subtle immunologic lesions which give rise to human misery.

KERMAN: Dr. Dean, in support of Drs. Bellanti and McCoy, the question that I think we all need to ask ourselves is: Is the government necessarily willing to accept the problems of 1) We have no real good data clinically in terms of defining normal, clinical, immune response; 2) What is the consequence of a longitudinal study on the same individuals across the United States under different environments, different pollutants, different influences of stress; and then definition of populations at risk vis-a-vis industries, and a longitudinal study of them. This is not a one-year study; it's not a three-year study; it's potentially a 20- or 30-year study! And if somebody doesn't start it today, we're not going to have an opportunity 30 years from now because by then we will be suffering the consequences. The questions raised by Drs. Bellanti and McCoy, I think, go to the heart of the issue, and I'm not sure that it's a question of whether we have the tools to do it. I think we do. It's a matter of whether we've got the guts to do it and say to the government: We're not going to give you an answer tomorrow and there's not going to be a publication six, nine, or eighteen months from now. We're going to begin right now to accumulate data and a record book on ourselves!

DEAN: Very good point.

STEVENSON: Dr. Bellanti's remark about the echo viruses strikes a very responsive chord as I was involved in work at the bench during that period. One of the things that was apparent was that the epidemiologists, who were interested in poliovirus, hepatitis, and the more severe enteric virus problems, with their tools, could not identify any health problems existing with these so-called orphan viruses. The reason was that the kinds of problems that these viruses caused were usually not life-threatening. People came down with diarrhea for a day or two. They didn't present to the family physician because it was just the "summer bug" that they were going to get over anyhow. I'm sure that there were literally hundreds of thousands of cases which one could pick up when one sampled sewage. We did this in a study at a boy's camp, and traced these viruses passing in and out of the population; however, they were not at a level of concern to the epidemiological community. I'm sure you have the same thing in immunotoxicology. People who work in plants get atopic dermatitis and have problems of this type. Yes, they're inconvenienced; but their lives are generally not threatened and, unless a severe allergy develops, they may not even present to the company nurse.

So one has a whole system here to look at and, if you are going to get down to the fairly low levels that Dr. Sigel was describing, the real doses that you find in the environment, you will have to sharpen your levels of sensitivity.

SIGEL: Dr. Dean, in direct response to your question about the validity of the model that you discussed, i.e., tumor resistance, and so on, I think this type of model is quite valuable. In fact, it probably should be the point of reference for all other models, because if we are going to look at macrophages, suppressor cells, blastogenic transformations, or whatever, *in vitro* or even *in vivo* (skin reactivity), we must relate them to something: the patient, an outbreak of an unusual problem in an industrial plant, experimental infections, or an animal tumor. Only then can we really ascertain which of our various parameters are relevant to the real world. So your model is important as part of the total testing system.

LaVIA: Dr. Dean, I have a central question in relation to your comment. You said something about host defense, and I don't know that we have a difinition of that yet since it is very complex. I've been here a day-and-a-half listening very carefully and what I will say may be redundant after what Drs. Bellanti, Kerman, and Kateley have said. We are confronted by a population of humans who have various diseases and who are affected by environmental agents. In the clinical laboratory, we have the means to study these things. You've done a lot of work together with people at NCI and know this well. We have these techniques and we would like to apply them. How do we do it? It's going to take maybe 10 or 15 years to start getting patterns. Definitely, it is not going to be a short-term thing. It's not going to be something publishable in a hurry. And the question is perhaps the same one that Dr. Kerman raised: Is a commitment going to be made?

DEAN: I sense that some members of the panel are proposing that we should test exposed people for immune alterations in order to accumulate a data base. I do not feel we are ready for large-scale testing or that it would be dollar-effective. I feel Dr. Bellanti's approach is better. First, do good epidemiology studies to select groups for immunologic alterations.

I think that in the meantime we have to validate the assays and show better correlation between alterations and host resistance and changes in immunologic parameters. We cannot afford to do all the tests that have been proposed here.

In summation, then, I think that Dr. Bellanti's approach to human studies is probably the correct one. First, collect the epidemiology data and the animal data in order to validate assays. Begin to show relationships! Then when these tasks are complete, we might select patient populations or exposed groups to examine for immunologic defects.

KERMAN: In answer to that, in discussion with Dr. Bekesi in regard to his studies in Michigan, Wisconsin, and New York, he stated that in fact normals in New York are not comparable with normals in Wisconsin. I think that we perhaps have a naive view of controls, and I do not believe that we have a medical history or historical point of view of immunology in terms of whatever tools we have at hand. We have to start and I think that, in terms of epidemiology, there are reasons why there is more breast cancer in New York and Chicago than in Los Angeles, and there are reasons why there is more of some other carcinoma in some areas of the country and not in others. We have not approached this question. In the short run, infectious disease and tumor challenge are fine. I'm not saying not to do that. But somebody has got to take the perspective and long view. Otherwise we'll never have the information.

DEAN: I think your suggestion to examine immunologic profiles of individuals on sustained immunotherapy in order to maintain a transplant would provide very useful information in order to evaluate groups exposed to a chemical with suspect immunologic effects.

KERMAN: The question that's being raised by Dr. Bellanti in terms of hypersensitive disease is: Does the fact that people who have hypersensitive diseases or even subclinical hypersensitive states lead subsequently to a serious lesion 5 or 20 years from now? We don't know the answer to that.

BELLANTI: That's not the question I'm asking, though. I'm just content knowing whether it leads to hypersensitivity disease—period! If it leads to more prolonged disease of course it's more important.

But the point I was trying to make was very clearly summarized by Dr. Dean, and I won't repeat it. He said it much better than I.

DEAN: That wouldn't be possible! Let's take a question from the floor, please.

STEELE: I'm a clinical immunotoxicologist—if there is such a vocation! I've been guided in all my studies with a clinical correlate and I have to agree, certainly, with Dr. Bellanti's eloquent presentation that this should be the guide, at least for me, personally. For instance, I can tell you that children with the fetal alcohol syndrome, and alcohol is certainly an immunotoxicant, have meningitis sepsis and also seroviral infections. So the assays I would like to do would be to examine both cellular immunity and humoral immunity.

I would like to go back to the presentations here, however, to get specific, and to talk about some of the clinical correlates that perhaps we've glossed over. For instance, someone talked about the tumor incidence in renal transplant patients, and whether this was induced by azathioprine or by steroids; but it's not tumors that are the primary problem we deal with with those patients; it's a set of megalovirus infections. So shouldn't we, with these patients, be examining respones to viruses, latency, and this sort of thing? And I think if we're going to have a battery of tests, it should be fairly basic, but then we should be guided by clinical correlate, and examine these particular entities in more detail.

Most of the presentations with diethylstilbesterol dealt with reactions against tumors and I think that's appropriate. The alkylating agents, for instance, are almost never used alone clinically. Now they are used in combination, and I have to present information on the immunologic aspects of these kinds of chemotherapeutic agents to the Southwest Oncology group, and I would like very much to have the data, either my own or anybody who is dealing with this, on the combinations of chemo-therapeutic agents being used, and then that could be correlated probably better with the clinical problems that patients have; albeit infection, et cetera. Expanding the assays, the basic assays, into the specific area of immune function, once garnered by clinical correlates, I think would in the long run provide more meaningful data.

HELLMAN: I think the credibility of the various tests that have been discussed here depend very much on whether you go in with a shovel or with a needle! And most of the things, at least that I've heard today, were performed by shovels rather than needles!

There is human exposure data available to be evaluated to determine whether some of these environmental parameters are in fact really that detrimental. We then need to question, as a nation not as scientists: Can we really afford to worry about whether someone gets a rash so that in our exuberance we do not shut down our chemical industry, as one example. We have to consider these questions as responsible citizens, not just as scientists wishing to obtain results.

ZWILLING: I think we're really looking at three separate problems here and the first one is what kind of effects on the immune response occurs when one has an environmental disaster; it seems to me, in that case, we depend on a sick patient to tell us that there has been an environmental disaster before we're capable of detecting it experimentally.

And another question is: What are the effects of new substances, as our chemical industries manufacture them, in terms of whether the people are directly exposed to them on an occupational level or whether people are being exposed to them in the course of their everyday lives?

Next, I think that one has to ask the question: What kind of subtle changes are occurring, if we are capable of analyzing them at all, in the immune response from those substances that (we might say) occur in our environment as a result of our automobile or gasoline combustion or the burning of coal; furthermore, what are the subtle interactions that take place within the host concerning gaseous substances and particulate substances, and what effect have they in combination not necessarily alone on the host?

MAO: I would like to make a comment about dose levels of test material used in the immunological tests. It is my impression that it would be easier for us to find out LD_{50}, LC_{50}, or ED_{50}, in either acute or chronic studies within a certain period of time and in a specific animal model. However, I do feel that it is relatively or rather difficult to estimate or to make a definite judgment on the so-called "NOEL," (no observable effect level). A no effect level may be defined as the level (quantity) of a substance administered to a group of experimental animals at which there are those effects observed, or measured at higher levels, are absent and at which no significant differences between the group of animals exposed to the quantity of test material and an unexposed control group of animals maintained under tests.

The establishment of a NOEL, based on close effect relationships in toxicological tests including immunotoxicological investigations, is essential to present tolerance setting. There are few factors which may be considered to determine the NOEL. But I would like to discuss only the duration of time for experimental design. Very recently we learned of a chemical compound (please forgive me that we cannot name this compound, but it is a pesticide) which did not exhibit the adverse immunological effect in a short-term (6 months) rat feeding experiment. The immunotoxicological effect (a chemically induced autoimmune hemolytic anemia) showed up in a long-term (2 years) beagle dog feeding study, but the same adverse immunological effect did not appear in a short-term (approximately one year) investigation with the same test compound and in the same test animal model. Therefore, the time factor may contribute to the "building-up" of test compound through the process of *in vivo* bio-accumulation even though this slow process started with a very low level of chemical compound at the beginning.

KERMAN: I would like to respond to Dr. Steele's very cogent remark. While we are trying to determine the importance of immunotoxicology and play various tunes to our particular prejudices and interests, we really should consider the immediate needs. Dr. Steele pointed out a beautiful example with kidney transplants with CMV virus. CMV is probably more prevalent and a larger problem at the moment than neoplasia, at least in frequency.

HADDEN: While it's true that transplant recipients have incidence of CMV infections, most of them do not die from it; we can pull the kidney, treat the CMV infection, and support the patient. So again I think it gets to the question that Dr. Hellman raised, i.e., is it a problem if somebody gets a rash? What is the relevance of it and should we be concerned about it? Not that we need to overlook the CMV infection or infectious episodes as an endpoint, but in reality, that may not be the main problem. The main problem for instance in kidney transplantation is still rejection, and that's where we lose most of our grafts; not from CMV.

PADARATHSINGH: I would like to add one final comment: We should really be thinking in terms of the prohost immunologic theory as described by Dr. Hadden earlier in the symposium, i.e., the many different ways and means that we can be affected by immune suppression as induced by genetic, therapeutic, and environmental factors. However, huge gaps exist as far as epidemiologic information and methods for correlating patterns of disease with exposure to environmental chemicals. Our understanding of teratogenesis, mutagenesis and/or carcinogenesis and ability to rapidly and economically test for health hazards need further development. Moreover, methods for correlating results from mouse to man also need wider elucidation. There is no time to waste. The public is becoming more concerned about the environment and health and, to this end, some government agency must take the groundwork as laid out by symposia such as this one and support efforts to attract and to help fund the work of the many scientists who, by their track record, are prepared to dedicate themselves to undertake problems in the field of environmental health research. The future is now.

LOOSE: Since this is my last chance to get on the tape, I'm going to have to give a few words of wisdom, I hope!

First of all, I'd like to respond to Dr. Bellanti's initial definition of immunotoxicology. I would recommend, rather than calling it the toxic effect or the effect of toxic chemicals on the immune responses that it be considered the interaction of the toxic chemical with the immune system. This would encompass not only the deleterious effect but also the metabolizing effect of the immunocompetent cells on the chemical in use.

In response to Dr. Dean's question regarding overt legislation, I think we must be aware that we may price ourselves out of the agrichemical market in the United States, relative to a world market if we don't put the immunotoxicological data in perspective. I think that's one of the things that was the aim of this meeting but in my opinion fell a little bit short. What is the relevance of the immunosuppression that we see both clinically and experimentally? I don't think we really addressed ourselves to that as well as we should have. All of us, aware of the bureaucratic morass, know that if we don't present this information clearly, it will be incorrectly extrapolated by legislators and/or regulatory agencies. Then we will end up with a lot of regulation which was not the initial intent.

DEAN: Maybe that's the charge to go home with!

We have a number of papers and experiments dealing with a variety of compounds which show that at certain dose levels one gets an alteration in the immune response. However, when one really sits down in the corner and asks oneself: What does this portend? The answer is: We don't yet know. I think Dr. Bekesi's human clinical immunology data from his small PBB-exposed population in Michigan puts it squarely where it's at. He looked at a group of exposed people and found what he termed immunologic alterations based on his clinical immunology experience with relation to neoplasia. These people fell out of his norms. Those people, to my knowledge, aren't dying of overwhelming infectious disease or any other thing that might be related to it at this stage in time. That isn't to say they may not develop altered host resistance in the future.

I think one of the reasons the NIEHS picked up on that phenomenon is that indeed it is a phenomenon which suggested that there was an alteration in what we thought was the normal response and we didn't know what that meant, or whether it was related to PBB or not related to PBB. I think that's the best example I am aware of where we are trying to make a correlate between an environmental chemical exposure and clinical changes in a human population.

MOORE: With regard to what can we do and whether we are pricing ourselves out of the market with immunotoxicology, I guess you could pick almost any other area of safety assessment and raise the same concern.

I feel that the immunotoxicity of chemicals should be investigated, not because we have definite answers one way or the other, but so that when one finally sits down to make a decision regarding safety of a chemical, that decision can be based on fact rather than on innuendo.

DEAN: My thanks to all attendees, particularly the speakers: I think it has been an excellent and informative workshop.

List of Participants

Dr. Bernard Adkins, Jr.
Manager
Inhalation Toxicology Program
Northrop Services, Inc.
P.O. Box 12313
Research Triangle Park, NC 27709

Dr. Leigh Anderson
Building 202
Argonne National Laboratories
9700 Cass Avenue
Argonne, IL 60439

Dr. Angelo Andrese
Eastman Kodak Company
Health Safety and Human Factors
 Laboratory
Rochester, NY 14605

Dr. Douglas L. Archer
Food and Drug Administration
Bureau of Foods
1090 Tusculum Avenue
Cincinnati, OH 45226

Dr. Nancy J. Balter
International Center for Interdisciplinary
 Studies of Immunology
Georgetown University Medical Center
3800 Reservoir Road, NW
Washington, DC 20007

Dr. J. G. Bekesi
The Mount Sinai Medical Center
1 Gustave L. Levy Place
New York, NY 10029

Dr. Joseph J. Bellanti
Professor and Director
International Center for Inter-
 disciplinary Studies of Immunology
Georgetown School of Medicine
Washington, DC 20057

Dr. Anna Barker
Battelle Memorial Institute
Columbus Laboratories
505 King Avenue
Columbus, OH 43201

Dr. Jerry A. Bash
Assistant Professor Pediatrics
Immunologic Oncology Division
Georgetown University School
 of Medicine
Box 63 Med-Dent Building
3900 Reservoir Road
Washington, DC 20007

Dr. Zeb Bell
PPG Industries
1 Gateway Center
Pittsburgh, PA 15222

Dr. Alan Blandamer
Manager of Marketing
Immunology Testing
Litton Bionetics, Inc.
5516 Nicholson Lane
Kensington, MD 20795

Dr. David Bice
Inhalation Toxicology Research Institute
Lovelace Biomedical and Environmental
 Research Institute, Inc.
P.O. Box 5890
Albuquerque, NM 87115

Dr. R. K. Bourne
Lehn and Fink Products Company
225 Summit Avenue
Montvale, NJ 07645

Dr. David Brusick
Director, Department of Genetics
 and Cell Biology
Litton Bionetics, Inc.

5516 Nicholson Lane
Kensington, MD 20795

Dr. Kirby I. Campbell
6119 Webbland Place
Cincinnati, OH 45213

Dr. Grace Cannon
Department of Immunology
Litton Bionetics, Inc.
5516 Nicholson Lane
Kensington, MD 20795

Dr. Charles E. Carter
Scientific Director
NIEHS
P.O. Box 12233
Research Triangle Park, NC 27709

Dr. Ronald V. Citarella
American Cyanamid Company
Medical Research Division
Lederle Laboratories
Pearl River, NY 10965

Ms. Janette R. Cushman
Department of Animal, Dairy, and
   Veterinary Sciences
Utah State University
UMC-46
Logan, UT 84322

Dr. Jack H. Dean
Head, Immunology Section
Environmental Biology Branch
National Institutes of Environmental
   Health Sciences
P.O. Box 12233
Research Triangle Park, NC 27709

Dr. Anthony J. Dennis
Battelle Memorial Institute
Columbus Laboratories
505 King Avenue
Columbus, OH 43201

Dr. Preston Dorsett
Associate Professor of Microbiology
University of Tennessee Center for
   the Health Sciences
Room 643
858 Madison Avenue
Memphis, TN 38163

Dr. Mario R. Escobar
Medical College of Virginia

MCV Station
Richmond, VA 23298

Dr. Donald Fish
Frederick Cancer Research Center
Building 522
P.O. Box B
Frederick, MD 21701

Dr. David A. Fuccillo
Director
Advanced Testing and Developing
   Laboratory
Litton Bionetics, Inc.
5516 Nicholson Lane
Kensington, MD 20795

Dr. Joseph Gainer
Food and Drug Administration
HFV-500
Building 328-A
Beltsville, MD 20705

Dr. Donald E. Gardner
US Environmental Protection Agency
Health Effects Research Laboratory
Research Triangle Park, NC 27711

Dr. James Gerson
Department of Pediatrics
Hershey Medical Center
Hershey, PA 17033

Dr. Abdul Ghaffar
University of South Carolina
Department of Microbiology and
   Immunology
Columbia, SC 29208

Dr. Ron Gillette
Meloy Laboratories, Inc.
6715 Electronic Drive
Springfield, VA 22151

Mr. Harvey Giss
Manager, Program Development
Litton Bionetics, Inc.
5516 Nicholson Lane
Kensington, MD 20795

Dr. Irving Gray
Department of Biology and International
   Center for Interdisciplinary Studies
   of Immunology
Georgetown University
3800 Reservoir Road
Washington, DC 20007

Dr. Nathan D. Greene
Southwest Foundation for Research
and Education
P.O. Box 28147
8848 West Commerce Street
San Antonio, TX 78284

Dr. John W. Hadden
Director, Department of
Immunopharmacology
Sloan Kettering Institute
for Cancer Research
New York, NY 10021

Dr. Shirley Harder
Environmental Protection Agency
Medical Research Building
224-H
Chapel Hill, NC 27514

Mr. R. W. Hartgrove
C R & D
Haskell Laboratory
E. I. du Pont
1007 Market Street
Wilmington, DE 19898

Dr. Manfred M. Hein
7 Rockeby Court
Kensington, MD 20795

Eugene R. Heise, Ph.D.
Director
Medical Immunology Laboratory
Wake Forest University
Bowman Gray School of Medicine
300 South Hawthorne Road
Winston-Salem, NC 27103

Dr. K. B. Hellman
Food and Drug Administration
Bureau of Radiological Health
Twinbrook Parkway
Rockville, MD 20857

Dr. Alfred Hellman
National Institutes of Health
National Cancer Institute
Building 41, Room A108
Bethesda, MD 20205

Dr. Evan M. Hersh
MD Anderson Medical College and
Tumor Institute
6732 Burthner Street
Houston, TX 77030

Dr. Ronald D. Hinsdill
Director, Center for Environmental
Toxicology
University of Wisconsin
1550 Linden Drive
Madison, WI 53706

Dr. J. L. Hudson
Cell Biology Program
HFT-164
Food and Drug Administration
National Center for Toxicological
Research
Jefferson, AR 72079

Dr. Nelson Irey
Armed Forces Institute of Pathology
Registry of Tissue Reaction to Drugs
Walter Reed Hospital
Washington, DC 20306

Dr. Richard D. Irons
CIIT
P.O. Box 12137
Research Triangle Park, NC 27709

Dr. Keith E. Jensen
Executive Director
Pfizer, Inc.
199 Maywood Avenue
Maywood, NJ 07607

Dr. A. Bennett Jenson
National Institutes of Health
Building 30, Room 228
Bethesda, MD 20014

Dr. Terje Kalland
Institute of Anatomy
University of Bergen
N5000 Bergen
Norway

Dr. John Kateley
Director, Immunodiagnostics
Laboratory
Edward W. Sparrow Hospital
1215 East Michigan Avenue
Lansing, MI 48909

Dr. Meir Kende
Frederick Cancer Research Center
National Cancer Institute
Building 533
P.O. Box B
Frederick, MD 21701

Dr. Nancy Isaacson Kerkvliet
School of Veterinary Medicine
Oregon State University
Corvallis, OR 97331

Dr. Ronald Kerman
Department of Surgery
Division of Organ Transplantation
University of Texas Medical School
Houston, TX 77030

Dr. Florence K. Kinoshita
Hercules Incorporated
910 Market Street
Wilmington, DE 19899

Dr. Loren D. Koller
School of Veterinary Medicine
University of Idaho
Moscow, ID 83843

Dr. Samuel Kushner
American Cyanamid Company
Medical Research Division
Lederle Laboratories
Pearl River, NY 10965

Dr. Stanley Lang
American Cyanamid Company
Medical Research Division
Lederle Laboratories
Pearl River, NY 10965

Dr. Mariano F. Lavia
Medical University of South Carolina
171 Ashley Avenue
Charleston, SC 29403

Dr. Leland D. Loose
Albany Medical College
New Scotland Avenue
Albany, NY 12208

Dr. Edmund J. Lovett III
Assistant Professor
Department of Surgery
The University of Connecticut
  Health Center
School of Medicine
Farmington, CT 06032

Dr. Michael I. Luster
National Institutes of Health
NIEHS
P.O. Box 12233
Research Triangle Park, NC 27711

Dr. Thomas S. S. Mao
P.O. Box 5774
Bethesda, MD 20014

Dr. James L. McCoy
Laboratory of Immunodiagnosis
Building 10, Room 8811
National Cancer Institute
Bethesda, MD 20014

Dr. James B. McMahon
P.O. Box B
Frederick, MD 21701

Dr. Elizabeth Miller
710-B
A. N. Richards Medical Research
  Building
University of Pennsylvania
Philadephia, PA 19104

Dr. John A. Moore
Deputy Director, National
  Toxicology Program
National Institute of
  Environmental Health Sciences
P.O. Box 12233
Research Triangle Park, NC 27709

Dr. Sally Mulhern
Food and Drug Administration
Bureau of Foods
200 C Street, SW
Washington, DC 20204

Dr. Albert Munson
Department of Pharmacology
Medical College of Virginia
Richmond, VA 23298

Mr. James C. Nance
President
Litton Bionetics, Inc.
5516 Nicholson Lane
Kensington, MD 20795

Dr. Gordon W. Newell
National Academy of Sciences
2101 Constitution Avenue
Washington, DC 20418

Dr. Richard A. Nicklas
Food and Drug Administration
Bureau of Drugs
5600 Fishers Lane
Rockville, MD 20857

Dr. Martin Padarathsingh
Director
Department of Immunology
Litton Bionetics, Inc.
5516 Nicholson Lane
Kensington, MD 20795

Dr. D. Elliot Parks
Immunopathology
Scripps Clinic and Research Foundation
10666 North Torrey Pines Road
La Jolla, CA 92037

Dr. M. Peterson
Environmental Protection Agency
Medical Research Building C
224-H
Chapel Hill, NC 27514

Dr. Diana Post
Veterinary Medical Officer, HFV, 216
Bureau of Veterinary Medicine
Food and Drug Administration
5600 Fishers Lane
Rockville, MD 20857

Dr. Ken Powers
Food and Drug Administration
HFV-500
Building 328-A
Beltsville, MD 20705

Dr. Dean Roberts
Food and Drug Administration
NCTR
Jefferson, AR 72079

Dr. Julia P. Roboz
Research Associate
Department of Neoplastic Disease
Mt. Sinai Medical Center
1 Gustave L. Levy Place
New York, NY 10029

Dr. Georgia B. Schuller
HFX 120
Bureau of Radiological Health
Food and Drug Administration
5600 Fisher Lane
Rockville, MD 20857

Mr. J. T. Seawell
Chemical Manufacturers Association
1825 Connecticut Avenue, NW
Washington, DC 20009

Dr. Irving J. Selikoff
Director, Environmental Sciences
Laboratory
Mt. Sinai School of Medicine
5th Avenue and 100th Street
New York, NY 10029

Dr. Kenneth Sell
Director of Intramural Research
Building 5, Room 137
National Institute of Allergy
and Infectious Diseases
Bethesda, MD 20014

Dr. Ronald Shiotsuka
USAMBRDL
Building 568
Fort Detrick, MD 21701

Dr. Michael Sigel
Chairman
Department of Microbiology and
Immunology
University of South Carolina
School of Medicine
Columbia, SC 29208

Dr. John Silva
Department of Surgery
Box 3966
Duke University Medical Center
Durham, NC 27710

Dr. Paul Siminoff
Director of Immunology
Bristol Laboratories
P.O. Box 657
Syracuse, NY 13201

Dr. Myron B. Slomka
Shell Oil Company
Health, Safety, and Environment
P.O. Box 4320
Houston, TX 77210

Dr. Federico Spreafico
Head, Department of Oncology
and Immunology
Instituto Di Ricerche
Farmacologiche "Mario Negri"
Via Eritrea, 62
20157 Milano
ITALY

Dr. Russell Steele
HFT-164

Food and Drug Administration
National Center for Toxicological
  Research
Jefferson, AR 72079

Dr. Kent R. Stevens
Manager of Toxicology
Booz, Allen, and Hamilton
Foster D. Snell Division
66 Hanover Road
Florham Park, NJ 07932

Dr. Robert E. Stevenson
Vice President and General Manager
Biomedical Research Division
Litton Bionetics, Inc.
5516 Nicholson Lane
Kensington, MD 20795

Ms. Carol Terminelli
Schering Corporation
B5-215
60 Orange Street
Bloomfield, NJ 07003

Dr. Gary Thurman
Department of Biochemistry
Ross Hall, Room 554
George Washington University Medical
  Center
2300 Eye Street, NW
Washington, DC 20037

Dr. John Thurston
National Animal Disease Center
P.O. Box 70
Ames, IA 50010

Dr. Ann Tucker
Department of Pharmacology
Medical College of Virginia
Richmond, VA 23298

Dr. Virginia Utermohlen
Cornell University
N-204B-MVR
Ithaca, NY 14853

Dr. Robert J. Van Ryzin
Director
Toxicology and Pathology
Pharmaceutical Research and
  Development
Sandoz, Incorporated
East Hanover, NJ 07936

Dr. Frizell Vaughan
1620 School of Public Health I
University of Michigan
Ann Arbor, MI 48109

Dr. Adele Vessey
Food and Drug Administration
HFF-268
200 C Street, SW
Washington, DC 20204

Dr. Philip Watanabe
Dow Chemical USA
1803 Building
Toxicology Research Laboratory
Midland, MI 48640

Joel Warren, Ph.D.
Director
Leo Goodwin Institute for Cancer
  Research, Inc.
3301 College Avenue
Fort Lauderdate, FL 33314

Dr. Carrie Whitmire
National Institutes of Health
National Cancer Institute
Landow Building, Room 3C25
7910 Woodmont
Bethesda, MD 20014

Mr. David Williams
US Environmental Protection Agency
Office of Toxic Substance Assessment
  Division
TS-792
401 M Street, SW
Washington, DC 20024

Dr. D. Williams
Disease Control, EE
Michigan Department of Public Health
3500 North Logan
P.O. Box 30035
Lansing, MI 48909

J. Henry Wills, Ph.D.
National Institute for Occupational
  Safety and Health
Room 8A53
5600 Fishers Lane
Rockville, MD 20857

Dr. Craig K. Wood
Haskell Laboratory

DuPont de Nemours & Company
Newark, DE 19711
Dr. Edmond Yunis
Harvard Medical School
Sidney Farber Cancer Institute
44 Binney Street
Boston, MA 02115
Dr. Arian Zarkower
Pennsylvania State University

Department of Veterinary Sciences
115 Animal Industries Building
University Park, PA 16802
Dr. Bruce S. Zwilling
Ohio State University
Department of Microbiology
484 West 12th Avenue
Columbia, OH 43210

Index